Advances in Experimental Medicine and Biology

Volume 1007

Advances in Experimental Medicine and Biology presents multidisciplinary and dynamic findings in the broad fields of experimental medicine and biology. The wide variety in topics it presents offers readers multiple perspectives on a variety of disciplines including neuroscience, microbiology, immunology, biochemistry, biomedical engineering and cancer research. Advances in Experimental Medicine and Biology has been publishing exceptional works in the field for over 30 years and is indexed in Medline, Scopus, EMBASE, BIOSIS, Biological Abstracts, CSA, Biological Sciences and Living Resources (ASFA-1), and Biological Sciences. The series also provides scientists with up to date information on emerging topics and techniques. 2015 Impact Factor: 1.953

More information about this series at http://www.springer.com/series/5584

Sherif El-Khamisy
Editor

Personalised Medicine

Lessons from Neurodegeneration to Cancer

EXTRAS ONLINE

Springer

Editor
Sherif El-Khamisy
Krebs Institute and Sheffield Institute for Nucleic Acids
Department of Molecular Biology and Biotechnology
Firth Court, University of Sheffield
Sheffield, UK

Center for Genomics
Helmy Institute for Medical Sciences
Zewail City of Science and Technology
Giza, Egypt

Additional material to this book can be downloaded from http://extras.springer.com.

ISSN 0065-2598 ISSN 2214-8019 (electronic)
Advances in Experimental Medicine and Biology
ISBN 978-3-319-60731-3 ISBN 978-3-319-60733-7 (eBook)
DOI 10.1007/978-3-319-60733-7

Library of Congress Control Number: 2017948659

Printed on acid-free paper

This Springer imprint is published by Springer Nature
The registered company is Springer International Publishing AG
The registered company address is: Gewerbestrasse 11, 6330 Cham, Switzerland

Preface

The individual variability in response to therapy has inspired the unified vision for the utmost need to personalise medical decisions. It has led to the development of the concept of personalised medicine, which is a rapidly growing field aimed at delivering more precise and tailored therapies than conventional approaches. The recent advances in this field are driven by the fast-evolving technologies in genomics, proteomics and metabolomics, gene--editing tools and the use of genetically retractable model organisms. In this book, we review and discuss recent advances that served to translate personalised medicine from concept to practice with an up-to-date current status, ranging from lessons learned from DNA repair (Chaps. 1, 2, and 3), the emerging role of proteomics and metabolomics (Chaps. 4 and 5), targeting specific cellular processes such as RNA export (Chap. 6) or specific cell types such as astrocytes (Chap. 7), the role of mitochondria (Chap. 8), how model organisms such as yeast and zebrafish pushed the frontiers in this field (Chaps. 9 and 10) and examples from successful drug discovery efforts (Chap. 11) to recent developments in stem cell and gene therapeutics (Chaps. 12 and 13).

Sheffield, UK
Giza, Egypt

Sherif El-Khamisy

Contents

Approaches for Identifying Novel Targets in Precision Medicine: Lessons from DNA Repair

1

Dean T. Williams and Christopher J. Staples

Abstract

Genome stability is maintained by a number of elegant mechanisms, which sense and repair damaged DNA. Germline defects that compromise genomic integrity result in cancer predisposition, exemplified by rare syndromes caused by mutations in certain DNA repair genes. These individuals often exhibit other symptoms including progeria and neurodegeneration. Paradoxically, some of these deleterious genetic alterations provide novel therapeutic opportunities to target cancer cells; an excellent example of such an approach being the recent development of poly (ADP-ribose) polymerase inhibitors as the first 'synthetic lethal' medicine for patients with BRCA-mutant cancers. The therapeutic exploitation of synthetic lethal interactions has enabled a novel approach to personalised medicine based on continued molecular profiling of patient and tumour material. This profiling may also aid clinicians in the identification of specific drug resistance mechanisms following relapse, and enable appropriate modification of the therapeutic regimen. This chapter focuses on therapeutic strategies designed to target aspects of the DNA damage response, and examines emerging themes demonstrating mechanistic overlap between DNA repair and neurodegeneration.

Keywords

PARP • DNA repair • Synthetic lethality • Cancer • Mitochondria • Ageing

D.T. Williams
School of Medical Sciences, Bangor University, Bangor, Gwynedd LL57 2DG, UK

Department of Vascular Surgery, Ysbyty Gwynedd, Bangor LL57 2PW, UK

C.J. Staples (✉)
School of Medical Sciences, Bangor University, Bangor, Gwynedd LL57 2DG, UK
e-mail: c.staples@bangor.ac.uk

1.1 Introduction

Personalised medicine is a broad and rapidly evolving field that is becoming increasingly important in the targeted prevention, diagnosis and treatment of human disease. The development and introduction of a range of targeted

S. El-Khamisy (ed.), *Personalised Medicine*, Advances in Experimental Medicine and Biology 1007,
DOI 10.1007/978-3-319-60733-7_1

cancer therapies has in many cases improved patient response rates and enhanced patient outcomes, while the identification of disease risk genes allows clinicians to employ screening programmes to identify patients who are at a high risk of developing disease, allowing them to make informed decisions and lifestyle choices.

The treatment of cancer and neurodegeneration is changing as a consequence of personalised medicine. The histological characterisation and differentiation of human cancers is well established, and more recently these processes have been enhanced by the advent of next-generation sequencing and informed sub-classification of cancer types. Parallel to this, the development of novel therapeutic approaches targeting each cancer type and subtype has led to the development of new bespoke therapies and the optimisation of existing regimens. Modern approaches to the treatment of particular cancer types are being increasingly influenced by molecular profiling. Among these success stories are the use of anti-oestrogens in hormone receptor-positive breast cancers, monoclonal antibodies such as Herceptin in HER2-positive breast cancer [1] and cetuximab for cancers housing a mutant EGFR gene [2], tyrosine kinase inhibitors in chronic myeloid leukaemia (CML), Raf inhibitors such as Vemurafenib for malignant melanoma [3], and PARP inhibitors in ovarian, breast and prostate cancers [4].

Many cancer therapies induce tumour cell death by causing DNA damage; this includes the use of therapeutic radiation, topoisomerase inhibitors like etoposide, and agents that chemically modify the DNA strand such as cisplatin and temozolomide. The capacity of the cancer cell to repair this damage is a crucial determinant of patient response, and the development of novel medicines that target 'synthetic lethal' interactions between components of the DNA Damage Response (DDR) to selectively kill DNA repair-deficient cancer cells serves as an excellent example of how knowledge of the biology of mammalian DNA repair can translate into the full implementation of a personalised medicine strategy to improve outcomes for cancer patients.

Neurodegenerative diseases are typified by progressive death of nerve cells, resulting eventually in varying degrees of ataxia (loss of motor functions) and/or dementia. The most highly-studied of these include Alzheimer's Disease (AD), Parkinson's Disease (PD), Huntington Disease (HD) and Amyotrophic Lateral Sclerosis (ALS). The accumulation of DNA damage is also an important factor in the pathogenesis of neurodegeneration [5]. Defects in DNA repair lead to genomic instability and activation of damage response pathways, which ultimately induce cell cycle checkpoints and may lead to senescence or cell death – these cellular phenotypes are associated with both aging and tumour suppression. Indeed, the cellular capacity to repair DNA damage is inversely correlated with age. This chapter will focus on the central DNA repair pathways and how DNA repair defects may be exploited to develop more bespoke, personalised medicine strategies to improve outcomes for cancer patients. We will also explore the emerging overlap between aspects of the DNA repair machinery and the pathology of neurodegeneration.

1.2 DNA Damage-Specific Repair Mechanisms

Nucleic acids, proteins and lipids are all subject to damage. DNA is constantly damaged by endogenous reactive species, exogenous chemicals, radiation, and spontaneous nucleotide decay. Reactive oxygen species (ROS) alone are thought to cause up to 50,000 lesions per cell, per day – these include various types of damage including base modifications, single and double-strand breaks (DSBs) and interstrand cross-links (ICLs). These distinct forms of damage are repaired by specific repair pathways; Non-Homologous End-Joining (NHEJ) and Homologous Recombination (HR) which repair double-strand breaks [6], Base Excision Repair (BER) which repairs single-strand breaks [7] (SSBs) as well as numerous forms of base modification, Nucleotide Excision Repair (NER) which repairs helix-distorting lesions such as UV-induced pyrimidine dimers [8], and Mismatch Repair (MMR) which repairs errors introduced during replication [9]. The Fanconi Anaemia (FA) pathway co-operates with components of the HR and NER machinery to repair replication-blocking lesions induced by interstrand cross-links [10, 11]. Collectively, these pathways function to ensure that DNA damage is corrected in a timely manner. Therefore, the DNA Damage Response (DDR) also involves the induction of checkpoints, which halt cell cycle progression so that mutations and other forms of damage are not inherited by daughter cells. If DNA damage proves irreparable, or levels of damage are too high, DDR mechanisms can function to eliminate these cells by inducing apoptosis.

Amongst the most toxic and dangerous of DNA lesions is the Double-Strand Break (DSB); if left unrepaired DSBs cause catastrophic chromosome rearrangements and genome instability, promoting tumourigenesis [11]. This is reflected by the observation that the detection of even one single DSB by the cell is sufficient to induce cell cycle arrest until repair has taken place. DSBs are repaired via either NHEJ (which involves error-prone direct re-ligation), or HR, which is error-free but limited to S and G2 phase by the requirement for an intact sister chromatid template. During NHEJ, the DSB is recognised by the Ku70/80 heterodimer, which binds and activates the Phosphatidyl Inositol 3-Kinase-related Kinase (PIKK) enzyme DNA-dependent Protein Kinase (DNA-PK) [12]. DNA-PK phosphorylates a number of NHEJ proteins including Artemis [13] and the scaffold XRCC4, which orchestrate repair of the break site, the final religation being performed by DNA ligase IV. NHEJ operates independently of cell-cycle phase. In contrast, during HR repair the initial damage recognition is by the Mre11-Rad50-Nbs1 (MRN) complex, which in turn activates the master regulator PIKK Ataxia-Telangiectasia Mutated [14] (ATM), driving cell cycle arrest via p53 and the mediator kinase Chk2. The break site is resected by the co-ordinated action of Mre11 and Exo1 nucleases [15], and then Replication Protein A (RPA) coats the subsequent stretch of ssDNA formed. This resection is considered a 'licensing step', which commits the cell to HR-mediated repair. RPA is then displaced by BRCA2-dependent loading of Rad51 [16], which forms a nucleofilament designed to search the intact sister chromatid for the correct repair template to initiate error-free repair.

The lifetime cancer risk of the individual is increased by the inheritance of mutations in DNA repair genes, and indeed genes encoding components of the DNA repair machinery are among the most frequently mutated in human cancers. This is most notably exemplified by the high likelihood of breast and ovarian cancer development in carriers of BRCA1 or BRCA2 mutations; both proteins function to promote HR repair of DNA DSBs, preventing the toxic action of error-prone genome-destabilising NHEJ [17]. Patients with inherited mutations in other DSB repair genes such as ATM and Rad51 genes also display elevated cancer risk [18, 19], and somatic mutations in these genes and other components of the damage sensing and signal transduction machinery such as CHEK2 and Rad50 have also been reported in human cancers. A polymorphism in the gene encoding the BER polymerase DNA Polβ results in a low-activity enzyme that promotes transformation and is associated with an aggressive mutator phenotype [20]. Overexpression of DNA repair factors is also thought to play a significant role in tumour biology. Many tumours overexpress Rad51, an event associated with the rescue of recombination defects in BRCA-null cells. Therefore, it has been hypothesised that elevation of Rad51 levels in repair-deficient tumour cells limits genome instability during tumour progression [21]. In certain instances, elevated expression of DNA repair genes correlates with increasing tumour grade and therapeutic resistance. For example, the ICL repair protein FancD2 is re-expressed in high-grade gliomas, and pharmacological inhibition of the Fanconi Anaemia pathway acutely sensitises glioma cell lines to the alkylating agents temozolomide and carmustine [22].

1.3 Targeting DNA Repair Mechanisms

The response of patients to DNA-damaging therapies such as radiation, platinum agents and alkylating agents is in part determined by the ability of cancer cells to repair the damage induced during therapy. The pharmacological inhibition of DNA repair enzymes therefore has the potential to increase cancer cell sensitivity to these agents, thereby improving the tumour response to therapy and bettering patient outcomes. The most readily targetable of these enzymes are the PIKKs, and indeed specific and potent ATP-competitive inhibitors of DNA-PK, ATM and ATR have been developed over the past two decades, though there is considerable variation in the likelihood of these molecules progressing to clinical trials [23]. Since these kinases induce DNA damage-dependent cell cycle checkpoints, following inhibition the cell progresses into mitosis even in the presence of DNA damage, leading to mitotic catastrophe and cell death. Furthermore, many cancers exhibit high levels of replication stress [24] – therefore inhibiting the DDR checkpoint kinases alone has the potential to act as an effective anti-cancer therapy.

Among the first molecules known to inhibit PIKKs was caffeine, a methylxanthine compound that inhibits all PIKKs at a relatively high dose [25]. Since then, specificity and potency have been greatly refined, culminating in the development of a number of exciting compounds. The specific ATM inhibitors KU-55933, CP466722 and KU-60019 initially showed promise in vitro, though unfortunately these compounds did not prove clinically useful as they displayed a limited bioavailability profile [26–28]. However, these drugs had proven that ATM inhibition could sensitise cancer cells to DNA damage such as ionising radiation, and damaging therapies such as etoposide and camptothecin. Interestingly, cancer xenografts lacking p53 were considerably more sensitive to KU-60019 and radiation than xenografts using isogenic cells with functional p53 [27]. This suggested that ATM inhibitors might be especially effective in combination with DNA-damaging agents in cancers with defective p53. The compound KU-559403 shows greatest clinical promise, based on a good solubility and tissue distribution profile in vivo. KU-559403 increased the cytotoxic effects of camptothecin and etoposide in vitro, as well as in colorectal cancer murine xenografts [29]. However, in contrast to KU-60019, this effect was independent of p53 status. This observation may reflect differences between colon cancer and glioblastoma cells in xenograft experiments. The AtoM phase I trial has now begun to test the AstraZeneca ATM inhibitor AZD0156 both as monotherapy and in combination with other agents including the PARP inhibitor Olaparib (Lynparza) (Clinical Trial Identifier: NCT02588105). We await additional evidence from these clinical trials to gain some perspective on the true potential of these compounds as future therapies.

One of the hallmarks of cancer is increased replication stress, a complex phenomenon that is in part responsible for the increased genome stability present in many cancers. When aberrant replication fork structures are formed or replication forks stall, stretches of single-stranded DNA are formed. This ssDNA is coated by the protein Replication Protein A (RPA), which in turn promotes activation of the PIKK kinase ATM- and Rad3-related (ATR) [30]. ATR and its downstream targets such as the checkpoint kinase Chk1 function to stabilise stalled replication forks, repress firing of dormant replication origins and aid in replication fork restart. This has the cumulative effect of preventing DNA damage and subsequent genome instability. Various DNA lesions trigger ATR signalling in addition to stalled replication forks, such as resected DNA ends at DSBs. As a gene essential for survival, it has been suggested that the clinical use of ATR inhibitors may be overtly toxic to patients. To counter this, there are a number of recent studies showing that tumour cells are markedly more sensitive to ATR inhibition compared to untransformed cells, and furthermore a growing list of synthetic lethal interactions involving ATR and other proteins lost in certain cancers is emerging [31]. The first ATR inhibitor that demonstrated specificity and potency was VE-821 (Vertex Pharmaceuticals), which facilitates bypass of the

G2/M checkpoint and sensitises cancer cell lines to radiation, or treatment with damaging therapies such as cisplatin, etoposide, gemcitabine and camptothecin [32, 33]. A refined analogue of VE-821, VE-822 also sensitised pancreatic and lung cancer cell lines and xenografts to radiation and chemotherapies [34]. VE-822 is currently being tested as a combination therapy with gemcitabine, cisplatin, or etoposide in a phase I clinical trial. Pre-clinical data from trials of VX-970 demonstrated increased sensitivity of lung cancer cells to replication stress-inducing agents such as gemcitabine and cisplatin [35]. Trials combining VX-970 with other damaging chemotherapies such as topotecan and gemcitabine are ongoing (NCT02157792, NCT02487095 and NCT02157792), with initial results showing positive responses in patients with tumours resistant to other chemotherapies. We await the full results of these trials with interest.

1.4 Synthetic Lethality and Cancer Therapy

Though mutations in DNA repair genes predispose the individual to cancer, DNA repair deficiencies in cancer cells also yield opportunities for therapeutic intervention. The phenomenon of synthetic lethality has been exploited and developed in recent years to reveal a number of genetic interactions that provide novel opportunities to achieve selective cancer cell kill. Synthetic lethality occurs when the inactivation of one pathway allows survival, but inactivation of a second pathway leads to extensive cell death. In cancers with specific genetic alterations, the second pathway can be targeted using a small molecule inhibitor, culminating in the desired specific toxicity. This approach is theoretically generally applicable across a range of tumour types. In this regard, ATR is a promising personalised medicine target; multiple studies in recent years have demonstrated that ATR inhibitors selectively target cancer cells with particular genetic backgrounds. Early studies demonstrated a synthetic lethal interaction between ATR and ATM or p53 in cancer cells exposed to DNA-damaging chemotherapies [33, 36]. This observation fits well with the known co-operative tumour suppressor roles of ATM and p53 [37]. Since p53 is among the most disrupted genes in human cancers, this study suggested that ATR inhibition in combination with DNA damage could have therapeutic benefit in a wide range of cancer types. Subsequent studies using ATR inhibitors have demonstrated synthetically lethal interactions between ATR and a number of other genes associated with aspects of the DNA damage response. Work carried out in Srinivasan Madhusudan's lab showed that ATR is synthetically lethal in XRCC1-deficient ovarian cancer cells [38], while David Cortez' group demonstrated lethality between ATR and the structure-specific repair endonuclease ERCC4 in osteosarcoma cells [39]. A synthetic lethal screen using the ATR knock-in model of DLD1 colorectal cancer cells identified a synthetic lethal interaction between ATR and DNA Polymerase Delta [40] (POLD1). POLD1 depletion in the absence of ATR results in reduced DNA repair, increased DNA damage, and caspase-dependent apoptosis following a defective checkpoint. Loss-of-function POLD1 mutations have recently been identified in small subsets of colorectal and endometrial cancers [41, 42]. There is also increasing evidence that cancer cells lacking ATM (such as a subset of mantle cell lymphomas) are sensitive to ATR inhibitors [43]. Among the major functional ATR targets is the checkpoint kinase CHK1, for which kinase inhibitors are currently in clinical trials. One exciting study found that replication stress induced by the investigational CHK1 inhibitor AZD7762 causes extensive apoptosis, but only in combination with VE-821 [44]. Mechanistic analysis revealed that simultaneous ATR and CHK1 inhibition causes severe and persistent replication fork stalling and subsequent ssDNA accumulation that eventually leads to replication fork collapse. This synthetic lethal interaction was reversed via chemical inhibition of cyclin-dependent kinases, indicating that the initial synthetic interaction was caused by misregulated origin firing. This is a rare example of a cancer-specific synthetic lethal interaction between two components of the same repair pathway and suggests that ATR and CHK1 inhibitors

Table 1.1 List of DNA repair genes

Gene	Process	Associated cancers	Repair syndromes associated	SLIs	Inhibitor	Mitophagy or ND?
ATM	HR	Leukaemia, breast	Ataxia telangiectasia	PARP1	KU-559403	Mitophagy defect and ND
				p53		
ATR	HR, Replisome		Seckel syndrome	Chk1	VX-970	
	Stability			XRCC1	VE-821	
				ERCC4		
				POLD1		
				ATM		
Mre11	HR	Colorectal	AT-Like Disease		Mirin	ND
53BP1	NHEJ		RIDDLE syndrome	ATR + cisplatin	UNC2170	
BRCA1	HR	Breast, ovarian		PARP1		
BRCA2	HR	Breast, ovarian		PARP1		
Rad51	HR	Ovarian			B-02	
BLM	HR	Various	BLM syndrome			
WRN	NHEJ, HR, BER	Osteosarcoma	WRN syndrome			Progeria, ND
		Melanoma				
XPA	NER	Skin cancers	Xeroderma pigmentosum			Mitophagy defect and ND
FA genes	ICL	Leukaemia	Fanconi anaemia	ATM		Mitophagy defect
		HNSCC				

Selected DNA repair genes are listed in this table, alongside corresponding repair processes, associated cancers, repair syndromes, synthetic lethal interactions (SLIs) and the most therapeutically relevant inhibitors for each protein. The presence of a role in mitophagy and prevention of neurodegeneration (ND) is also indicated

could form the basis of a novel combination therapy. Table 1.1 summarises DNA repair genes and associated synthetic lethal interactions and syndromes.

1.5 PARP Inhibitors: Personalised Medicine for Patients with DNA Repair-Deficient Cancers

The most clinically advanced and highly-studied example of the therapeutic exploitation of synthetic lethality is the development of Poly (ADP-ribose) polymerase (PARP) inhibitors such as Olaparib (Lynparza) in patients carrying germline BRCA1 or BRCA2 mutations who have developed breast, prostate or ovarian cancer. In 2005, a preclinical study clearly demonstrated the striking effect of PARP1 inhibitors in *BRCA1*- and *BRCA2*-defective cells – a source of great excitement in the scientific community [45]. PARP is a DNA damage sensor involved in SSBR, BER and the alternative pathway of end-joining [46]. Patients that carry a single-hit BRCA mutation have a greatly elevated lifetime breast, prostate and ovarian cancer risk, resulting from the acquisition of a 'second-hit' that compromises the function of the healthy BRCA allele [47]. BRCA1 and BRCA2 both have crucial roles in HR repair, and components of the HR machinery also have major roles in the restart of stalled replication forks [48], as does PARP itself [49]. There are several proposed mechanisms for the selective toxicity of PARP inhibitors in HR-deficient cells. PARP inhibition impairs BER, leading to an increased number of DNA single-strand breaks – these are converted to DSBs that remain unrepaired in HR-deficient cells, leading to toxicity (see Fig. 1.1). This idea is countered by the failure to detect increases in SSB levels in PARP inhibitor-treated cells in the

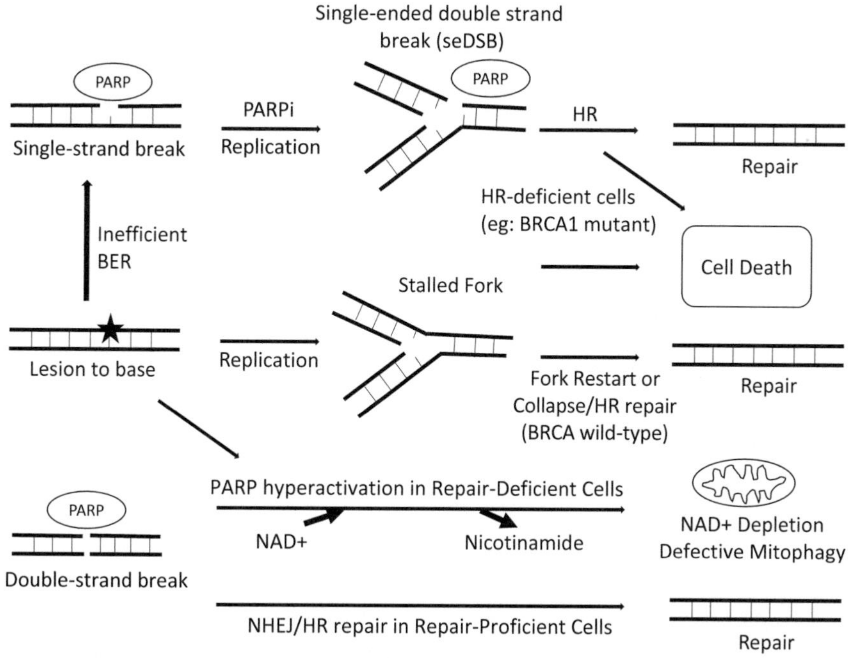

Fig. 1.1 The role of PARP in DNA repair and mitophagy. PARP1 binds to various forms of damaged DNA to assist repair, including single and double-strand breaks. The repair machinery in HR-proficient cells repairs single-ended DSBs generated during replication. Cancer cells defective in HR repair fail to repair these breaks, leading to cell death. Additionally, PARP has an active role in binding stalled replication forks and assisting in their restart. Trapping of PARP on DNA may also be an important determinant of the sensitivity of HR-deficient cells to PARP inhibitors (not shown). PARP is often hyperactivated in cells defective for DNA repair proteins – this is thought to lead to defective mitophagy via depletion of the cellular NAD+ pool

absence of an exogenous source of DNA damage. Alternative models suggest that PARP inhibition causes 'trapping' of PARP on the DNA, leading to replication fork blockage and impaired transcription and repair. This theory is supported by evidence that PARP itself drives toxicity in PARP inhibitor-treated cells [50]. Follow-up studies have demonstrated clearly that compromised function of numerous other DNA repair genes including ATM, ATR, CHEK1, FANCD2, RAD51 and RPA1 leads to PARP inhibitor sensitivity, implying that HR repair and replication fork stability are major determinants of this response [51]. The extensive data demonstrating that mutation, downregulation or loss of numerous DNA repair proteins leads to cellular PARP inhibitor sensitivity raises the possibility that DNA sequence analysis and proteomic profiling of tumour material could be used predictively to identify differential patient responses to PARP inhibition.

Phase I clinical trials of Olaparib proceeded rapidly, and the study cohort was intentionally biased to include patients with a BRCA1 or BRCA2 mutation. These trials were a great success, as it was quickly apparent that Olaparib was tolerable and safe, with side effects such as fatigue and gastrointestinal symptoms being relatively mild [52]. The results of these trials showed effective anti-tumour activity in BRCA-mutant breast, ovarian and prostate cancers [53–55], and leant support to the idea that drugs targeting synthetic lethal interactions could prove successful in the clinic. A later phase II trial testing olaparib in platinum-sensitive relapsed ovarian cancer was conducted, but no overall survival benefit was noted, leading to a delay in clinical development [56]. However, further analysis demonstrated that patients with *BRCA1*- or *BRCA2*-mutant ovarian cancers displayed the greatest response to olaparib [57]. This led to new phase III trials such as SOLO-2 – a Phase III, multicentre trial intended to determine the efficacy of oral maintenance Olaparib as monotherapy in patients with platinum-sensitive recurrent BRCA-mutant ovarian cancer (NCT01874353). In SOLO-2, patients with either germline or somatic BRCA mutations were enrolled, and randomised to receive Olaparib tablets or placebo until disease progression was observed. The trial reported a clinically meaningful improvement of progression-free survival (PFS) among patients treated with Olaparib tablets compared to placebo. In 2014, the European Commission (EC) granted authorisation for Olaparib capsules as the first therapy for the maintenance treatment of patients with platinum-sensitive relapsed *BRCA*-mutated platinum-responsive epithelial ovarian, fallopian tube, and primary peritoneal cancer.

Following encouraging in vitro data [58], the PARP inhibitor BMN-673 is also being tested in patients with solid tumours housing mutations in *BRCA1* or *BRCA2*, and who have experienced disease progression following at least one current therapy. In addition to these single-agent trials, PARP inhibitors are also being evaluated as part of combination therapies for advanced solid cancers. A number of trials are currently validating the PARP inhibitor ABT-888 (Veliparib) in combination with other DNA-damaging chemotherapies. For example, ABT-888 is being evaluated in combination with the alkylating agent temozolomide in solid tumour patients. The effect of adding ABT-888 to an existing combination of carboplatin and paclitaxel in HER2-negative metastatic and inoperable BRCA mutant breast cancer is also being assessed in Phase III clinical trials.

1.6 Identifying Defective DNA Repair in Tumours

The clinical application of tools for rapid patient stratification is fast becoming a reality. The advent of affordable and rapid sequencing and proteomics now provides oncologists with in-depth profiles of the genetic and proteomic alterations found in patients' tumours. In the past, the sensitivity of cancers to platinum agents has been used as a crude marker of HR-deficiency. This is unreliable, as some cancers that respond to platinum compounds do not respond to PARP inhibition; reflected in the observation that in some clinical trials PARP inhibitors yielded positive responses in patients with platinum-resistant cancers. Some alterations may have a epigenetic origin – the BRCA1 gene promoter is hypermethylated in around 15% of sporadic ovarian carcinomas [59, 60] and suppression of BRCA2 has been associated with methylation and silencing of its regulator FANCF [61]. Indeed, methylation of the BRCA1 promoter is linked with therapeutic resistance and a negative prognosis in ovarian cancer [60, 62]. However, cellular alterations that lead to repair deficiency or PARP inhibitor sensitivity may not always be a consequence of mutations in DNA repair genes, and in some cases may not be detectable even by whole-proteome analysis. Direct assessments of DNA repair in human tumours are potentially an excellent biomarker – however this presents scientists with a number of technical challenges, as any protocol would require a tissue sample treated with an appropriate DNA-damaging agent. The formation of RAD51 foci is an excellent readout of HR repair activity [63] and indeed reduced numbers of RAD51 foci per nucleus in ascites from ovarian cancers have been correlated broadly with reduced HR repair [64], and a more positive response to chemotherapy. HR deficiency also causes elevated PARP activation, suggesting that hyper-activated PARP could predict how cancers may respond to PARP inhibition [65]. However, considerable variability in PARP activity from patient to patient has been observed [66], and this may seriously compromise the possibility that PARP activity could serve as a useful biomarker.

Multiplex sequencing can be used to identify mutations in DNA repair genes that result in increased or decreased HRR – this could prove a useful clinical tool. Whole-exome sequencing provides targeted sequencing of most exons, including DNA repair genes, but is not commonly applied in clinical practice at present. A PARP inhibitor clinical trial employed whole-exome sequencing in prostate cancer patients, finding a high response rate in the subset of patients with a HR-defective cancer [67]. An alternative strategy involves profiling gross aberrations in chromosome structure, a feature common to HRR-deficient cancers. Markers of this phenotype include loss of heterozygosity (LOH), allelic imbalance near telomeres (TAI); and large-scale state transitions (LSTs – chromosomal breaks between adjacent sections of greater than 10 megabases. LOH, TAI and LST scores correlate with each other and predict platinum response in ovarian and breast cancers [68]. Several HRR deficiency biomarkers that involve the assessment of patterns of loss of heterozygosity (LOH) are being tested in clinical trials of PARP inhibitors. Following treatment of patients with recurrent ovarian cancers with PARP inhibitors, those with germline BRCA mutations displayed the greatest response, followed by patients with high LOH but lacking a BRCA mutation. Patients lacking either LOH or a BRCA mutation responded most poorly [69]. This data implies that LOH has the potential to predict PARP inhibitor response.

1.7 Personalised Medicine Strategies for Therapy-Resistant Cancers

The efficacy of anti-cancer drugs is too often limited by the development of acquired or inherent therapeutic resistance. Despite the enormous advances made in our understanding of DNA repair mechanisms, and the encouraging clinical data emerging, it is apparent that some patients exhibit a better initial response to PARP inhibitors than others, and that in many patients cancers eventually become refractory to therapy.

Hope comes however, from the therapeutic potential of personalised medicine for patients with drug-resistant cancers. With a complete molecular understanding of the biology of drug cytotoxicity and the mechanisms that lead to resistance comes the ability to identify non-responsive or relapsed patients with tumours that have developed a specific inherent or acquired resistance mechanism. This approach would enable stratification of patients to allow administration of the optimal therapeutic strategy, followed by continual molecular evaluation of the tumour biology prior to and during treatment. One hopes that in the future, personalised molecular profiling of drug resistance might allow clinicians to draw on pharmacological resources to specifically resensitise different types of drug-resistant cancers.

An important mechanism of PARP inhibitor resistance involves the down regulation of factors that normally repress HR repair in favour of error-prone NHEJ. Factors implicated thus far include REV7, 53BP1 and JMJD1C [70–72]. A number of these factors are routinely lost in breast and ovarian cancers, suggesting the importance of screening patients for loss of these proteins prior to, and during treatment with PARP inhibitors. An extremely interesting recent study highlighted an alternative resistance mechanism, demonstrating that the loss of the repair protein PTIP protects BRCA-deficient cells from DNA damage [51]. Despite its similarity to Rev7 and 53BP1 in regulating the balance between HR and NHEJ, PTIP loss has no effect on HR activity in BRCA-deficient cells. Surprisingly, loss of PTIP inhibits MRE11 nuclease binding to stalled replication forks, thereby protecting the DNA from nuclease degradation. The study noted that in more general terms, the development of resistance to PARP inhibitors and platinum compounds correlates with replication fork protection.

The mechanisms via which some cells are able to avoid ATR inhibitor-induced toxicity are also under investigation. Notably, one CRISPR-Cas9-based study identified CDC25A as an important determinant of ATR inhibitor sensitivity. Cells lacking CDC25A resist high doses of ATR inhibitors, as they fail to prematurely enter mitosis following inhibitor treatment [73]. Using WEE1 inhibitors to force mitotic entry re-sensitises CDC25A-deficient cells to ATR inhibition.

Genetic heterogeneity is a feature of most cancers that drives therapeutic resistance, and is itself a consequence of elevated genome instability. Sequence analysis of single breast cancer cells has clearly demonstrated that resistance is driven by the generation of extensive clonal diversity within tumours [74]. In the context of defective repair and PARP inhibition, the inference is that subpopulations of tumour cells harbour alterations in regulators of repair pathway choice, and that these repair-proficient clones expand following therapy [58–61]. Encouraging preliminary work has demonstrated that targeting a heterogenous population composed of repair-deficient and repair-proficient cells by depleting BRCA2 prevented selective expansion of resistant cells following Olaparib treatment [75]. These studies are crucial to our understanding of how resistance arises and why many patients treated with synthetic medicines might fail to respond or quickly relapse. The identification of a wide range of synthetic lethal interactions could have profound clinical implications related to personalised medicine, more specifically the introduction of tumour genotype-based cancer therapy. As cancer researchers gradually add to their knowledge of lethal interactions and increase the number of targeted therapies in their arsenal, one might envisage a future where a synthetic medicine library could be drawn on to target a large subset of human cancers following tumour sequencing and proteomic analysis.

1.8 DNA Repair Syndromes and Neurodegeneration

Repair of DNA damage is a crucial tumour suppressor mechanism – this is exemplified by the fact that a range of rare genetic cancer predisposition disorders are caused by mutations in DNA repair genes. Interestingly, patients suffering from these diseases often exhibit a neurodegenerative phenotype, amongst other symptoms. Ataxia Telangiectasia (A-T) is a human syndrome caused by a defect in DSB repair resulting from mutations in the ATM gene [76]. A-T patients exhibit ataxia, and neurodegeneration of granule and Purkinje cells in the cerebellum. Other symptoms include telangiectasia, increased incidence of lymphoma, leukaemia and other tumours, and diabetes later in life [77]. Werner Syndrome (WS) results from mutations in the WRN gene [78], which encodes a RecQ family helicase that plays important roles at DNA replication forks, in BER, in both NHEJ and HR pathways at DSBs, and is crucial for maintenance of telomere stability and length [79]. WRN is not frequently found mutated in cancers, though many cancers express low levels of WRN due to extensive promoter hypermethylation [80]. WS patients exhibit accelerated aging (progeria) and ultimately die from cancer or cardiovascular defects as a consequence of progressive neurodegeneration. Exposure to the ultraviolet component of sunlight causes DNA damage, largely in the form of pyrimidine dimers. These lesions are removed by two forms of nucleotide excision repair (NER) – Global Genome Repair (GG-NER) that is dependent on XPA, and Transcription-Coupled Repair (TC-NER), which is dependent on CSA and CSB [8]. Xeroderma Pigmentosum (XP) is an inherited autosomal recessive condition resulting from mutation of one of a number of NER factors [81]. The disease is characterized by severe photosensitivity, altered skin pigmentation and a greatly increased risk of skin basal and squamous cell carcinoma. Approximately 30% of patients also suffer from neurological abnormalities including abnormal motor control, ataxia, neuropathy, dementia, atrophy and microcephaly. The symptoms vary in severity between patients, but are generally progressive, chronic, and are caused by gradual neurodegeneration as a consequence of neuronal apoptosis. Collectively, these findings demonstrate a clear mechanistic link between unrepaired DNA damage and neurodegeneration.

Defects in SSB repair (SSBR) are also associated with disease, and neurodegeneration [82]. During SSBR, PARP1 binds to the break to recruit the LIG3α-XRCC1 complex required for repair [83]. The neurodegenerative diseases Ataxia-Oculomotor Apraxia-1 (AOA1) and SpinoCerebellar Ataxia with axonal Neuropathy-1 (SCAN1) are autosomal-recessive disorders associated with defects in SSB repair caused by mutations in the Aprataxin (APTXN) and Tyrosyl-DNA phosphodiesterase-1 (TDP-1) genes, respectively [84, 85]. APTXN is a nucleotide hydrolase that can remove obstructive termini from DNA strand breaks that block repair and religation of these sites [86]. Interestingly, patients do not exhibit many of the typical features of DNA repair disorders like radiation sensitivity and increased cancer incidence; instead, symptoms are limited to neurodegenerative phenotypes. SCAN1 patients suffer progressive cerebellar ataxia, areflexia, peripheral neuropathy and loss of pain and touch sensation in the hands and legs. AOA1 is characterized by progressive cerebellar ataxia, then oculomotor apraxia and peripheral axonal motor neuropathy. These observations suggest that the neuronal system is sensitive to defects in the repair of DNA SSBs relative to the rest of the body.

Unlike the symptoms of cancer predisposition and aging, DNA damage does not appear to account entirely for the neurodegenerative phenotypes observed in patients with defective DDR syndromes. In fact, the neurological phenotypes closely mimic symptoms of patients with organ failure related to mitochondrial disorders; namely cerebellar degeneration, seizures and neuropathy. Mitochondria are vital organelles that mediate a range of cellular functions including energy production, apoptosis and calcium homeostasis. It is now well accepted that altered mitochondrial function plays a significant role in the pathology of AD, PD, ALS and HD [87–89] This may be a result of increased ROS production resulting from defects in components of the electron transport chain (ETC), or mutations in either mitochondria DNA or nuclear DNA that encodes proteins involved in mitochondrial function. As examples, nuclear mutations in the PARK2 and PTEN-Inducible Kinase 1 (PINK1) genes are associated with the neurodegenerative features of PD [90]. These genes encode proteins essential for mitophagy, a selective organelle autophagy pathway that functions to remove defective mitochondria. Autophagy is a degradative process via which the cell can remove defective organelles like mitochondria, as well as having additional functions in turnover of long-lived proteins, recycling of nutrients, and survival during conditions of severe nutrient starvation. In the initiation of mitophagy, PINK1 accumulates on the surface of dysfunctional mitochondria where it functions to recruit Parkin, an E3 Ubiquitin ligase [91]. The activity of Parkin drives a series of events that results in the engulfment of damaged mitochondria by autophagosomes, followed by their degradation in lysosomes.

1.9 PARP is Hyperactivated in DNA Repair-Deficient Cells and in Neurodegeneration

Intriguingly, cells defective in ATM, XPA, and multiple FA pathway components all share a common feature – they display a defect in mitophagy [92–94]. ATM and FA proteins are present in mitochondria while XPA and CS proteins are not, and it appears that mitochondrial effects in these cells are a secondary consequence of the disruption to genome stability caused by loss of these proteins. There is, however, a common feature which links cells defective for each of these repair proteins; namely, the hyperactivation of PARP enzymes. PARP is activated by intracellular stresses linked with both cancer and neurodegenerative disorders, such as DNA damage and elevated ROS levels [65]. PARP activity involves the conversion of Nicotinamide Adenine Dinucleotide (NAD+) to mono-(ADP-ribose), resulting in release of free nicotinamide (see Fig. 1.1). These monomeric units are then polymerised into PAR chains and added to substrate proteins. The net effect of PARP activity is to consume NAD+, eventually depleting cellular stocks of this essential activated carrier molecule. NAD+ is a cofactor for the sirtuin deacetylases, and consequently PARP hyperactivation results in inhibition of sirtuins. Sirtuins are NAD+ -dependent enzymes that regulate metabolism, DNA repair and ageing. Sirtuin 1 (SIRT1) is thought to have a central role in regulation of mitophagy via the transcription factor PGC-1α, the loss of which results in neurodegeneration [95].

Recent studies suggest the possibility of targeted therapeutic intervention to restore NAD+ levels either via supplementation or inhibition of

PARP enzymes. NAD+ supplementation is neuroprotective in Parkin mutant flies, as is co-mutation of PARP [96]. Administration of PARP inhibitors in a mouse model of HD resulted in increased lifespan, and reduction of the symptoms of neurological dysfunction [98]. It appears that ongoing unrepaired DNA damage induces signalling between the nucleus and the mitochondria, and this is consistent with new evidence demonstrating that rescuing NAD+/SIRT1 signalling in ATM-null cells partially reverses neurological defects and increases lifespan. Interestingly, in this context replenishing NAD+ actually stimulates both DNA repair and mitophagy [97]. The crucial role of PARP in these processes is further highlighted by evidence for the importance of negative regulation of PARylation, which is mediated in part via the deconstruction of PAR chains by the enzyme Poly (ADP-Ribose) Glycohydrolase (PARG). Consistent with a role for altered PARylation in neurodegeneration, Sharifi and colleagues have described a link between impaired PAR degradation and neurodegeneration [99]. Studies in worms have also convincingly demonstrated that PARG promotes nerve regeneration in damaged motor neurons [100]. In contrast, PARP activity inhibited axonal regeneration, and in this model pharmacological PARP inhibitors were also neuroprotective.

Collectively, these findings highlight important links between DNA damage, mitochondrial function and neurodegeneration. Furthermore, evidence is building that strategies designed to increase intracellular NAD^+ concentrations via dietary supplementation, or the pharmacological inhibition of PARP, could prove useful in a subset of patients with neurodegenerative disorders.

1.10 Summary

The advent of personalised medicine is a very exciting time for clinicians and basic scientists alike, with the prospect that genetics and cell biology will increasingly inform the development of bespoke approaches to maintaining health and treating disease. Nonetheless, tumour heterogeneity and inherent or acquired drug resistance represent a formidable barrier to the development of successful therapies. The recent generation of a prolific amount of tumour-specific genetic and proteomic data has resulted in identification of novel potential targets and added a new dimension to medical research. The continuing challenge in medical research is how to utilise identified molecular idiosyncrasies to create a therapeutic advantage in managing disease.

The process of translating potential therapies from bench to bedside is complex and peppered with frustration and disappointments as well as successes. The development of therapies from basic molecular discoveries to clinical practice is inherently costly. The provision of treatments at a reasonable cost is a constant challenge, particularly if these are to be provided as maintenance therapies. Similarly, long-term treatment may result in unwanted adverse events or loss of efficacy. To expedite these difficult processes, advances in personalised medicine strategies should be coupled with appropriate modifications to clinical trial design to permit the assessment and verification of putative patient selection strategies and properly reflect the co-morbidities and genetic variation of the target population.

References

1. Gu G, Dustin D, Fuqua SA (2016) Targeted therapy for breast cancer and molecular mechanisms of resistance to treatment. Curr Opin Pharmacol 31:97–103. doi:10.1016/j.coph.2016.11.005
2. Kassouf E, Tabchi S, Tehfe M (2016) Anti-EGFR therapy for metastatic colorectal cancer in the era of extended RAS gene mutational analysis. BioDrugs 30:95–104. doi:10.1007/s40259-016-0166-5
3. Boespflug A, Thomas L (2016) Cobimetinib and vemurafenib for the treatment of melanoma. Expert Opin Pharmacother 17:1005–1011. doi:10.1517/14656566.2016.1168806
4. Cerrato A, Morra F, Celetti A (2016) Use of poly ADP-ribose polymerase [PARP] inhibitors in cancer cells bearing DDR defects: the rationale for their inclusion in the clinic. J Exp Clin Cancer Res 35:179. doi:10.1186/s13046-016-0456-2
5. Maynard S, Fang EF, Scheibye-Knudsen M, Croteau DL Bohr VA (2015) DNA damage, DNA repair, aging, and neurodegeneration. Cold Spring Harb Perspect Med 5, doi:10.1101/cshperspect.a025130
6. Chapman JR, Taylor MR, Boulton SJ (2012) Playing the end game: DNA double-strand break repair pathway choice. Mol Cell 47:497–510. doi:10.1016/j.molcel.2012.07.029

7. Robertson AB, Klungland A, Rognes T, Leiros I (2009) DNA repair in mammalian cells: base excision repair: the long and short of it. Cell Mol Life Sci 66:981–993. doi:10.1007/s00018-009-8736-z
8. Marteijn JA, Lans H, Vermeulen W, Hoeijmakers JH (2014) Understanding nucleotide excision repair and its roles in cancer and ageing. Nat Rev Mol Cell Biol 15:465–481. doi:10.1038/nrm3822
9. Li GM (2008) Mechanisms and functions of DNA mismatch repair. Cell Res 18:85–98. doi:10.1038/cr.2007.115
10. Ceccaldi R, Sarangi P, D'Andrea AD (2016) The Fanconi anaemia pathway: new players and new functions. Nat Rev Mol Cell Biol 17:337–349. doi:10.1038/nrm.2016.48
11. Pierce AJ et al (2001) Double-strand breaks and tumorigenesis. Trends Cell Biol 11:S52–S59
12. Gottlieb TM, Jackson SP (1993) The DNA-dependent protein kinase: requirement for DNA ends and association with Ku antigen. Cell 72:131–142
13. Soubeyrand S et al (2006) Artemis phosphorylated by DNA-dependent protein kinase associates preferentially with discrete regions of chromatin. J Mol Biol 358:1200–1211. doi:10.1016/j.jmb.2006.02.061
14. Lee JH, Paull TT (2005) ATM activation by DNA double-strand breaks through the Mre11-Rad50-Nbs1 complex. Science 308:551–554. doi:10.1126/science.1108297
15. Shibata A et al (2014) DNA double-strand break repair pathway choice is directed by distinct MRE11 nuclease activities. Mol Cell 53:7–18. doi:10.1016/j.molcel.2013.11.003
16. Thorslund T et al (2010) The breast cancer tumor suppressor BRCA2 promotes the specific targeting of RAD51 to single-stranded DNA. Nat Struct Mol Biol 17:1263–1265. doi:10.1038/nsmb.1905
17. Escribano-Diaz C et al (2013) A cell cycle-dependent regulatory circuit composed of 53BP1-RIF1 and BRCA1-CtIP controls DNA repair pathway choice. Mol Cell 49:872–883. doi:10.1016/j.molcel.2013.01.001
18. Thompson D et al (2005) Cancer risks and mortality in heterozygous ATM mutation carriers. J Natl Cancer Inst 97:813–822. doi:10.1093/jnci/dji141
19. Song H et al (2015) Contribution of germline mutations in the RAD51B, RAD51C, and RAD51D genes to ovarian cancer in the population. J Clin Oncol 33:2901–2907. doi:10.1200/JCO.2015.61.2408
20. Donigan KA, Hile SE, Eckert KA, Sweasy JB (2012) The human gastric cancer-associated DNA polymerase beta variant D160N is a mutator that induces cellular transformation. DNA Repair (Amst) 11:381–390. doi:10.1016/j.dnarep.2012.01.004
21. Schild D, Wiese C (2010) Overexpression of RAD51 suppresses recombination defects: a possible mechanism to reverse genomic instability. Nucleic Acids Res 38:1061–1070. doi:10.1093/nar/gkp1063
22. Patil AA et al (2014) FANCD2 re-expression is associated with glioma grade and chemical inhibition of the Fanconi Anaemia pathway sensitises gliomas to chemotherapeutic agents. Oncotarget 5:6414–6424. doi:10.18632/oncotarget.2225
23. Brown JS, O'Carrigan B, Jackson SP, Yap TA (2017) Targeting DNA repair in cancer: beyond PARP inhibitors. Cancer Discov 7:20–37. doi:10.1158/2159-8290.CD-16-0860
24. Boyer AS, Walter D, Sorensen CS (2016) DNA replication and cancer: from dysfunctional replication origin activities to therapeutic opportunities. Semin Cancer Biol 37-38:16–25. doi:10.1016/j.semcancer.2016.01.001
25. Sarkaria JN et al (1999) Inhibition of ATM and ATR kinase activities by the radiosensitizing agent, caffeine. Cancer Res 59:4375–4382
26. Hickson I et al (2004) Identification and characterization of a novel and specific inhibitor of the ataxia-telangiectasia mutated kinase ATM. Cancer Res 64:9152–9159. doi:10.1158/0008-5472.CAN-04-2727
27. Biddlestone-Thorpe L et al (2013) ATM kinase inhibition preferentially sensitizes p53-mutant glioma to ionizing radiation. Clin Cancer Res 19:3189–3200. doi:10.1158/1078-0432.CCR-12-3408
28. Rainey MD, Charlton ME, Stanton RV, Kastan MB (2008) Transient inhibition of ATM kinase is sufficient to enhance cellular sensitivity to ionizing radiation. Cancer Res 68:7466–7474. doi:10.1158/0008-5472.CAN-08-0763
29. Batey MA et al (2013) Preclinical evaluation of a novel ATM inhibitor, KU59403, in vitro and in vivo in p53 functional and dysfunctional models of human cancer. Mol Cancer Ther 12:959–967. doi:10.1158/1535-7163.MCT-12-0707
30. Zeman MK, Cimprich KA (2014) Causes and consequences of replication stress. Nat Cell Biol 16:2–9. doi:10.1038/ncb2897
31. Andrs M et al (2016) Small molecules targeting ataxia telangiectasia and Rad3-related (ATR) kinase: an emerging way to enhance existing cancer therapy. Curr Cancer Drug Targets 16:200–208
32. Charrier JD et al (2011) Discovery of potent and selective inhibitors of ataxia telangiectasia mutated and Rad3 related (ATR) protein kinase as potential anticancer agents. J Med Chem 54:2320–2330. doi:10.1021/jm101488z
33. Reaper PM et al (2011) Selective killing of ATM- or p53-deficient cancer cells through inhibition of ATR. Nat Chem Biol 7:428–430. doi:10.1038/nchembio.573
34. Fokas E et al (2012) Targeting ATR in vivo using the novel inhibitor VE-822 results in selective sensitization of pancreatic tumors to radiation. Cell Death Dis 3:e441. doi:10.1038/cddis.2012.181
35. Hall AB et al (2014) Potentiation of tumor responses to DNA damaging therapy by the selective ATR inhibitor VX-970. Oncotarget 5:5674–5685. doi:10.18632/oncotarget.2158
36. Kwok M et al (2016) ATR inhibition induces synthetic lethality and overcomes chemoresistance in TP53- or ATM-defective chronic lymphocytic leukemia cells. Blood 127:582–595. doi:10.1182/blood-2015-05-644872
37. Turenne GA, Paul P, Laflair L, Price BD (2001) Activation of p53 transcriptional activity requires

ATM's kinase domain and multiple N-terminal serine residues of p53. Oncogene 20:5100–5110. doi:10.1038/sj.onc.1204665
38. Sultana R et al (2013) Ataxia telangiectasia mutated and Rad3 related (ATR) protein kinase inhibition is synthetically lethal in XRCC1 deficient ovarian cancer cells. PLoS One 8:e57098. doi:10.1371/journal.pone.0057098
39. Mohni KN, Kavanaugh GM, Cortez D (2014) ATR pathway inhibition is synthetically lethal in cancer cells with ERCC1 deficiency. Cancer Res 74:2835–2845. doi:10.1158/0008-5472.CAN-13-3229
40. Hocke S et al (2016) A synthetic lethal screen identifies ATR-inhibition as a novel therapeutic approach for POLD1-deficient cancers. Oncotarget 7:7080–7095. doi:10.18632/oncotarget.6857
41. Bellido F et al (2016) POLE and POLD1 mutations in 529 kindred with familial colorectal cancer and/or polyposis: review of reported cases and recommendations for genetic testing and surveillance. Genet Med 18:325–332. doi:10.1038/gim.2015.75
42. Church DN et al (2013) DNA polymerase epsilon and delta exonuclease domain mutations in endometrial cancer. Hum Mol Genet 22:2820–2828. doi:10.1093/hmg/ddt131
43. Menezes DL et al (2015) A synthetic lethal screen reveals enhanced sensitivity to ATR inhibitor treatment in mantle cell lymphoma with ATM loss-of-function. Mol Cancer Res 13:120–129. doi:10.1158/1541-7786.MCR-14-0240
44. Sanjiv K et al (2016) Cancer-specific synthetic lethality between ATR and CHK1 kinase activities. Cell Rep 17:3407–3416. doi:10.1016/j.celrep.2016.12.031
45. Bryant HE et al (2005) Specific killing of BRCA2-deficient tumours with inhibitors of poly(ADP-ribose) polymerase. Nature 434:913–917. doi:10.1038/nature03443
46. Beck C, Robert I, Reina-San-Martin B, Schreiber V, Dantzer F (2014) Poly(ADP-ribose) polymerases in double-strand break repair: focus on PARP1, PARP2 and PARP3. Exp Cell Res 329:18–25. doi:10.1016/j.yexcr.2014.07.003
47. Rubinstein WS (2008) Hereditary breast cancer: pathobiology, clinical translation, and potential for targeted cancer therapeutics. Familial Cancer 7:83–89. doi:10.1007/s10689-007-9147-7
48. Kolinjivadi AM et al (2017) Moonlighting at replication forks: a new life for homologous recombination proteins BRCA1, BRCA2 and RAD51. FEBS Lett. doi:10.1002/1873-3468.12556
49. Bryant HE et al (2009) PARP is activated at stalled forks to mediate Mre11-dependent replication restart and recombination. EMBO J 28:2601–2615. doi:10.1038/emboj.2009.206
50. Murai J et al (2012) Trapping of PARP1 and PARP2 by clinical PARP inhibitors. Cancer Res 72:5588–5599. doi:10.1158/0008-5472.CAN-12-2753
51. Ray Chaudhuri A et al (2016) Replication fork stability confers chemoresistance in BRCA-deficient cells. Nature 535:382–387. doi:10.1038/nature18325
52. Fong PC et al (2009) Inhibition of poly(ADP-ribose) polymerase in tumors from BRCA mutation carriers. N Engl J Med 361:123–134. doi:10.1056/NEJMoa0900212
53. Tutt A et al (2010) Oral poly(ADP-ribose) polymerase inhibitor olaparib in patients with BRCA1 or BRCA2 mutations and advanced breast cancer: a proof-of-concept trial. Lancet 376:235–244. doi:10.1016/S0140-6736(10)60892-6
54. Audeh MW et al (2010) Oral poly(ADP-ribose) polymerase inhibitor olaparib in patients with BRCA1 or BRCA2 mutations and recurrent ovarian cancer: a proof-of-concept trial. Lancet 376:245–251. doi:10.1016/S0140-6736(10)60893-8
55. Sandhu SK et al (2013) Poly (ADP-ribose) polymerase (PARP) inhibitors for the treatment of advanced germline BRCA2 mutant prostate cancer. Ann Oncol 24:1416–1418. doi:10.1093/annonc/mdt074
56. Ledermann J et al (2012) Olaparib maintenance therapy in platinum-sensitive relapsed ovarian cancer. N Engl J Med 366:1382–1392. doi:10.1056/NEJMoa1105535
57. Ledermann J et al (2014) Olaparib maintenance therapy in patients with platinum-sensitive relapsed serous ovarian cancer: a preplanned retrospective analysis of outcomes by BRCA status in a randomised phase 2 trial. Lancet Oncol 15:852–861. doi:10.1016/S1470-2045(14)70228-1
58. Andrei AZ et al (2015) Increased in vitro and in vivo sensitivity of BRCA2-associated pancreatic cancer to the poly(ADP-ribose) polymerase-1/2 inhibitor BMN 673. Cancer Lett 364:8–16. doi:10.1016/j.canlet.2015.04.003
59. Yang HJ, Liu VW, Wang Y, Tsang PC, Ngan HY (2006) Differential DNA methylation profiles in gynecological cancers and correlation with clinico-pathological data. BMC Cancer 6:212. doi:10.1186/1471-2407-6-212
60. Wiley A et al (2006) Aberrant promoter methylation of multiple genes in malignant ovarian tumors and in ovarian tumors with low malignant potential. Cancer 107:299–308. doi:10.1002/cncr.21992
61. Lim SL et al (2008) Promoter hypermethylation of FANCF and outcome in advanced ovarian cancer. Br J Cancer 98:1452–1456. doi:10.1038/sj.bjc.6604325
62. Patch AM et al (2015) Whole-genome characterization of chemoresistant ovarian cancer. Nature 521:489–494. doi:10.1038/nature14410
63. Baumann P, Benson FE, West SC (1996) Human Rad51 protein promotes ATP-dependent homologous pairing and strand transfer reactions in vitro. Cell 87:757–766
64. O'Donnell RL et al (2016) Advanced ovarian cancer displays functional intratumor heterogene-

ity that correlates to ex vivo drug sensitivity. Int J Gynecol Cancer 26:1004–1011. doi:10.1097/IGC.0000000000000745
65. Gottipati P et al (2010) Poly(ADP-ribose) polymerase is hyperactivated in homologous recombination-defective cells. Cancer Res 70:5389–5398. doi:10.1158/0008-5472.CAN-09-4716
66. Zaremba T et al (2011) Poly(ADP-ribose) polymerase-1 (PARP-1) pharmacogenetics, activity and expression analysis in cancer patients and healthy volunteers. Biochem J 436:671–679. doi:10.1042/BJ20101723
67. Mateo J et al (2015) DNA-repair defects and Olaparib in metastatic prostate cancer. N Engl J Med 373:1697–1708. doi:10.1056/NEJMoa1506859
68. Telli ML et al (2016) Homologous recombination deficiency (HRD) score predicts response to platinum-containing neoadjuvant chemotherapy in patients with triple-negative breast cancer. Clin Cancer Res 22:3764–3773. doi:10.1158/1078-0432.CCR-15-2477
69. Swisher EM et al (2017) Rucaparib in relapsed, platinum-sensitive high-grade ovarian carcinoma (ARIEL2 Part 1): an international, multicentre, open-label, phase 2 trial. Lancet Oncol 18:75–87. doi:10.1016/S1470-2045(16)30559-9
70. Hong R et al (2016) 53BP1 depletion causes PARP inhibitor resistance in ATM-deficient breast cancer cells. BMC Cancer 16:725. doi:10.1186/s12885-016-2754-7
71. Xu G et al (2015) REV7 counteracts DNA double-strand break resection and affects PARP inhibition. Nature 521:541–544. doi:10.1038/nature14328
72. Watanabe S et al (2013) JMJD1C demethylates MDC1 to regulate the RNF8 and BRCA1-mediated chromatin response to DNA breaks. Nat Struct Mol Biol 20:1425–1433. doi:10.1038/nsmb.2702
73. Ruiz S et al (2016) A genome-wide CRISPR screen identifies CDC25A as a determinant of sensitivity to ATR inhibitors. Mol Cell 62:307–313. doi:10.1016/j.molcel.2016.03.006
74. Wang Y et al (2014) Clonal evolution in breast cancer revealed by single nucleus genome sequencing. Nature 512:155–160. doi:10.1038/nature13600
75. Rytelewski M et al (2016) Reciprocal positive selection for weakness – preventing olaparib resistance by inhibiting BRCA2. Oncotarget 7:20825–20839. doi:10.18632/oncotarget.7883
76. Savitsky K et al (1995) A single ataxia telangiectasia gene with a product similar to PI-3 kinase. Science 268:1749–1753
77. Boder E, Sedgwick RP (1958) Ataxia-telangiectasia; a familial syndrome of progressive cerebellar ataxia, oculocutaneous telangiectasia and frequent pulmonary infection. Pediatrics 21:526–554
78. Yu CE et al (1996) Positional cloning of the Werner's syndrome gene. Science 272:258–262
79. Oshima J, Sidorova JM, Monnat RJ Jr (2017) Werner syndrome: clinical features, pathogenesis and potential therapeutic interventions. Ageing Res Rev 33:105–114. doi:10.1016/j.arr.2016.03.002
80. Agrelo R et al (2006) Epigenetic inactivation of the premature aging Werner syndrome gene in human cancer. Proc Natl Acad Sci U S A 103:8822–8827. doi:10.1073/pnas.0600645103
81. Lehmann AR, McGibbon D, Stefanini M (2011) Xeroderma pigmentosum. Orphanet J Rare Dis 6:70. doi:10.1186/1750-1172-6-70
82. Reynolds JJ, Stewart GS (2013) A single strand that links multiple neuropathologies in human disease. Brain 136:14–27. doi:10.1093/brain/aws310
83. El-Khamisy SF, Masutani M, Suzuki H, Caldecott KW (2003) A requirement for PARP-1 for the assembly or stability of XRCC1 nuclear foci at sites of oxidative DNA damage. Nucleic Acids Res 31:5526–5533
84. El-Khamisy SF et al (2005) Defective DNA single-strand break repair in spinocerebellar ataxia with axonal neuropathy-1. Nature 434:108–113. doi:10.1038/nature03314
85. Hirano M et al (2007) DNA single-strand break repair is impaired in aprataxin-related ataxia. Ann Neurol 61:162–174. doi:10.1002/ana.21078
86. Reynolds JJ et al (2009) Defective DNA ligation during short-patch single-strand break repair in ataxia oculomotor apraxia 1. Mol Cell Biol 29:1354–1362. doi:10.1128/MCB.01471-08
87. Cha MY et al (2015) Mitochondrial ATP synthase activity is impaired by suppressed O-GlcNAcylation in Alzheimer's disease. Hum Mol Genet 24:6492–6504. doi:10.1093/hmg/ddv358
88. Smigrodzki RM, Khan SM (2005) Mitochondrial microheteroplasmy and a theory of aging and age-related disease. Rejuvenation Res 8:172–198. doi:10.1089/rej.2005.8.172
89. Lezi E, Swerdlow RH (2012) Mitochondria in neurodegeneration. Adv Exp Med Biol 942:269–286. doi:10.1007/978-94-007-2869-1_12
90. Verstraeten A, Theuns J, Van Broeckhoven C (2015) Progress in unraveling the genetic etiology of Parkinson disease in a genomic era. Trends Genet 31:140–149. doi:10.1016/j.tig.2015.01.004
91. Vives-Bauza C et al (2010) PINK1-dependent recruitment of Parkin to mitochondria in mitophagy. Proc Natl Acad Sci U S A 107:378–383. doi:10.1073/pnas.0911187107
92. Valentin-Vega YA et al (2012) Mitochondrial dysfunction in ataxia-telangiectasia. Blood 119:1490–1500. doi:10.1182/blood-2011-08-373639
93. Fang EF et al (2014) Defective mitophagy in XPA via PARP-1 hyperactivation and NAD(+)/SIRT1 reduction. Cell 157:882–896. doi:10.1016/j.cell.2014.03.026
94. Sumpter R Jr et al (2016) Fanconi anemia proteins function in mitophagy and immunity. Cell 165:867–881. doi:10.1016/j.cell.2016.04.006
95. Lagouge M et al (2006) Resveratrol improves mitochondrial function and protects against metabolic

disease by activating SIRT1 and PGC-1alpha. Cell 127:1109–1122. doi:10.1016/j.cell.2006.11.013
96. Lehmann S, Costa AC, Celardo I, Loh SH, Martins LM (2016) Parp mutations protect against mitochondrial dysfunction and neurodegeneration in a PARKIN model of Parkinson's disease. Cell Death Dis 7:e2166. doi:10.1038/cddis.2016.72
97. Fang EF et al (2016) NAD+ replenishment improves lifespan and healthspan in ataxia telangiectasia models via mitophagy and DNA repair. Cell Metab 24:566–581. doi:10.1016/j.cmet.2016.09.004
98. Cardinale A, Paldino E, Giampa C, Bernardi G, Fusco FR (2015) PARP-1 inhibition is neuroprotective in the R6/2 mouse model of Huntington's disease. PLoS One 10:e0134482. doi:10.1371/journal.pone.0134482
99. Sharifi R et al (2013) Deficiency of terminal ADP-ribose protein glycohydrolase TARG1/C6orf130 in neurodegenerative disease. EMBO J 32:1225–1237. doi:10.1038/emboj.2013.51
100. Byrne AB et al (2016) Inhibiting poly(ADP-ribosylation) improves axon regeneration. Elife 5:e12734. doi:10.7554/eLife.12734

Nucleotide Excision Repair: From Neurodegeneration to Cancer

2

Anastasios Liakos, Matthieu D. Lavigne, and Maria Fousteri

Abstract

DNA damage poses a constant threat to genome integrity taking a variety of shapes and arising by normal cellular metabolism or environmental insults. Human syndromes, characterized by increased cancer pre-disposition or early onset of age-related pathology and developmental abnormalities, often result from defective DNA damage responses and compromised genome integrity. Over the last decades intensive research worldwide has made important contributions to our understanding of the molecular mechanisms underlying genomic instability and has substantiated the importance of DNA repair in cancer prevention in the general population. In this chapter, we discuss Nucleotide Excision Repair pathway, the causative role of its components in disease-related pathology and recent technological achievements that decipher mutational landscapes and may facilitate pathological classification and personalized therapy.

Keywords

NER deficiency syndromes • Genotype-phenotype relationship • DNA damage responses • Cancer genomics • NER-associated somatic mutation landscapes • Synthetic lethality

2.1 Introduction

Genome integrity is a vital component of all life forms. However, it is constantly challenged by a multitude of genotoxic agents, which produce diverse DNA lesions that alter DNA chemistry, structure and integrity. Such genotoxic agents can be found in the environment and consist of ultraviolet (UV) radiation, ionizing radiation (IR), and many pharmaceuticals, notably anticancer drugs (e.g.: cisplatin, Topoisomerase I and II inhibitors). In addition, threats can rise from endogenous metabolic products or by-products such as reactive oxygen species (ROS), alkylating agents and errors during replication (see [1–3] for review).

A. Liakos • M.D. Lavigne (✉) • M. Fousteri (✉)
Biomedical Sciences Research Center
'Alexander Fleming', 34 Fleming st.,
16672 Vari, Athens, Greece
e-mail: lavigne@fleming.gr; fousteri@fleming.gr

S. El-Khamisy (ed.), *Personalised Medicine*, Advances in Experimental Medicine and Biology 1007,
DOI 10.1007/978-3-319-60733-7_2

Cells regularly respond to these challenges by rapidly inducing pathways/networks of molecular switches that consist of specialized DNA repair mechanisms and signaling cascades, which control DNA and cell status after genotoxic insult. DNA Damage Responses (DDR), as a whole, thus guarantees the durability and maintenance of accurate genomic information. On the other hand, overload in damages or deficient repair mechanisms leave unrepaired lesions and trigger the activation of "no-return" pathways, such as apoptosis, enforcing cell elimination [4], or favor the development of cancer [5].

Among the plethora of DNA repair mechanisms, NER is the one responsible for the removal of bulky, helix distorting DNA adducts. NER efficiency relies in the extreme versatility in the type of recognized DNA lesions. It senses the distortion caused to the DNA double helix indifferently of the lesion chemical structure and excises a short oligonucleotide spanning the lesion (see below).

NER defects result in a large clinical spectrum of human pathologies including neurodevelopmental abnormalities, premature ageing, neurodegeneration and cancer-prone phenotypes. This review aims to clarify and unify some of the most recent models deciphering NER involvement in keeping cells healthy. In particular, we highlight studies that help to understand how DNA damage, differences in genetic background, stress load and cell micro-environment all contribute to determine cell-fate and clinical consequences of different NER diseases. Finally, in line with a clearer understanding of NER-related molecular, cellular and systemic mechanistic details, we describe advances that can facilitate clinical management of NER syndromes and NER-related disorders.

2.2 NER: Target Lesions, Pathways and NER Deficiency Syndromes

We only give here a brief overview of NER topics that have been extensively discussed recently in very comprehensive and detailed reviews [6, 7].

2.2.1 Versatility of DNA Lesions Handled by NER

To achieve versatility NER sensing enzymes do not focus on the lesions per se and this characteristic also contributes to explain the broad range of NER-related patho-physiology. NER senses and repairs DNA double helix-distorting lesions and by virtue can recognize an extraordinarily wide range of substrates with varying chemical structures. A collective feature of NER substrates is that they thermodynamically destabilize the DNA duplex and are bulky. Together with UV light induced toxic cyclopurines (6-4 pyrimidine-pyrimidone photoproducts (6-4PPs) and cyclobutane-pyrimidine dimers (CPDs)), platinated adducts helix distorting lesions are the most common adducts and are handled exclusively by NER.

2.2.2 NER Pathways

The complexity of NER repair mechanism is due to both the size of the molecular scaffolds and the fact that the actions of the involved factors need to be well-orchestrated in a multi-stage process. NER relies on the enzymatic activities or on the stabilizing and regulating interactions of about 30 proteins [8]. Two different modes of NER, namely Global Genome NER (GG-NER or GGR) and Transcription-Coupled NER (TC-NER or TCR), operate the recognition of distorted DNA and determine both spatial- and time-related preferences.

2.2.2.1 Following the DDR Rule of Rs: Recognize, Repair, Restore

Lesion Sensing

NER DNA sensing proteins do not rely on a "lesion-binding" pocket that should fit to a specific type of chemical lesion, but they rather recognize multiple shapes of aberrant bulks in the DNA helix. Briefly, in GG-NER, damage recognition operates throughout the whole genome and depends on the rather random action of XPC-RAD23B or UV-DDB1/2 (XPE) complex [9–11].

In TC-NER, it is the stalling of RNA polymerase II (RNAPII) on DNA adducts and the impairing of RNA synthesis reaction that triggers the alarm. TC-NER occurs faster than GG-NER, but is exclusively limited to the transcribed strand of expressed genes. Importantly, the recruitment of Cockayne Syndrome B (CSB) and Cockayne Syndrome A (CSA) proteins is essential in humans and other eukaryotes for completion of the subsequent core NER reaction at sites of damage stalled RNAPII (see [12, 13] and references therin).

DNA Melting, Lesion Check, and Nucleotide Excision

After damage recognition, the two subpathways converge to recruit TFIIH complex and promote the opening/melting of the lesion containing DNA by the action of its subunits XPB and XPD (reviewed exhaustively in [14]). In turn, XPA, RPA and XPG proteins are recruited. XPA serves to verify the presence of an impairing DNA damage and signals to the 5′ DNA endonuclease XPF-ERCC1 complex whereas RPA binds and protects the single-stranded DNA opposite the damage facilitating the coordination of repair and the correct orientation of the DNA endonucleases. DNA endonuclease XPG associates with and confers stability to TFIIH [15]. It has been shown that incision 5′ to the damage by XPF-ERCC1 precedes the 3′ incision by XPG [16].

De Novo Synthesis and DNA Sealing

Excision of the lesion-containing DNA is followed by de novo synthesis of the 25–30 nt resulting gap by the DNA repair synthesis factors using the undamaged strand as a template. Notably, the identity of the enzymes operating gap filling and ligation depends on the cell cycle status [17]. PCNA, RFC1 and DNA polymerases (DNA pol) delta and kappa fill in the gap in non-cycling cells whereas in dividing cells DNA pol epsilon is also engaged in NER DNA synthesis [18]. Finally, repaired DNA strand is sealed by either XRCC1-DNA ligase IIIa complex or DNA ligase I, in non-cycling and dividing cells, respectively [19].

Chromatin Restoration

Noteworthy, NER acts on DNA in the context of chromatin, and for this reason a mechanism of "access – repair – restore" had been proposed [20]. Recent dramatic advances in our understanding of how NER requires the concordant activity of histone modifying and ATP-dependent remodeling enzymes to transiently "open" a repair bubble, and ensure a full reassembly of the repaired DNA into chromatin after NER completion are very important, but cannot be discussed here due to space constrains. We invite the reader to consult reviews by Peterson and Almouzni [21] and Scharer [7] for more information. It is therefore anticipated that defects in chromatin reorganization after DNA damage could also favor NER pathologies.

2.2.3 NER Deficiency Syndromes

NER deficiencies rise from germ-line mutations in genes encoding the factors involved at any step of the pathway. Hence, defects are inheritable and the associated consequences are systemic and directly impact on human health. As detailed in this section, various diseases have been thoroughly described. Mutations that affect functionality of NER proteins cause mild to extreme photosensitivity, cancer, neurodevelopmental defects and neurodegeneration (reviewed in [22]). However, many other symptoms exist and there is a particularly complex relationship of clinical diseases to NER mutations. In important reviews, Kraemer and co-workers [23] and Rapin [24] present a thorough analysis of the genotype to phenotype characteristics that highlight both the heterogeneous physiological consequences of one or several mutations in NER genes, but also the complexity for clinicians to detect and classify patients based only on the phenotypes.

2.2.3.1 Xeroderma Pigmentosum (XP)

XP is an autosomal recessive disorder characterized by sun and other environmental stresses sensitivity that increase their predisposition for skin, eye and tongue cancers and to lesser extent to other various internal tumors (see review by

Marteijn and colleagues [2] and Spivak [12]). XP patients show a 2000-fold increased incidence of melanoma and 10,000-fold in non-melanoma skin cancers [25]. In 25% of the patients progressive neurological degeneration is also detected. Seven complementation groups with defects in the NER pathway have been assigned genetically in XP (XP-A to -G). An eighth one, XP variant (-V) is proficient in NER, but carries mutations in *POLH* gene that encodes for DNA polymerase η (eta), a translesion synthesis (TLS) polymerase that specializes in error-free replication of DNA containing UV lesions [26]. These findings provided important insights in the genotype/phenotype relationship in XP patients. Nevertheless, systematic examination and long term follow-up of 89 XP patients in the UK, has revealed much larger clinical heterogeneity than anticipated dependent on the affected gene and the exact mutation [27]. Although they do not develop abnormal neurological phenotypes, the TC-NER proficient groups of XP-C, XP-E and XP-V patients, due to relatively normal sunburn reactions, are diagnosed much later than other XP groups and they develop considerable high levels of skin cancer. Surprisingly, among these three XP groups only XP-C patients show in addition progressive ocular damage that is increased with the age. On the other hand, XP-F and XP-G patients have much smaller incidence of skin cancer than the rest of the XP groups. XP patients with different mutations in *XPA, XPB, XPD* or *XPG* gene display none or progressive neurodegeneration with variable severity depending on the exact mutation. In the severely affected cases, XP-related neurologic disease is considered a primary neurodegenerative disease that is mainly characterized by the loss of large neurons throughout the brain, spinal cord, and peripheral nervous system [28].

2.2.3.2 Cockayne Syndrome (CS)

Cockayne Syndrome was firstly reported in 1936 [29] for two siblings with dwarfism, retinal atrophy and deafness and its progression was analyzed [30]. Another case-study of two other siblings described phenotypes linked to progeria [31]. In Western Europe the incidence of Cockayne Syndrome has been estimated to be 2.7 per million live births [32]. Genetic studies uncovered that the two genes that encode for the two TC-NER indispensable proteins, CSA and CSB, are implicated in classical Cockayne Syndrome [33, 34]. Among CS patients almost 60 % carries mutations in *CSB* gene while the rest 40 % in *CSA*. CS is a multisystem disorder characterized among others by cutaneous photosensitivity, deafness, cataracts, large cold extremities, growth and developmental abnormalities, microcephally, dysmyelination, demyelination, increased brain calcification and vasculopathy, progressive neurodegeneration, and mental retardation (for a review with most up-to-date clinical features of CS- related diseases, see [35]). In addition, a large comprehensive clinical description of CS and recommendations for care has been reported by Wilson and co-workers [36].

Combined Phenotype of XP/CS

Specific mutations in *XPB*, *XPD* or *XPG* genes were identified in patients diagnosed with XP and these patients were classified with the rare XP/CS phenotype as they present skin sensitivity similar to XP patients, but also severe developmental abnormalities such as short stature, deficient sexual development and retinal atrophy similar to CS patients [23].

Cerebro-oculo-facio-skeletal Syndrome (COFS)

COFS syndrome (reviewed in [37]) belongs to the spectrum of inherited defects in NER resulting in acute photosensitivity. It is a rare autosomal recessive inherited disorder characterized by congenital microcephaly, congenital cataracts and/or microphthalmia, arthrogryposis, severe developmental delay, severe postnatal growth failure and facial dysmorphism. COFS that carry mutations in the CSB gene belong to the most severely affected CS patients and show a prenatal onset of the symptoms. In addition to *CSB*, mutations have been identified in *XPD*, *XPG* and *ERCC1* genes. Similarly to CS, cells from COFS patients have impaired TC-NER pathway, and they are GG-NER proficient.

2.2.3.3 UV Sensitive Syndrome (UVSS)

UVSS, which was firstly reported in 1994 [38], is an autosomal recessive disorder. UVSS causative mutations have been identified on *CSA* or *CSB* gene (three affected patients) [39, 40], while the rest of the cases were attributed to mutations of the recently identified *UVSSA* (UV-stimulated scaffold protein A) gene [41–43]. UVSSA protein interacts with RNAPII and it is stable associated with TC-NER complexes in response to UV [41, 43]. UVSSA forms a complex with the ubiquitin-specific protease USP7 and upon UV irradiation prevents degradation of CSB protein at the early steps of repair [42, 44].

UVSS patients share some clinical features with the CS patients such as cutaneous photosensitivity, freckling and telangiectasia. However, this syndrome lacks the severe growth and neurological abnormalities characterizing CS patients (as reviewed by Spivak [45]). The phenotypic difference of the two syndromes seems quite striking considering that cells from both UVSS and CS patients are characterized by defective TC-NER and are unable to restore gene expression after UV stress [46]. Although the molecular mechanism that underlies the clinical differences seen in the two syndromes is not known, several hypotheses have been proposed based on the additional molecular functions of CS proteins beyond TC-NER (reviewed in Schwertman and co-workers [47]).

2.2.3.4 Trichothiodystrophy (TTD)

Specific mutations in *XPB*, *XPD* and *TTDA* genes result in TTD, a disease that is characterized by sulfur deficient brittle hair and ichthyosis. In addition, mental retardation and demyelination have been reported, as well as skeletal abnormalities [23, 32]. Interestingly, increased cancer susceptibility is lacking from these patients and this results in an overlap of clinical prognosis between CS and TTD. However, the two conditions show distinct clinical features such as cachexia, optic atrophy and deafness that are absent in TTD [24].

2.2.3.5 Clinical Features and Mutation Position Effect

As illustrated in Fig. 2.1, mutations in one gene of NER pathway could lead to different diseases. For example, different mutations in the *XPD* gene cause six different NER disorders (XP, XP/CS, XP/TTD, COFS, XP with neurological disease, TTD). Reciprocally, each clinical disorder may be the result of mutations in different NER genes as is the case of UVSS and COFS syndromes. The position of the mutation and thus the amount and stability of the protein produced could provide explanation for this complexity. For example, a missense but simultaneously tolerated mutation could result in milder phenotypes compared to a nonsense mutation, which results in truncated often nonfunctional protein. Also, given that NER acts as a molecular cascade where interactions of different proteins are vital for the completion of DNA repair, mutations that affect crucial protein regions for interaction with other NER partners could be deleterious compared to other mutations that do not. However, the fact that the same mutation could cause two distinct NER related phenotypes [48] implies that the genetic background or other unidentified factors may play a crucial role for unraveling the genotype/phenotype correlations of NER disorders.

Considering these features and depending on cells microenvironment, a wide range of symptoms could arise at the organism level when NER pathway is not functional. Moreover, since NER factors are shared with other pathways the etiology of NER-related diseases is complicated (see below for details). For instance, to efficiently overcome ICLs, Fanconi Anaemia (FA) pathway combines NER components, nuclease pathways, TLS polymerase activity, and Homologous Recombination (HR) (see review by Dietlein and co-workers [49]).

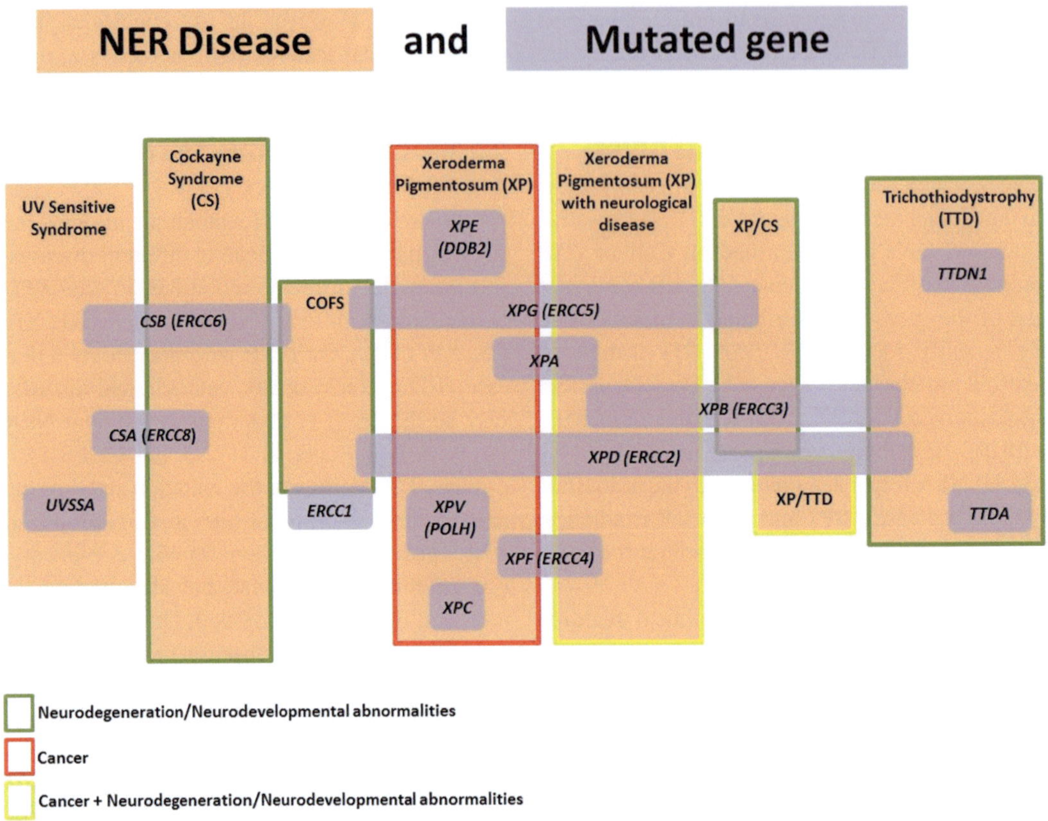

Fig. 2.1 Genotype/phenotype relationships between NER disorders highlighting the overlap with observed neurological and cancer abnormalities (Adapted from [50])

2.3 Molecular, Cellular and Systemic Consequences of NER Alteration

In cells presenting NER deficiencies, environmental exposure and endogenous stress accelerate the age-dependent accumulation of somatic mutations. Age-related diseases such as cancer or neurodegeneration, which characterize NER patients, therefore present common molecular bases for their onset and progression although they seem clinically opposed. In fact, both pathologies develop faster and more frequently in these patients [51]. The consequences of poor DNA damage management by the cell can either be increased cell-death, which is a hallmark of neuropathology, or uncontrolled proliferation, a hallmark of cancer. A fine line separates how DNA damages infer on cell survival or death [3, 52]. NER molecular deficiencies may impact on key decision-making nodes that can drive the cell into one path or the other (Fig. 2.2). Consequences are modulated by the genetic, epigenetic and environmental contexts, developmental stage and cell identity and microenvironment that directly act on these switches.

2.3.1 From DNA Damage to Cell Death Driven Neuropathologies

Neurodegeneration and neurodevelopmental phenotypes result both from extensive cell death of either the post-mitotic division-resistant neurons, or from the impairment of neuronal cell differentiation during development. Neuronal development requires extensive proliferation of neural progenitor cells, which in turn gradually

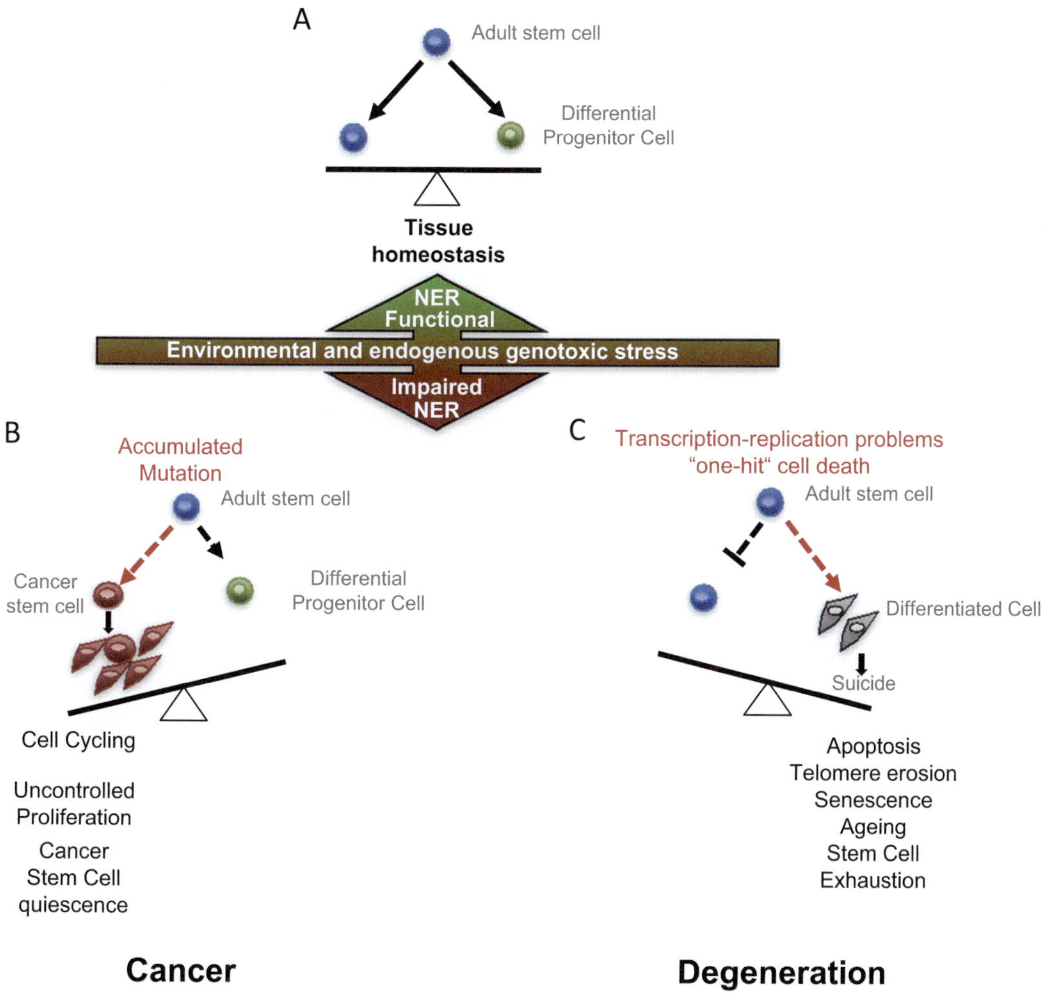

Fig. 2.2 (**a**) Genotoxic stress is managed by functional NER in normal cells. The consequences of impaired NER on exposed cells balance between cancer (**b**) and Degeneration (**c**) depending on endogenous and exogenous parameters

differentiate in order to generate a wide spectrum of specialized neuronal and glial cells. During different stages of neural development, the nervous system is challenged by different types of DNA damage. At the first stages of neurogenesis, it seems that the main type of DNA damage that cells need to overcome is the replication stress due to the extensive expansion of neural progenitor cells. As neural progenitor cells differentiate and maturate, oxidative damage and transcription deregulation become the major threats for neuronal genomic stability [53]. Importantly, cells micro-environment and physiology greatly impact on the clinical outcome of NER impairment with regards to neurodegeneration and neurodevelopmental abnormalities. Acknowledging these important parameters, new studies are being designed and pursued and aim to decipher the versatility in NER components molecular functions in different environments. It is beyond any doubt that, the multiple roles of some of the NER factors beyond the classic DNA repair context could help to further understand the cause of NER neuropathologies and lead to targeted therapeutic strategies.

2.3.1.1 Neuropathologies Derived from Misregulation of Transcription

Several lines of evidence support a crucial role of CSB in both RNA pol II [54–59] and RNA pol I mediated transcription [60, 61]. Apart from CSB and the basal transcription factor TFIIH, other NER components have been shown to have a role in RNA pol II transcription among them XPG [15, 62] and CSA [63]. Similar to CSB, TFIIH components, XPB and XPD, as well as XPG, but also CSA have been shown to be important for RNA pol I transcription and mutations in these NER factors result in reduction of rRNA synthesis [60, 64, 65]. These observations could provide a link between the molecular defects caused by the absence of any of these factors and the phenotype in CS or XP/CS patients. For example, defects in RNA pol I transcription will severely impair ribosome synthesis, which is fundamental for normal growth rate and neurodevelopment. Thus, a number of phenotypic neurological characteristics of CS patients, such as dysmyelination, microcephally and abnormal development of the brain, could be indirect consequences of such dysfunctions [28].

Interestingly, CSB has been shown to be necessary for the trans-differentiation of fibroblasts to neurons. Indeed, absence of CSB affects the expression of more than 1200 genes in human fibroblasts, many of which are related to neural development [66]. A follow-up study [67] pointed that the abnormal neurotrophin signaling could be the cause of defective neurogenesis in CSB patients.

2.3.1.2 The Transcription/Replication Collision Problem in Neuropathology

Many disorders caused by aberrant response to replication stress are characterized by growth failure and neurological problems [68]. In line with this, it has been shown that NER factors (endonucleases XPF and XPG) require CSB in order to process R loops resulting in DSB formation and trigger of DDR [69]. An R-loop is a three-strand nucleic acid structure and consists of an RNA-DNA hybrid plus a displaced ssDNA. R loops are naturally occurring and are considered to be byproducts of transcription activity [70]. In a recent study, which identifies and characterizes interacting partners of a tagged CSB [71], CSB was found to be co-purified with topoisomerase I (Topo I). Loss of Topo I has been linked to increased R-loop formation and increased interference between transcription and replication [72, 73]. Thus, an important role for CSB could be to recruit topo I at sites of R-loop formation or to facilitate its action by proper chromatin remodeling at the respective genomic sites. In the brain, increased genotoxic stress could be sufficient to facilitate R-loop formation as RNAPII will be stalled during repair of bulky lesions [13, 74].

Finally, R-loops could act as a barrier for replication fork progression leading to replication stress and genomic instability, factors that promote cancer formation [68, 75, 76]. Nonetheless, as mentioned before, during neurogenesis there are high rates of DNA replication. Also, even though the vast majority of mature brain cells do not replicate, there are regions in the adult brain where neuronal progenitor replication still occurs such as hippocampus and lateral ventricle [77]. Thus, neuronal cells ability to resolve possible transcription/replication collisions coordinated by the actions of a functional TC-NER machinery in the early stages of neural development, but also in the adult life may be critical for proper development of neuronal system.

2.3.1.3 Autophagy and Neurodegeneration

The word autophagy derives from the Greek words "auto", which means "self" and "phagy", which means "eating". Autophagy is a natural occurring regulated cellular process through which cellular components such as proteins or even whole organelles are degraded and recycled. This mechanism plays a crucial role in cell homeostasis. Mitochondria are vital cellular organelles that, besides their energy-supplying role in the cell, have the ability of releasing hazardous byproducts (such as ROS). These moieties represent a threat for cellular life and stability. For this reason, mitophagy -a specialized type of autophagy is necessary to remove damage by

ROS or dysfunctional mitochondria. A striking functionality of neurons that rely on autophagy impairment has been correlated to neurodegenerative disorders such as Alzheimer and Parkinson diseases (see review [78]).

Interestingly, CSA and CSB proteins were found to be localized to mitochondria upon oxidative stress and to interact with mitochondrial proteins [79, 80]. In line with this, primary CS-A and CS-B human fibroblasts showed elevated levels of ROS productions [81]. Also, CS-B cells showed impaired mitophagy and this phenotype was rescued using stimulants of autophagy [82]. The same abnormality exists also in XP-A as well as Ataxia Telengiectasia (AT) cells linking neurodegeneration with impaired mitophagy [83].

A number of clinical features observed in CS patients are similar to those described for mitochondrial diseases [35]. The use of autophagy stimulants as therapeutic strategy for CS or XP patients seems promising and could lead in better management of these diseases [82]. However, the exact role of NER proteins in mitochondria and the causative link with patients' clinical features is still not clear.

2.3.1.4 Telomere Instability as an Ageing "Driver"

The stability of telomeres is vital for genome maintenance and NER efficiency in these genomic loci is expected to guarantee chromosomal integrity. However, the existing literature complicates rather than clarifies the role of NER in telomeres. While some studies [84] suggested that telomeres are less prone to UV lesions when compared to the rest of the genome, another study suggests that telomeres are hypersensitive to UV irradiation [85].

On the other hand, short telomere length has been correlated with ageing and neurodegenerative disorders [86] and factors such as oxidative stress can enhance telomere shortening. Interestingly, CSB was shown to interact with TRF2 a component of the telomere protective complex Shelterin [87]. The same study supports that CS-B cells show telomere shortening and deregulation of TERRA expression, a long non-coding RNA participating in their maintenance. The fact that CS cells show elevated ROS production compared to control cells [81] in combination with the absence of CSB-mediated protective interactions in telomeres could lead in extensive telomere shortening and thus ageing phenotype. Apart from CSB several other NER proteins have been associated with a role in telomere maintenance such as ERCC1/XPF, XPB, XPD and XPC (see review [88]), however their exact role remains unclear.

2.3.1.5 The "One Hit" Model Explanation

It has been proposed [28] that, many of the neurological features of CS, as retinal degeneration, fit the "one hit" model for inherited neuronal degeneration [89]. According to this model, it is not the accumulation of damages, which results eventually in cell death, but rather cells are constantly more prone to cell death due to certain molecular defects (in CS case, aberrant RNA pol I and pol II transcription or higher DNA damage levels) and a single catastrophic event can trigger cell death. Given that each tissue's microenvironment is different, the events that trigger cell death are variable and together could explain the multi-systemic abnormalities observed in CS and XP patients.

2.3.2 From DNA Damage to Uncontrolled Cell Proliferation (Cancer)

The development of cancer cells benefits from stochastic "driver" mutations in proto-oncogenes. In this respect, cancer risk is heavily influenced by extrinsic factors [90] and erroneous DNA repair, due to NER deficiency, is an important contributor to carcinogenesis. Understanding the nature, the cause, the time of formation and the localization of DNA damages that can be repaired by NER and defining the correlation between DNA damage formation and frequency of mutations in exposed genomes, is therefore an active area of ongoing research [2, 91–93].

2.3.2.1 Monitoring DNA Damage and NER Activity

Next-Generation Sequencing (NGS) derived technologies have provided new tools to analyze the presence and the repair of DNA damages by NER in a genome-wide manner. Excision-sequencing mapping of dipyrimidine [94] and the CPD-seq method [95], which relies on the recognition of CPD sites by the repair enzyme T4 Endonuclease V, were developed to measure NER targeted damage levels in stress exposed genomes. Although these studies report single-nucleotide resolution maps of NER damages, the applicability of these techniques to human samples is still hypothetic. Other techniques, relying on immunoprecipitation of pyrimidine dimers, can also provide information on the location of damages after genotoxic stress, however these methods, although applicable in human samples, still lack high-resolution [96–98]. Another active area of research concerns the monitoring of NER-specific repair activity. Two studies demonstrate how eXcision Repair-sequencing (XR-seq) can map excised CPD lesions at single-nucleotide resolution in human cells exposed to UV [99, 100]. These studies provide valuable information that could be used to correlate DNA damage and repair signatures with observed mutational signatures in cancer or normal genomes (described in detail below).

2.3.2.2 Genetic Consequences of NER Deficiency in the Next Generation of Cells

Deficient NER directly contributes to increased mutagenesis in exposed cells and favors their transformation into cancer [2, 93]. It is commonly accepted that NER-dependent mutations occur when the damaged/unrepaired DNA template is miss-replicated. As opposed to normal cells that are capable to replicate in an error free mode, NER-deficient cells accumulate so many damages that they may be forced to favor an error-prone pathway [101]. Interestingly, both biochemical and genomic studies established that CPDs occur with great preference at TpT dipyrimidines, followed by TpC, CpT, and CpC [100, 102, 103]. Nonetheless, early studies on UV mutagenicity established that in spite of being a major photoproduct, TpT sites do not represent mutational hotspots following UV stress. Instead, CpC photolesions have been shown to have high mutagenicity as confirmed by the high frequency of C > T (G > A) mutation in skin tumor samples of XP patients [103, 104]. The switch to error-prone TLS DNA polymerase ζ probably favours C > T mutations [93], and in agreement, the inactivation of error-free TLS DNA polymerase η that limits the occurrence of these cases leads to XP variant (XPV) syndrome, which displays hypermutability [26, 105].

2.3.2.3 Range of NER-Associated Cancers Is Growing

The discovery that NER protects against skin cancer raised almost instantly the question of whether its misregulation could possibly contribute to other types of environmentally induced cancer in humans [6]. Indeed, consistent with the fact that they raise in "sunlight exposed" tissues, skin, head-and-neck or tip-of-the-tongue cancers are the most commonly detected in NER-deficient patients, and they are related to their inherited incapability to deal with UV-stress. However, the fact that protection of other genotoxic stress such as oxidative stress or cigarette smoke largely depends on cell ability to perform NER, one could expect that patients with deficiencies in NER should also present signs of oncogenesis in internal organs. Little efforts have been made sofar in deciphering such occurrences in XP patients, most likely because they never appeared strikingly. A logic explanation for the prevalence of "sunlight"-related cancers consists in the high potency of UV radiation to create DNA adducts. In turn, the fast and aggressive life-threatening character of these carcinomas may precede the potential influence of damages/mutations in internal organs. In fact, although other types of cancers in NER patients have not been recorded systematically, interesting cases confirm this possibility. Three primary internal tumors (a neuroendocrine tumor of the thyroid, a gastric adenocarcinoma, and a glioma of the brain) were found in young XP children. All of them contained one mutation on the p53 gene, which were different from the ones found in patients' skin tumors and could have resulted from unrepaired lesions caused by oxidative damage [106]. Another early study reported that among the XP patients with internal cancer, there was a disproportionate representation of malignant neoplasms of the brain (especially sarcomas), and oral cavity (excluding tongue) [107]. Finally, after having developed several skin cancers, an XP-B patient that was proven to be a heavy smoker also developed a lung cancer, which led to her death at 55 years old [27]. Thus, it seems important to investigate more carefully the consequences of NER impairment in internal organs (see below).

2.3.2.4 Cancer Genomics Identifies NER-Dependent Somatic Mutation Landscapes

Next-generation sequencing (NGS) approaches allowed massive increases in the throughput of human genome analyses and have tremendously advanced the resolution of somatic mutation landscapes. The joined efforts of large consortiums such as The Cancer Genome Atlas (TCGA: https://cancergenome.nih.gov/) have brought huge expectations for a deeper understanding of both the molecular causes and the genetic/epigenetic characteristics of a multitude of cancer types. Advanced mathematical approaches [91, 108] are used to analyze all available genomic DNA sequences and allow the precise extraction of consensus mutational signatures (check http://cancer.sanger.ac.uk/cosmic/signatures for a comprehensive and updated list of signatures of mutational processes detected in Human Cancer). Such signatures are determined by the probability of each possible base substitution in a trinucleotide context, and are buried within cancer genomes. Powerful algorithms are capable of "de-mixing" the various mutational patterns that result from different mutational processes, which have operated through the life for each analyzed tissue/tumor. As a result, cancer geneticists are now able to distinguish cancers simply by looking for characteristics of mutational activities that can operate in different tissue types or in different environments [109, 110].

In other words, analysis of such somatic mutations catalogues can inform investigators on the possible mutagen sources providing insights into the mechanisms involved in the mutagenic processes that shape tumor DNA (see review [111]). In particular, and of interest here, UV light mutational signatures, which are associated to NER misfunction (C > T (or G > A on complementary strand) mutations, see above for molecular reasons) or tobacco smoke (C > A (or G > T on complementary strand) guanine substitutions occurring after exposure to benzo[a]pyrene contained in tobacco smoke) were detected in skin and lung cancers genomes [112, 113] and were assigned number 7 and 4, respectively [91] (Fig. 2.3).

Interestingly, these signatures showed strong transcriptional strand bias (as marked in Fig. 2.3) with less mutations on the transcribed strand than on the non-transcribed strand [112, 113]. Transcription activity and operation of TC-NER pathway were thus proposed to be directly involved in the generation of these signatures [91]. Accordingly, these signatures show a lower rate of mutagenesis in gene bodies as compared to intergenic regions.

It is thus evident that cancer genome sequencing offers great investigative power as a means to not only map mutation events, but also to understand the clinical prospects associated with this technology. Comparative diagnosis of tumor and normal biopsies can reveal where a specific repair activity has occurred (and potentially, has not), which were the repair processes that operated for years before the cancer became symptomatic, and what possible carcinogens promote a given cancer. In this way, novel mutational asymmetries such as (T > C vs. A > G) could prove to be NER-associated mechanisms of mutagenesis in liver cancer [92].

Mutation analyses also uncovered a reduced local mutation density within regulatory DNA, which was shown to depend on intact NER machinery, as cancers with NER mutations accumulate more mutations in regulatory regions [114]. Similarly, it was demonstrated that low mutation rate around transcription start site in squamous cell carcinoma (SCC) depends on intact XPC activity

NER Associated Signatures	Found In	Known Exposure/Aetiology
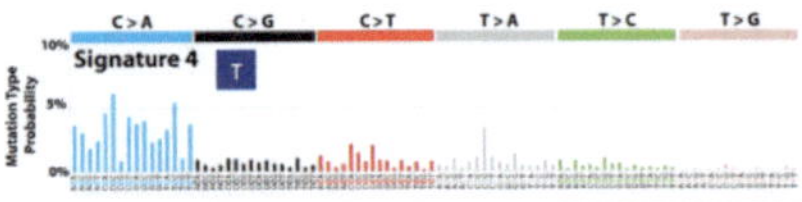	head and neck cancer liver cancer lung adenocarcinoma lung squamous carcinoma small cell lung carcinoma oesophageal cancer	tobacco carcinogens (e.g.: benzo[a]pyrene causing adducts on guanine)
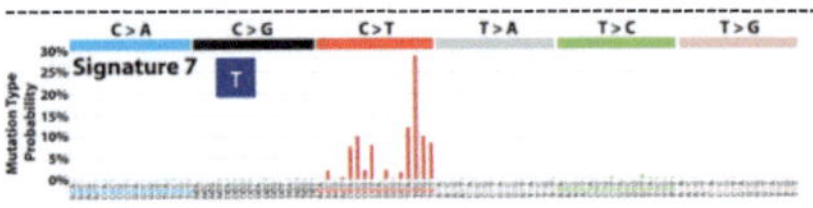	skin cancers cancers of the lip (categorized as: head and neck or oral squamous cancers)	prevalence in UV exposed areas
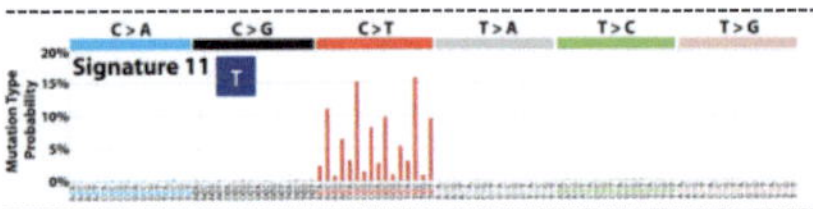	melanoma glioblastoma	alkylating agenttemozolomide
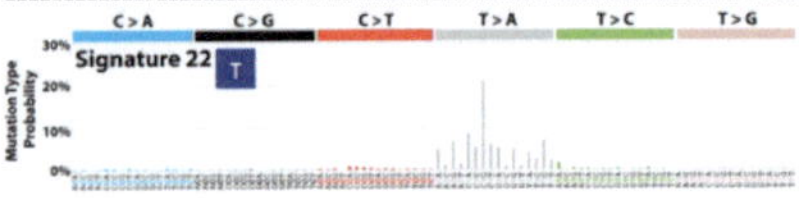	Urothelial (renal pelvis) carcinoma liver cancers	aristolochic acid
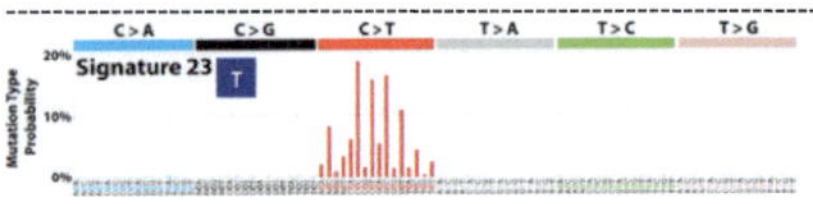	only in one single liver cancer sample	unknown
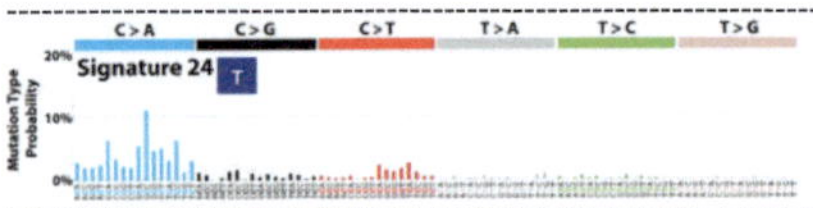	subset of Liver cancers	exposed to Aflatoxin causing adducts on guanine
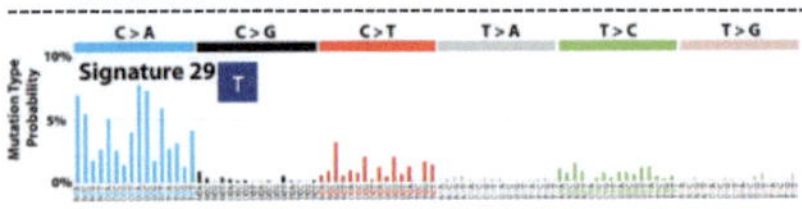	gingivo-buccal oral squamous cell carcinoma	individuals with a tobacco chewing habit*

Fig. 2.3 Mutational signatures recorded in various cancer genomes as extracted from COSMIC database show transcription strand bias (*blue T boxes*) and NER specific features. *: Different from signature 4 characteristic of tobacco smoking

[115]. Finally, in light of the findings that epigenetic silencing of DNA repair genes could be sufficient to promote tumorigenesis [116], we anticipate that looking for differences in mutational signatures and correlate them to mutational status in epigenetic genes or to epigenetic maps could advance our knowledge on the exact influence of chromatin reorganization in DNA repair.

Importantly, we note that the bioinformatics algorithms are particularly discriminative and can distinguish between C > T mutations that occurred because of the lack of NER operation or because of other activities like C deamination at CpGs [91]. Also, as mentioned above, they can be used to discover new signatures that fit NER or TC-NER specificity. For instance, the transcriptional bias in mutation profiles such as the one of Aflatoxin adducts on guanine (signature 24 (C > A or G > T) and Aristolochic Acid adducts on Adenine (Signature 22 (T > A or A > T)) (http://cancer.sanger.ac.uk/cosmic/signatures) could help to understand the reasons leading to liver or renal pelvis tumors (Fig. 2.3). All the signatures in Fig. 2.3 present a transcription bias that is compatible with increased NER efficiency via TC-NER. However, this bias does not necessarily imply that the cells are NER-deficient. Rather bursts of genotoxic stress might have overwhelmed them, leaving unrepaired lesions in an expected unbalanced manner, due to TC-NER improved yield vs GG-NER.

Cancer Genomics Identifies NER Somatic Mutations

An early report claimed the absence of mutations in NER genes in sporadic solid tumors possibly because their many other essential cellular functions outside NER could favor a negative selection process where cells would commit to cell death before being able to transform [117]. However, more recent studies performed with higher resolution point in the other direction. As mutations accumulate steadily in tissues that get older (see review for details [118]), acquired somatic mutations can rise within NER genes for patients that did dot inherit NER defects from birth. In turn, in these cells, lack of proficient NER facilitates carcinogenesis [2, 93]. Accordingly, enrichment of signature 5 that exhibits transcriptional strand bias for T > C substitutions was found in bladder cancers harboring inactivating mutations in ERCC2 [119]. Polak and coworkers reported that 9 out of 29 (~30 %) studied melanoma genomes harbored nonsynonymous mutations in NER genes [114]. In particular, they identified a mutation in CETN2, a protein known to recognize DNA distortions in GG-NER preferentially, and showed accordingly an intact strong suppression of mutations in transcribed regions. In sharp contrast, genomes carrying mutations in important core NER subunits, *XPG*/ERCC5 and *XPF*/*ERCC4*, showed high mutation density also in transcribed regions, demonstrating that defects in both TC-NER and GG-NER cancels mutation landscape heterogeneities and as expected they significantly increase mutagenesis. As explained below, the latter could be used as a therapeutic means. An interesting review by Dietlein and coworkers, explains how in general genes involved in different DNA damage repair pathways are frequently altered in cancer, and highlights accumulated inactivating somatic mutations within NER pathway in prostate cancer [49]. In addition, a DDB1 mutation was reported in diffuse large B-cell lymphomas [120], and a recent study inquiring the mutational landscape of DNA repair genes in cancer reports that CSB mutations are acquired in lung, breast and skin tumors, and that, among others, *ERCC2*, *LIG1* and *POLE* are also frequently mutated in various cancers [121]. These results should be put in perspective with the findings that CSB repair factor is overexpressed in cancer cells to increase apoptotic resistance and promote tumor growth [122].

2.3.2.5 NER-Linked Molecular Defects Leading to Cancer

Transcription-Replication Collisions and Cancer

Impaired NER and TC-NER activity can leave unprocessed repair bubbles that represent barriers to replication fork progression. For instance, cancer genomic analyses in correlation with NER activity mapping demonstrated that late-repaired regions are associated with a higher level of cancer-linked mutations [99]. In line with this, human mutation rate has been shown to correlate with DNA replication timing [92, 123]. Increased frequency of transcription-replication collisions can overwhelm the cell, and increase DNA DSB, rearrangements, chromosome fusions, which are all features known to promote carcinogenesis [124].

Autophagy and Cancer

It was recently shown that deficiency in autophagy reduces XPC expression and inhibits DDB2 recruitment at damage sites [125]. Authors hypothesized that as XPC and DDB2 are key players for damage recognition by GG-NER pathway, this abnormality could result in decreased DNA repair, accumulation of mutations and cancer development. Indeed, pharmacological inhibition of autophagy induced skin carcinogenesis in mice. It would be interesting to test if whether UVRAG, an inducer of autophagy [126], which is known to help in recruiting NER via its association with DDB1 at damage sites to protect cells against UV irradiation [127] is involved in this process.

Although autophagy role in cancer is controversial [128], it seems that autophagy deregulation represents a bridge between cancer and neurodegeneration and that the crosstalk between NER proteins and autophagy has a clear protective role against both diseases. Further research in this field could uncover the exact mechanisms through which this crosstalk is mediated and a possible evaluation and targeting of NER proteins as regulators of autophagy could lead to specific treatment strategies against cancer and neurodegeneration.

2.4 NER Proteins as Markers and Targets for Personalized Therapeutics

Following the recent discoveries showing that DNA-repair deficiency is correlated to better prognosis in cancer, researchers and clinicians began to see DNA repair pathways as "Achille's heel of cancer" [129]. Together they have intensified efforts to develop biomarkers in DNA repair pathways to predict tumor response to therapy. In other words, deep-sequencing-based genetic diagnosis should be used to detect if, and which, genetic alterations in the DNA repair pathways are altered in each tumor to be treated. In parallel, the mapping of characteristic mutations in all sorts of cancer genomes (see above) of specific mutational landscapes and signatures should further inform on the potential status of DNA repair capabilities in specific tumors. This approach could help in predicting which DNA repair pathway could be affected in each patient and could be correlated to their clinical history. Along with revolutionary single-cell analyses techniques, researchers can also start to disentangle genetic heterogeneities of tumors and to understand cell-type specific genotype-phenotype relationships that must be well apprehended to maximize therapeutic target specificity. Overall, such strategies are still under development and will continue to facilitate customizing treatment for each patient. In turn, such precise and personalized medicine should limit the occurrence of unresponsive treatments. In case that a drug will benefit from a DNA-repair deficient environment, the doses to apply will be lower and this could limit known secondary of current anti-cancer drugs, which remain generally very uncomfortable to the patients. In addition to this therapeutic avenue, and in situations were patients do no not show repair deficiencies, the identification of potent DNA repair inhibitors could be used in synthetic-lethal combination therapies to artificially create an environment beneficial for the primary drug and guarantee better patient survival and quality of life (see also reviews for deeper understanding) [49, 130, 131]. As explained, impairment or deregulation of NER components predisposes cells to various diseases ranging from neuropathology to cancer. Nonetheless, at the same time, and as mentioned earlier, somatically acquired NER inhibition would offer opportunities in cancer management [2, 49, 131].

2.4.1 NER-Dependent p53 Loss-of-Function Facilitates Cancer Stem Cells Development

The molecular and cellular bases of tumor cell birth are intimately linked to NER activity. In the case of transformed cancer cells, important DNA damage response (DDR) checkpoints have been bypassed to allow tumour cell initiation, and proliferation. Hotspots of somatic mutations in key players ruling the cancer Stem Cell (CSC) theory, such as p53, are observed in about 25% of the human cancers [132], and justify its name "tumor-suppressor gene". p53 normal function imposes an essential barrier to CSC formation as it coordinates DDR in general and in particular its function is required for NER [133]. The gene *TP53* shows similar mutation spectra across different cancer types. The patterns of mutation were associated with known carcinogens such as the one we described above: UV light and tobacco smoke. These result in high frequency of C > T, and C > A substitutions respectively in p53 coding sequence [134]. Guaranteeing normal tissue homeostasis and coordinating adult stem cells (ASC) stock regeneration, p53 helps in tissue regeneration after injuries and coordinates the molecular regulation of stem cell quiescence [135, 136]. Therefore, NER deficiency driven mutations in p53 promotes the onset of a wide variety of cancers due to the multiplication of CSCs in an uncontrolled manner [136, 137]. Combining these observations with the fact that CSCs can acquire the potential to migrate, and therefore establish a metastasis, and with the discovery that CSCs are resistant to chemotherapy and radiation [138], one can anticipate that

CSC-rich tumors are associated with aggressive disease and poor prognosis. Thus, lack of efficient surveillance by NER is critical in the initiation of this "dark" path. Proliferating CSCs, which have developed resistance to DNA damage accumulate mutations at a fast rate and these are transferred to the next generation of self-renewing or differentiating cells [139]. In this vicious circle, p53 mutations accumulate with continued exposure to carcinogens, and cells acquire increasing resistance to apoptosis.

Interestingly, p53 restoration in CSCs has shown some therapeutic efficacy as it can suppress tumor growth. Nonetheless, these effects could be limited by the lack of tumor regression in p53 missense mutations genetic background, which could produce a dominant-negative effect [140, 141]. Nonetheless, as described below possibilities of combinatorial approaches with traditional cancer therapies aiming at the bulk of the tumor could be promising avenues to reduce tumor size. For instance, p53-based differentiation-inducing therapies can target CSCs that tend to remain in a dormant state and are not sensitive to chemo or radiation therapies [142].

2.4.2 Ways to Improve Therapy Efficiency

2.4.2.1 Differential Background of Accumulated Damages in Healthy and Cancer Cells

Although responses to traditional DNA-damaging anticancer therapy are limited in CSC rich tumors, the possibility to specifically target the differences in DNA repair capacity between normal and tumor cells is exciting. If CSCs and their progeny have accumulated high background levels of somatic mutations [143], promoting even more DNA damages in a context where these cells cannot rely on DDR can increase the chances that these cells reach a point of "no-return" before their neighbor normal cells. Indeed, normal cells rely on their proficient repair system, which contributes to maintain an overall lower mutation burden during their lifetime.

2.4.2.2 Increasing the Probability That NER Fails to Help Cancer Cells to Survive

The biomedical field seems to be rushing towards the investigation of novel markers of DNA repair pathways and apply focused efforts to identify potential drugable DNA repair targets [131]. Inhibition of NER in a personalized manner depending on patients' DNA repair abilities holds great promises for cancer therapy, especially considering that acquired tumor resistance to chemotherapy could be due to over expression of the NER elements [144]. Mouw and coworkers analyzed the frequency of mutations in NER genes in several solid tumor types [145]. They suggested the presence of underlying NER genes alterations in several epithelial cancer genomes including the ones of bladder, colorectal and renal cancers, and conclude that additional genomic studies may identify clinical contexts in which NER pathway alterations could be used to inform therapy selection. In fact, it would be interesting to study the contribution of all NER genes polymorphisms to cancer probability and test whether their associated drug efficacy could increase prognosis of certain cancers (reviewed in [146]). We list below some of the various promising markers and NER-related inhibitors that could be used in combination with established anti-cancer agents such as platinum-based drugs that damage DNA deliberately, but usually suffer from the counteracting effects of functional NER.

2.4.3 NER-Specific Synthetic Lethality Approaches

Synthetic lethality strategy aims to artificially achieve defects in two different genes or pathways which together result in cell death.

Cisplatins are alkylating agents that form intra strand crosslinks in DNA, as well as DNA-protein crosslinks, which are predominantly repaired via NER. Cisplatin can induce cell cycle arrest and cell death via various pathways [147] and it has been used for decades as an anticancer drug in many tumors such as testicular, ovarian, bladder and lung cancers. Nevertheless, the discovery of the molecular mechanisms of tumour resistance to these drugs and combination studies with resistance modulators brings back these chemotherapeutics at the centre of the cancer stage [148].

The increased sensitivity of XP-patients derived cells to cisplatin treatment revealed that NER pathway is implicated in the repair of cisplatin lesions [149]. Following this stepping-stone discovery, both NER and cancer fields intensified efforts to characterize more precisely, which impaired functionalities of NER pathway affect cancer cells. For example, compromised NER activity is frequent in several solid tumor types, and the assessment of XPG expression levels may be a useful marker to predict tumour sensitivity to the alkylating agent Irofulven [150]. In an attempt to personalize cancer therapy and take advantage of these observations, development of assays that could measure directly NER capacity of tumor samples have been performed [151], but optimization of these test is needed before routine clinical application. NGS approaches will be very useful for the diagnosis of uncommon NER related disorders [152]. By extension, NER deficiency could be monitored by signature changes or by somatic mutations in NER genes in tumor cells (see above). Thorough analysis of recently established, or yet to come, high-resolution cancer mutational profiles will help in this direction.

Inhibiting artificially NER can boost the efficiency of treatment, and prior knowledge of tumor repair capacity for each patient will lead to better planning of anti-cancer strategies. As detailed below, an increasing number of molecules of the NER pathway has been studied for their role in cisplatin therapy and response.

2.4.3.1 XPA-XPF/ERCC1

Early efforts to identify inhibitors that can disrupt XPA-XPF/ERCC1 interaction demonstrated promising results [153, 154]. Furthermore, tumors with low ERCC1 expression have been correlated to better responses in cisplatin treatment for various types of cancer as testicular [155, 156], ovarian [157] and non-small cell lung [158] cancers. XPA expression is associated with ovarian cancer [159]. Corroboratively, increased XPA levels have been correlated with cisplatin chemoresistance in non-small cell lung cancer [160] and lung cancer cell lines [161]. Nonetheless, XPA levels did not correlate with sensitivity to cisplatin treatment in testicular germ cell tumors [155].

2.4.3.2 XPF/ERCC1

Downregulation of XPF/ERCC1 complex through RNA interference resulted in increased cisplatin toxicity for various cancer cell lines [162]. Recently small molecule inhibitors that target XPF/ERCC1 complex have been identified and efficiently tested [163]. Moreover, low XPF expression in head-and-neck cancer patients is associated with better response to chemo-radiotherapy, while high XPF expression correlates with a worse response [164].

2.4.3.3 RPA

Apart from breaking NER protein-protein interactions, NER related cancer strategies, have also focused on protein-DNA interactions as many members of NER machinery show a direct binding to DNA. Inhibitors of RPA-DNA interactions were identified [165] and further studies led to the identification of TDRL-505, an inhibitor of RPA binding affinity, which prevents cell cycle progression and increases the efficiency of anticancer drugs in vitro [166]. Also, an analogue of TDRL-505, named TDRL-551, showed promising results in combinatorial platinum based therapy against ovarian and Non-small cell lung cancer [167].

2.4.3.4 ERCC2 (XPG)

In line with the idea that more NER-related conditions can impact cancer therapeutics, a study showed that ERCC2 loss-of-function correlates with cisplatin sensitivity of human cells [168] and on the contrary, ERCC2 overexpression leads to cisplatin resistance [169]. In a recent study, Van Allen and co-workers [170] reasoned that tumors with loss of ERCC2 function may exhibit increased cisplatin sensitivity and they took advantage of the observation that somatic ERCC2 mutations were found in a significant percentage of urothelial carcinomas [171, 172]. They performed whole-exome sequencing (WES) of urothelial carcinoma tumors from patients with extreme responses to cisplatin-based chemotherapy. By comparing tumour sequences to patient respective germ-line ERCC2 sequence, they identified 9 de novo mutations in ERCC2, probably caused by environmental stress, which were acquired during these patients' life. The study concludes that ERCC2 loss-of-function mutations correlates with cisplatin sensitivity and can help to treat urothelial carcinoma. Interestingly, a recent study [119] confirms that ERCC2 somatic mutations have strong consequences in urothelial tumors. These findings further explain how driver events may increase the frequency of a tobacco-related mutational signature, thus highlighting the role of NER in shaping tumor mutational landscape.

2.4.3.5 CSB (ERCC6)

A specific ERCC6-Q524* mutations was recently found to inhibit NER efficiency and sensitize cells to cisplatin [173]. In contrast, and as mentioned above, CSB repair factor encoded by ERCC6 has been found to be overexpressed in cancer cells [122]. In this way, damaged cancer cells may need to boost their TC-NER activity to cope with accumulated stress such as oxidation, especially in transcribed regions, and avoid transcription-replication collisions that could precipitate their apoptosis (see above). Another study identified colorectal carcinomas of an undefined genetic basis with variants in WRN and ERCC6 that reduce capacity for repair of DNA DSBs [174]. Notably, in a very informative study looking at many DDR genes, the authors investigated the relationship between (i) candidate gene mutation co-occurrence across a panel of 19,689 tumor sample, (ii) clinical outcomes, (iii) the tumours mutation burden as evaluated in TCGA and COSMIC databases. They report that ERCC6-mutated tumors display a significantly higher mutational burden than overall melanoma, compatible with the lack of active TC-NER preventing mutation accumulation. In addition, ERCC6 was found among the 20 top mutated genes in 3 different cancers with somatic changes in 1.8% of lung cancers, 1.1% of breast cancers and 3.9% of skin cancers [121].

2.4.3.6 TFIIH

It is known that cancer cells viability requires increased levels of transcription and several NER proteins play a role in transcription regulation. Based on the above, targeting of NER factors that play a role in both repair and transcription could be extremely beneficial in anti-cancer treatment. For instance, TFIIH relies on XPB and XPD for transcription initiation and Excision repair. Triptolide (Trp) is an inhibitor of the ATPase activity of XPB and thus leads to inhibition of TFIIH mediated transcription and repair [175]. Indeed, Trp induces death in multidrug resistant tumor cells [176]. Although its toxicity represents a real disadvantage [177], analogues of this drug could be tested and used for clinical application. However, a more promising approach could rely on a recent study that identified, in a small molecule screen, SP to be an inhibitor of NER, which induces the degradation of TFIIH and the chemosensitization of tumor cells to two platinum derivatives [178].

2.4.4 Other NER-Related Personalized Therapeutic Approaches

NER pathway alterations could also render tumors susceptible to the very promising anticancer immunotherapies. For instance, in non-small cell lung cancer, it was reported that a high somatic mutation burden correlates with better clinical outcomes from anti-PD-1/PD-L1 therapy [179]. This study shows that in two independent patient cohorts, the treatment efficacy of pembrolizumab, an antibody targeting programmed cell death-1 (PD-1), was associated with a higher number of mutations detected in the sequenced tumors. It is likely that, the production of a large set of immunogenic altered proteins, occurs when NER or other DNA repair pathways are not functional, and this could facilitate cancer cells clearance by the immune system that is unleashed by PD-1/PD-L1 blockade.

Finally, NER-deficient tumors are also particularly sensitive to cell cycle checkpoint inhibitors of the ATR-CHK1-WEE1 pathway, many of which are under clinical trial evaluation [145].

2.4.5 Limited Therapeutical Prospects for Neurological Conditions

Overall, NER alterations emerged as attractive biomarkers to define a subset of tumors or patients that are or could be sensitive to a wide range of cancer agents. Studies discussed here and future studies should inform more precisely on clinical contexts in which NER pathway alterations could be used to decide on patient-specific therapy selection. Nonetheless, therapeutical prospects in neurological conditions rising from NER impairment seem very poor in comparison. As explained above, neurodevelopmental diseases rise from abnormalities occurring during early development and have been considered irreversible in adulthood, but a recent review [180] points to results obtained in mice using targeted pharmacological treatments in combination with regimes of training that might alleviate or reverse the symptoms even after the end of critical developmental periods. As far as XP patients that only display neurodegenerative phenotypes, the use of stem-cell therapy approaches could represent a promising solution, however the technology is still at its infancy [181].

2.5 Conclusions

Great advances have been made in our understanding of NER molecular mechanisms and the versatile functions of its components in different environments. Acknowledging these important parameters will contribute to the characterization, cellular diagnosis and clinical management of NER related pathologies. Up to date technological achievements now provide a better basis to further translate basic knowledge of fundamental biological processes to clinical applications.

Most current standard-of-care oncology therapeutic options limit tumour growth via lowering its proliferation or vascularization, but have limited effects on CSCs. Recent progress in understanding how cancer cells bypass normal cellular rules could help in repurposing already available drugs, which were originally designed to shutdown non-cancer related processes. Evidently, a better understanding of the biological impact of potential NER inhibitors should facilitate the development of optimal synthetic lethal combinations, that force to switch off DNA repair and increases the overall level of damages accumulated in rapidly multiplying cancer cells. This approach represents a very promising therapeutic avenue and will improve, not only personalized treatment of NER syndrome patients with cancer, but also patients with cancer in general.

References

1. Jackson SP, Bartek J (2009) The DNA-damage response in human biology and disease. Nature 461:1071–1078
2. Marteijn JA, Lans H, Vermeulen W, Hoeijmakers JHJ (2014) Understanding nucleotide excision repair and its roles in cancer and ageing. Nat Rev Mol Cell Biol 15:465–481
3. Roos WP, Thomas AD, Kaina B (2015) DNA damage and the balance between survival and death in cancer biology. Nat Rev Cancer 16:20–33
4. Roos WP, Kaina B (2006) DNA damage-induced cell death by apoptosis. Trends Mol Med 12:440–450
5. Jeggo PA, Pearl LH, Carr AM (2016) DNA repair, genome stability and cancer: a historical perspective. Nat Rev Cancer 16:35–42
6. Nouspikel T (2009) DNA repair in mammalian cells: nucleotide excision repair: variations on versatility. Cell Mol Life Sci 66:994–1009
7. Scharer OD (2013) Nucleotide excision repair in eukaryotes. Cold Spring Harb Perspect Biol 5:a012609
8. Hanawalt PC, Spivak G (2008) Transcription-coupled DNA repair: two decades of progress and surprises. Nat Rev Mol Cell Biol 9:958–970
9. Gillet LCJ, Schärer OD (2006) Molecular mechanisms of mammalian global genome nucleotide excision repair. Chem Rev 106:253–276
10. Scrima A et al (2008) Structural basis of UV DNA-damage recognition by the DDB1–DDB2 complex. Cell 135:1213–1223
11. Tang J, Chu G (2002) Xeroderma pigmentosum complementation group E and UV-damaged DNA-binding protein. DNA Repair 1:601–616
12. Spivak G (2016) Transcription-coupled repair: an update. Arch Toxicol 90:2583–2594

13. Vermeulen W, Fousteri M (2013) Mammalian transcription-coupled excision repair. Cold Spring Harb Perspect Biol 5:a012625
14. Compe E, Egly J-M (2016) Nucleotide excision repair and transcriptional regulation: TFIIH and beyond. Annu Rev Biochem 85:265–290
15. Ito S et al (2007) XPG stabilizes TFIIH, allowing transactivation of nuclear receptors: implications for Cockayne syndrome in XP-G/CS patients. Mol Cell 26:231–243
16. Staresincic L et al (2009) Coordination of dual incision and repair synthesis in human nucleotide excision repair. EMBO J 28:1111–1120
17. Lehmann AR (2011) DNA polymerases and repair synthesis in NER in human cells. DNA Repair 10:730–733
18. Ogi T et al (2010) Three DNA polymerases, recruited by different mechanisms, carry out NER repair synthesis in human cells. Mol Cell 37:714–727
19. Moser J et al (2007) Sealing of chromosomal DNA nicks during nucleotide excision repair requires XRCC1 and DNA ligase IIIα in a cell-cycle-specific manner. Mol Cell 27:311–323
20. Smerdon MJ, Lieberman MW (1978) Nucleosome rearrangement in human chromatin during UV-induced DNA- repair synthesis. Proc Natl Acad Sci U S A 75:4238–4241
21. Peterson CL, Almouzni G (2013) Nucleosome dynamics as modular systems that integrate DNA damage and repair. Cold Spring Harb Perspect Biol 5:a012658
22. Cleaver JE, Lam ET, Revet I (2009) Disorders of nucleotide excision repair: the genetic and molecular basis of heterogeneity. Nat Rev Genet 10:756–768
23. Kraemer KH et al (2007) Xeroderma pigmentosum, trichothiodystrophy and Cockayne syndrome: a complex genotype-phenotype relationship. Neuroscience 145:1388–1396
24. Rapin I (2013) Handbook of clinical neurology (Dulac O, Lassonde M, Sarnat H, eds), vol 113. Elsevier, pp 1637–1650
25. Bradford PT et al (2011) Cancer and neurologic degeneration in xeroderma pigmentosum: long term follow-up characterises the role of DNA repair. J Med Genet 48:168–176
26. Masutani C et al (1999) The XPV (xeroderma pigmentosum variant) gene encodes human DNA polymerase eta. Nature 399:700–704
27. Fassihi H et al (2016) Deep phenotyping of 89 xeroderma pigmentosum patients reveals unexpected heterogeneity dependent on the precise molecular defect. Proc Natl Acad Sci 113:E1236–E1245
28. Brooks PJ (2013) Blinded by the UV light: how the focus on transcription-coupled NER has distracted from understanding the mechanisms of Cockayne syndrome neurologic disease. DNA Repair 12:656–671
29. Cockayne EA (1936) Dwarfism with retinal atrophy and deafness. Arch Dis Child 11:1–8
30. Cockayne EA (1946) Dwarfism with retinal atrophy and deafness. Arch Dis Child 21:52–54
31. Neill CA, Dingwall MM (1950) A syndrome resembling progeria: a review of two cases. Arch Dis Child 25:213–223
32. Kleijer WJ et al (2008) Incidence of DNA repair deficiency disorders in western Europe: xeroderma pigmentosum, Cockayne syndrome and trichothiodystrophy. DNA Repair 7:744–750
33. Lehmann AR (1982) Three complementation groups in Cockayne syndrome. Mutat Res Mol Mech Mutagen 106:347–356
34. Tanaka K, Kawai K, Kumahara Y, Ikenaga M, Okada Y (1981) Genetic complementation groups in Cockayne syndrome. Somatic Cell Genet 7:445–455
35. Karikkineth AC, Scheibye-Knudsen M, Fivenson E, Croteau DL, Bohr VA (2017) Cockayne syndrome: clinical features, model systems and pathways. Ageing Res Rev 33:3–17
36. Wilson BT et al (2016) The Cockayne Syndrome Natural History (CoSyNH) study: clinical findings in 102 individuals and recommendations for care. Genet Med 18:483–493
37. Suzumura H, Arisaka O (2010) In: Ahmad SI (ed) Diseases of DNA repair. Springer, New York, pp 210–214. doi:10.1007/978-1-4419-6448-9_19
38. Itoh T, Ono T, Yamaizumi M (1994) A new UV-sensitive syndrome not belonging to any complementation groups of xeroderma pigmentosum or Cockayne syndrome: siblings showing biochemical characteristics of Cockayne syndrome without typical clinical manifestations. Mutat Res Repair 314:233–248
39. Horibata K et al (2004) Complete absence of Cockayne syndrome group B gene product gives rise to UV-sensitive syndrome but not Cockayne syndrome. Proc Natl Acad Sci U S A 101:15410–15415
40. Nardo T et al (2009) A UV-sensitive syndrome patient with a specific CSA mutation reveals separable roles for CSA in response to UV and oxidative DNA damage. Proc Natl Acad Sci 106:6209–6214
41. Nakazawa Y et al (2012) Mutations in UVSSA cause UV-sensitive syndrome and impair RNA polymerase IIo processing in transcription-coupled nucleotide-excision repair. Nat Genet 44:586–592
42. Schwertman P et al (2012) UV-sensitive syndrome protein UVSSA recruits USP7 to regulate transcription-coupled repair. Nat Genet 44:598–602
43. Zhang X et al (2012) Mutations in UVSSA cause UV-sensitive syndrome and destabilize ERCC6 in transcription-coupled DNA repair. Nat Genet 44:593–597
44. Fei J, Chen J (2012) KIAA1530 protein is recruited by Cockayne syndrome complementation group protein A (CSA) to participate in Transcription-coupled Repair (TCR). J Biol Chem 287:35118–35126
45. Spivak G (2005) UV-sensitive syndrome. Mutat Res Mol Mech Mutagen 577:162–169

46. Spivak G et al (2002) Ultraviolet-sensitive syndrome cells are defective in transcription-coupled repair of cyclobutane pyrimidine dimers. DNA Repair 1:629–643
47. Schwertman P, Vermeulen W, Marteijn JA (2013) UVSSA and USP7, a new couple in transcription-coupled DNA repair. Chromosoma 122:275–284
48. Oh K-S et al (2006) Phenotypic heterogeneity in the XPB DNA helicase gene (ERCC3): xeroderma pigmentosum without and with Cockayne syndrome. Hum Mutat 27:1092–1103
49. Dietlein F, Thelen L, Reinhardt HC (2014) Cancer-specific defects in DNA repair pathways as targets for personalized therapeutic approaches. Trends Genet 30:326–339
50. DiGiovanna JJ, Kraemer KH (2012) Shining a light on xeroderma pigmentosum. J Invest Dermatol 132:785–796
51. Jeppesen DK, Bohr VA, Stevnsner T (2011) DNA repair deficiency in neurodegeneration. Prog Neurobiol 94:166–200
52. Driver JA (2012) Understanding the link between cancer and neurodegeneration. J Geriatr Oncol 3:58–67
53. McKinnon PJ (2013) Maintaining genome stability in the nervous system. Nat Neurosci 16:1523–1529
54. Balajee AS, May A, Dianov GL, Friedberg EC, Bohr VA (1997) Reduced RNA polymerase II transcription in intact and permeabilized Cockayne syndrome group B cells. Proc Natl Acad Sci U S A 94:4306–4311
55. van den Boom V et al (2004) DNA damage stabilizes interaction of CSB with the transcription elongation machinery. J Cell Biol 166:27
56. Dianov GL, Houle JF, Iyer N, Bohr VA, Friedberg EC (1997) Reduced RNA polymerase II transcription in extracts of Cockayne syndrome and xeroderma pigmentosum/Cockayne syndrome cells. Nucleic Acids Res 25:3636–3642
57. van Gool AJ, van der Horst GT, Citterio E, Hoeijmakers JH (1997) Cockayne syndrome: defective repair of transcription? EMBO J 16:4155–4162
58. Selby CP, Sancar A (1997) Cockayne syndrome group B protein enhances elongation by RNA polymerase II. Proc Natl Acad Sci 94:11205–11209
59. Tantin D, Kansal A, Carey M (1997) Recruitment of the putative transcription-repair coupling factor CSB/ERCC6 to RNA polymerase II elongation complexes. Mol Cell Biol 17:6803–6814
60. Bradsher J et al (2002) CSB Is a component of RNA Pol I transcription. Mol Cell 10:819–829
61. Yuan X, Feng W, Imhof A, Grummt I, Zhou Y (2007) Activation of RNA polymerase I transcription by Cockayne syndrome group B protein and histone methyltransferase G9a. Mol Cell 27:585–595
62. Lee S-K, Yu S-L, Prakash L, Prakash S (2002) Requirement of yeast *RAD2*, a homolog of human *XPG* gene, for efficient RNA polymerase II transcription: implications for Cockayne syndrome. Cell 109:823–834
63. Groisman R et al (2003) The ubiquitin ligase activity in the DDB2 and CSA complexes is differentially regulated by the COP9 signalosome in response to DNA damage. Cell 113:357–367
64. Assfalg R et al (2012) TFIIH is an elongation factor of RNA polymerase I. Nucleic Acids Res 40:650–659
65. Koch S et al (2014) Cockayne syndrome protein A is a transcription factor of RNA polymerase I and stimulates ribosomal biogenesis and growth. Cell Cycle 13:2029–2037
66. Wang Y et al (2014) Dysregulation of gene expression as a cause of Cockayne syndrome neurological disease. Proc Natl Acad Sci 111:14454–14459
67. Wang Y et al (2016) Pharmacological bypass of Cockayne syndrome B function in neuronal differentiation. Cell Rep 14:2554–2561
68. Zeman MK, Cimprich KA (2014) Causes and consequences of replication stress. Nat Cell Biol 16:2–9
69. Sollier J et al (2014) Transcription-coupled nucleotide excision repair factors promote R-loop-induced genome instability. Mol Cell. doi:10.1016/j.molcel.2014.10.020
70. Aguilera A, García-Muse T (2012) R loops: from transcription byproducts to threats to genome stability. Mol Cell 46:115–124
71. Nicolai S et al (2015) Identification of novel proteins co-purifying with Cockayne Syndrome Group B (CSB) reveals potential roles for CSB in RNA metabolism and chromatin dynamics. PLoS One 10:e0128558
72. El Hage A, French SL, Beyer AL, Tollervey D (2010) Loss of topoisomerase I leads to R-loop-mediated transcriptional blocks during ribosomal RNA synthesis. Genes Dev 24:1546–1558
73. Tuduri S et al (2009) Topoisomerase I suppresses genomic instability by preventing interference between replication and transcription. Nat Cell Biol 11:1315–1324
74. Sollier J, Cimprich KA (2015) Breaking bad: R-loops and genome integrity. Trends Cell Biol 25:514–522
75. Groh M, Gromak N (2014) Out of balance: R-loops in human disease. PLoS Genet 10:e1004630
76. Mazouzi A, Velimezi G, Loizou JI (2014) DNA replication stress: causes, resolution and disease. DNA Damage Repair 329:85–93
77. Ming G, Song H (2011) Adult neurogenesis in the Mammalian brain: significant answers and significant questions. Neuron 70:687–702
78. Nixon RA (2013) The role of autophagy in neurodegenerative disease. Nat Med 19:983–997
79. Aamann MD et al (2010) Cockayne syndrome group B protein promotes mitochondrial DNA stability by supporting the DNA repair association with the mitochondrial membrane. FASEB J 24:2334–2346

80. Kamenisch Y et al (2010) Proteins of nucleotide and base excision repair pathways interact in mitochondria to protect from loss of subcutaneous fat, a hallmark of aging. J Exp Med 207:379–390
81. Pascucci B et al (2012) An altered redox balance mediates the hypersensitivity of Cockayne syndrome primary fibroblasts to oxidative stress: alterations in oxidative metabolism in Cockayne. Aging Cell 11:520–529
82. Scheibye-Knudsen M et al (2012) Cockayne syndrome group B protein prevents the accumulation of damaged mitochondria by promoting mitochondrial autophagy. J Exp Med 209:855–869
83. Fang EF et al (2014) Defective mitophagy in XPA via PARP-1 hyperactivation and NAD+/SIRT1 reduction. Cell 157:882–896
84. Kruk PA, Rampino NJ, Bohr VA (1995) DNA damage and repair in telomeres: relation to aging. Proc Natl Acad Sci U S A 92:258–262
85. Rochette PJ, Brash DE (2010) Human telomeres are hypersensitive to UV-induced DNA damage and refractory to repair. PLoS Genet 6:e1000926
86. Kota LN et al (2015) Reduced telomere length in neurodegenerative disorders may suggest shared biology. J Neuropsychiatr Clin Neurosci 27:e92–e96
87. Batenburg NL, Mitchell TRH, Leach DM, Rainbow AJ, Zhu X-D (2012) Cockayne syndrome group B protein interacts with TRF2 and regulates telomere length and stability. Nucleic Acids Res 40:9661–9674
88. Jia P, Her C, Chai W (2015) DNA excision repair at telomeres. DNA Repair 36:137–145
89. Clarke G et al (2000) A one-hit model of cell death in inherited neuronal degenerations. Nature 406:195–199
90. Wu S, Powers S, Zhu W, Hannun YA (2015) Substantial contribution of extrinsic risk factors to cancer development. Nature 529:43–47
91. Alexandrov LB et al (2013) Signatures of mutational processes in human cancer. Nature 500:415–421
92. Haradhvala NJ et al (2016) Mutational strand asymmetries in cancer genomes reveal mechanisms of DNA damage and repair. Cell 164:538–549
93. Helleday T, Eshtad S, Nik-Zainal S (2014) Mechanisms underlying mutational signatures in human cancers. Nat Rev Genet 15:585–598
94. Bryan DS, Ransom M, Adane B, York K, Hesselberth JR (2014) High resolution mapping of modified DNA nucleobases using excision repair enzymes. Genome Res 24:1534–1542
95. Mao P, Meas R, Dorgan KM, Smerdon MJ (2014) UV damage-induced RNA polymerase II stalling stimulates H2B deubiquitylation. Proc Natl Acad Sci 111:12811–12816
96. Powell JR et al (2015) 3D-DIP-chip: a microarray-based method to measure genomic DNA damage. Sci Rep 5:7975
97. Teng Y et al (2011) A novel method for the genome-wide high resolution analysis of DNA damage. Nucleic Acids Res 39:e10
98. Zavala AG, Morris RT, Wyrick JJ, Smerdon MJ (2014) High-resolution characterization of CPD hotspot formation in human fibroblasts. Nucleic Acids Res 42:893–905
99. Adar S, Hu J, Lieb JD, Sancar A (2016) Genome-wide kinetics of DNA excision repair in relation to chromatin state and mutagenesis. Proc Natl Acad Sci 113:E2124–E2133
100. Hu J, Adar S, Selby CP, Lieb JD, Sancar A (2015) Genome-wide analysis of human global and transcription-coupled excision repair of UV damage at single-nucleotide resolution. Genes Dev 29:948–960
101. McGregor WG, Wei D, Maher VM, McCormick JJ (1999) Abnormal, error-prone bypass of photoproducts by xeroderma pigmentosum variant cell extracts results in extreme strand bias for the kinds of mutations induced by UV light. Mol Cell Biol 19:147–154
102. Mitchell DL, Jen J, Cleaver JE (1992) Sequence specificity of cyclobutane pyrimidine dimers in DNA treated with solar (ultraviolet B) radiation. Nucleic Acids Res 20:225–229
103. Douki T, Cadet J (2001) Individual determination of the yield of the main UV-induced dimeric pyrimidine photoproducts in DNA suggests a high mutagenicity of CC photolesions †. Biochemistry (Mosc) 40:2495–2501
104. Dumaz N, Drougard C, Sarasin A, Daya-Grosjean L (1993) Specific UV-induced mutation spectrum in the p53 gene of skin tumors from DNA-repair-deficient xeroderma pigmentosum patients. Proc Natl Acad Sci 90:10529–10533
105. Stary A, Kannouche P, Lehmann AR, Sarasin A (2003) Role of DNA polymerase η in the UV mutation spectrum in human cells. J Biol Chem 278:18767–18775
106. Giglia G et al (1998) p53 mutations in skin and internal tumors of xeroderma pigmentosum patients belonging to the complementation group C. Cancer Res 58:4402
107. Kraemer KH, Lee MM, Scotto J (1984) DNA repair protects against cutaneous and internal neoplasia: evidence from xeroderma pigmentosum. Carcinogenesis 5:511–514
108. Lawrence MS et al (2013) Mutational heterogeneity in cancer and the search for new cancer-associated genes. Nature 499:214–218
109. Martincorena I, Campbell PJ (2015) Somatic mutation in cancer and normal cells. Science 349:1483–1489
110. Petljak M, Alexandrov LB (2016) Understanding mutagenesis through delineation of mutational signatures in human cancer. Carcinogenesis 37:531–540
111. Hollstein M, Alexandrov LB, Wild CP, Ardin M, Zavadil J (2017) Base changes in tumour DNA have the power to reveal the causes and evolution of cancer. Oncogene 36:158–167
112. Pleasance ED et al (2010) A comprehensive catalogue of somatic mutations from a human cancer genome. Nature 463:191–196

113. Pleasance ED et al (2010) A small-cell lung cancer genome with complex signatures of tobacco exposure. Nature 463:184–190
114. Polak P et al (2013) Reduced local mutation density in regulatory DNA of cancer genomes is linked to DNA repair. Nat Biotechnol 32:71–75
115. Perera D et al (2016) Differential DNA repair underlies mutation hotspots at active promoters in cancer genomes. Nature 532:259–263
116. Lahtz C, Pfeifer GP (2011) Epigenetic changes of DNA repair genes in cancer. J Mol Cell Biol 3:51–58
117. Mombach JCM, Castro MAA, Moreira JCF, Almeida RMCD (2008) On the absence of mutations in nucleotide excision repair genes in sporadic solid tumors. Genet Mol Res 7:152–160
118. Alexandrov LB et al (2015) Clock-like mutational processes in human somatic cells. Nat Genet 47:1402–1407
119. Kim J et al (2016) Somatic ERCC2 mutations are associated with a distinct genomic signature in urothelial tumors. Nat Genet 48:600–606
120. de Miranda NF et al (2013) DNA repair genes are selectively mutated in diffuse large B cell lymphomas. J Exp Med 210:1729
121. Chae YK et al (2016) Genomic landscape of DNA repair genes in cancer. Oncotarget 7(17):23312–23321
122. Caputo M et al (2013) The CSB repair factor is overexpressed in cancer cells, increases apoptotic resistance, and promotes tumor growth. DNA Repair 12:293–299
123. Stamatoyannopoulos JA et al (2009) Human mutation rate associated with DNA replication timing. Nat Genet 41:393–395
124. Helmrich A, Ballarino M, Nudler E, Tora L (2013) Transcription-replication encounters, consequences and genomic instability. Nat Struct Mol Biol 20:412–418
125. Qiang L et al (2016) Autophagy positively regulates DNA damage recognition by nucleotide excision repair. Autophagy 12:357–368
126. Liang C et al (2006) Autophagic and tumour suppressor activity of a novel Beclin1-binding protein UVRAG. Nat Cell Biol 8:688–698
127. Yang Y et al (2016) Autophagic UVRAG promotes UV-induced photolesion repair by activation of the CRL4DDB2 E3 ligase. Mol Cell 62:507–519
128. White E (2012) Deconvoluting the context-dependent role for autophagy in cancer. Nat Rev Cancer 12:401–410
129. Velic D et al (2015) DNA damage signalling and repair inhibitors: the long-sought-after achilles' heel of cancer. Biomol Ther 5:3204–3259
130. Curtin NJ (2012) DNA repair dysregulation from cancer driver to therapeutic target. Nat Rev Cancer 12:801–817
131. Jackson SP, Helleday T (2016) Drugging DNA repair. Science 352:1178–1179
132. Olivier M, Hollstein M, Hainaut P (2010) TP53 mutations in human cancers: origins, consequences, and clinical use. Cold Spring Harb Perspect Biol 2:a001008
133. Ford JM, Hanawalt PC (1997) Expression of wild-type p53 is required for efficient global genomic nucleotide excision repair in UV-irradiated human fibroblasts. J Biol Chem 272:28073–28080
134. Alexandrov LB, Stratton MR (2014) Mutational signatures: the patterns of somatic mutations hidden in cancer genomes. Cancer Genom 24:52–60
135. Chen W, Dong J, Haiech J, Kilhoffer M-C, Zeniou M (2016) Cancer stem cell quiescence and plasticity as major challenges in cancer therapy. Stem Cells Int 2016:1–16
136. Cicalese A et al (2009) The tumor suppressor p53 regulates polarity of self-renewing divisions in mammary stem cells. Cell 138:1083–1095
137. White AC, Lowry WE (2015) Refining the role for adult stem cells as cancer cells of origin. Trends Cell Biol 25:11–20
138. Kreso A, Dick JE (2014) Evolution of the cancer stem cell model. Cell Stem Cell 14:275–291
139. Tomasetti C, Vogelstein B (2015) Variation in cancer risk among tissues can be explained by the number of stem cell divisions. Science 347:78
140. Ventura A et al (2007) Restoration of p53 function leads to tumour regression in vivo. Nature 445:661–665
141. Wang Y et al (2011) Restoring expression of wild-type p53 suppresses tumor growth but does not cause tumor regression in mice with a p53 missense mutation. J Clin Invest 121:893–904
142. Guinea-Viniegra J et al (2012) Differentiation-induced skin cancer suppression by FOS, p53, and TACE/ADAM17. J Clin Invest 122:2898–2910
143. Adams PD, Jasper H, Rudolph KL (2015) Aging-induced stem cell mutations as drivers for disease and cancer. Cell Stem Cell 16:601–612
144. Barakat K, Tuszynski J (2013) New research directions in DNA repair. InTech, Rijeka
145. Mouw KW, D'Andrea AD, Konstantinopoulos PA (2015) Nucleotide excision repair (NER) alterations as evolving biomarkers and therapeutic targets in epithelial cancers. Oncoscience 2:942
146. Liu J, He C, Xing C, Yuan Y (2014) Nucleotide excision repair related gene polymorphisms and genetic susceptibility, chemotherapeutic sensitivity and prognosis of gastric cancer. Mutat Res Mol Mech Mutagen 765:11–21
147. Wang D, Lippard SJ (2005) Cellular processing of platinum anticancer drugs. Nat Rev Drug Discov 4:307–320
148. Kelland L (2007) The resurgence of platinum-based cancer chemotherapy. Nat Rev Cancer 7:573–584
149. Chu G (1994) Cellular responses to cisplatin. The roles of DNA-binding proteins and DNA repair. J Biol Chem 269:787–790
150. Koeppel F et al (2004) Irofulven cytotoxicity depends on transcription-coupled nucleotide excision repair and is correlated with XPG expression in solid tumor cells. Clin Cancer Res 10:5604

151. Earley JN, Turchi JJ (2011) Interrogation of nucleotide excision repair capacity: impact on platinum-based cancer therapy. Antioxid Redox Signal 14:2465–2477
152. Calmels N et al (2016) Uncommon nucleotide excision repair phenotypes revealed by targeted high-throughput sequencing. Orphanet J Rare Dis 11:26
153. Barakat KH et al (2012) Virtual screening and biological evaluation of inhibitors targeting the XPA-ERCC1 interaction. PLoS One 7:e51329
154. Gentile F, Tuszynski JA, Barakat KH (2016) New design of nucleotide excision repair (NER) inhibitors for combination cancer therapy. J Mol Graph Model 65:71–82
155. Mendoza J et al (2013) Association between ERCC1 and XPA expression and polymorphisms and the response to cisplatin in testicular germ cell tumours. Br J Cancer 109:68–75
156. Welsh C et al (2004) Reduced levels of XPA, ERCC1 and XPF DNA repair proteins in testis tumor cell lines: NER proteins in testis tumor cells. Int J Cancer 110:352–361
157. Li Q et al (2000) Association between the level of ERCC-1 expression and the repair of cisplatin-induced DNA damage in human ovarian cancer cells. Anticancer Res 20:645–652
158. Olaussen KA et al (2006) DNA repair by ERCC1 in non–small-cell lung cancer and cisplatin-based adjuvant chemotherapy. N Engl J Med 355:983–991
159. Stevens EV et al (2005) Expression of xeroderma pigmentosum A protein predicts improved outcome in metastatic ovarian carcinoma. Cancer 103:2313–2319
160. Weaver DA et al (2005) ABCC5, ERCC2, XPA and XRCC1 transcript abundance levels correlate with cisplatin chemoresistance in non-small cell lung cancer cell lines. Mol Cancer 4:18
161. Liu Y, Bernauer AM, Yingling CM, Belinsky SA (2012) HIF1 regulated expression of XPA contributes to cisplatin resistance in lung cancer. Carcinogenesis 33:1187–1192
162. Arora S, Kothandapani A, Tillison K, Kalman-Maltese V, Patrick SM (2010) Downregulation of XPF–ERCC1 enhances cisplatin efficacy in cancer cells. DNA Repair 9:745–753
163. Arora S et al (2016) Identification of small molecule inhibitors of ERCC1-XPF that inhibit DNA repair and potentiate cisplatin efficacy in cancer cells. Oncotarget 7(46):75104–75117
164. Seiwert TY et al (2014) DNA repair biomarkers XPF and phospho-MAPKAP kinase 2 correlate with clinical outcome in advanced head and neck cancer. PLoS One 9:e102112
165. Andrews BJ, Turchi JJ (2004) Development of a high-throughput screen for inhibitors of replication protein A and its role in nucleotide excision repair. Mol Cancer Ther 3:385
166. Shuck SC, Turchi JJ (2010) Targeted inhibition of replication protein A reveals cytotoxic activity, synergy with chemotherapeutic DNA-damaging agents, and insight into cellular function. Cancer Res 70:3189–3198
167. Mishra AK, Dormi SS, Turchi AM, Woods DS, Turchi JJ (2015) Chemical inhibitor targeting the replication protein A – DNA interaction increases the efficacy of Pt-based chemotherapy in lung and ovarian cancer. Biochem Pharmacol 93:25–33
168. Furuta T et al (2002) Transcription-coupled nucleotide excision repair as a determinant of cisplatin sensitivity of human cells. Cancer Res 62:4899
169. Aloyz R et al (2002) Regulation of cisplatin resistance and homologous recombinational repair by the TFIIH subunit XPD. Cancer Res 62:5457
170. Van Allen EM et al (2014) Somatic ERCC2 mutations correlate with cisplatin sensitivity in muscle-invasive urothelial carcinoma. Cancer Discov 4:1140
171. Guo G et al (2013) Whole-genome and whole-exome sequencing of bladder cancer identifies frequent alterations in genes involved in sister chromatid cohesion and segregation. Nat Genet 45:1459–1463
172. Weinstein JN et al (2014) Comprehensive molecular characterization of urothelial bladder carcinoma. Nature 507:315–322
173. Ceccaldi R et al (2015) A unique subset of epithelial ovarian cancers with platinum sensitivity and PARP inhibitor resistance. Cancer Res 75:628–634
174. Arora S et al (2015) Genetic variants that predispose to DNA double-strand breaks in lymphocytes from a subset of patients with familial colorectal carcinomas. Gastroenterology 149:1872–1883.e9
175. Titov DV et al (2011) XPB, a subunit of TFIIH, is a target of the natural product triptolide. Nat Chem Biol 7:182–188
176. Yi J-M et al (2016) Triptolide induces cell killing in multidrug-resistant tumor cells via CDK7/RPB1 rather than XPB or p44. Mol Cancer Ther 15:1495–1503
177. Qu L et al (2015) Integrated targeted sphingolipidomics and transcriptomics reveal abnormal sphingolipid metabolism as a novel mechanism of the hepatotoxicity and nephrotoxicity of triptolide. J Ethnopharmacol 170:28–38
178. Alekseev S et al (2014) A small molecule screen identifies an inhibitor of DNA repair inducing the degradation of TFIIH and the chemosensitization of tumor cells to platinum. Chem Biol 21:398–407
179. Rizvi NA et al (2015) Mutational landscape determines sensitivity to PD-1 blockade in non–small cell lung cancer. Science 348:124–128
180. Castrén E, Elgersma Y, Maffei L, Hagerman R (2012) Treatment of neurodevelopmental disorders in adulthood. J Neurosci 32:14074
181. Sakthiswary R, Raymond AA (2012) Stem cell therapy in neurodegenerative diseases: from principles to practice. Neural Regen Res 7:1822–1831

Role of Protein Linked DNA Breaks in Cancer

3

Walaa R. Allam, Mohamed E. Ashour, Amr A. Waly, and Sherif El-Khamisy

Abstract

Topoisomerases are a group of specialized enzymes that function to maintain DNA topology by introducing transient DNA breaks during transcription and replication. As a result of abortive topoisomerases activity, topoisomerases catalytic intermediates may be trapped on the DNA forming topoisomerase cleavage complexes (Topcc). Topoisomerases trapping on the DNA is the mode of action of several anticancer drugs, it lead to formation of protein linked DAN breaks (PDBs). PDBs are now considered as one of the most dangerous forms of endogenous DNA damage and a major threat to genomic stability. The repair of PDBs involves both the sensing and repair pathways. Unsuccessful repair of PDBs leads to different signs of genomic instabilities such as chromosomal rearrangements and cancer predisposition. In this chapter we will summarize the role of topoisomerases induced PDBs, identification and signaling, repair, role in transcription. We will also discuss the role of PDBs in cancer with a special focus on prostate cancer.

Keywords

Protein linked DNA breaks • Topoisomerases • DAN repair • Topoisomerases poisons • Genome integrity

W.R. Allam (✉) • M.E. Ashour • A.A. Waly
Center for Genomics, Helmy Institute for Medical Sciences, Zewail City of Science and Technology, Giza, Egypt
e-mail: wallam@zewailcity.edu.eg

S. El-Khamisy (✉)
Krebs Institute and Sheffield Institute for Nucleic Acids, Department of Molecular Biology and Biotechnology, Firth Court, University of Sheffield, Sheffield S10 2TN, UK

Center for Genomics, Helmy Institute for Medical Sciences, Zewail City of Science and Technology, Giza, Egypt
e-mail: s.el-khamisy@sheffield.ac.uk

3.1 PDBs Identification and Signaling

3.1.1 PDBs Identification

Protein linked DNA breaks (PDBs) are considered as a major threat to genome integrity and overall cell survival. A good example here is topoisomerase cleavable complex (Topcc), that are produced by trapping the enzyme covalently

S. El-Khamisy (ed.), *Personalised Medicine*, Advances in Experimental Medicine and Biology 1007,
DOI 10.1007/978-3-319-60733-7_3

on the DNA, by topoisomerases inhibitors treatment such as camptothecin (CPT), doxorubicin and etoposide [1–4]. For example, CPT, covalently links Top1 to the 3′-end of DNA which in turn activates DNA damage response (DDR) [1, 3]. The DDR is regulated by three phosphatidylinositol-3 kinase-like protein kinases: ataxia telangiectasia and Rad3-related protein (ATR), ataxia-telangiectasia mutated (ATM), and DNA-dependent protein kinase (DNA-PKcs), which determine cell fate as one of three responses; repair, senescence, or apoptosis.

ATM activates DDR in response to replication-independent double strand breaks (DSBs), for example ionizing radiation (IR) exposure. The primary substrate of ATM is Checkpoint kinase 2 (Chk2) and ATM can induce apoptosis directly or indirectly through Chk2 [5–7].

Under normal conditions, ATM was reported to exist in an inactive form and upon DNA damage stimulation; it converts to active monomers [8]. When activated, ATM phosphorylates several proteins involved in check point control, DNA repair and apoptosis regulation including, among others, p53, BRCA1, CHK2, H2AX, Nbs1 [9]. This phosphorylation causes cell cycle arrest at certain checkpoints and promote DNA repair. Several studies reported Mre11/Rad50/Nbs1 (MRN) complex to be essential for ATM-dependent activation in response to DNA damage [10–12]. Consistently, MRN complex was shown to bind directly to ATM, inducing conformational changes that increases ATM affinity toward its substrate, also MRN complex increases p53 and CHK2 ATM-dependent activation [13].

ATR activates DDR in response to single strand-double strand (ssDNA-dsDNA) junctions which arise as a consequence of stalled replication fork by damaged DNA, nucleotide excision repair (NER) activity, or resection of DSB (produced by IR and topoisomerase 2 (Top2) poison), and the primary substrate of ATR is Chk1, which in turn targets a number of cell cycle regulator and DNA repair proteins [5, 6, 14]. DNA-PKcs has a well-defined role in DSB repair by non-homologous end joining (NHEJ), and checkpoint control [15].

It is important to highlight that there is a considerable overlapping between the ATM and ATR downstream targets [16, 17]; some studies suggest that cellular processing of DSBs, such as proteasomal degradation of enzyme from Topcc, to possess a determining role in the subsequent activation of DDR [18, 19]. Unlike ATR, ATM loss is not lethal, but ATM mutations cause a rare autosomal recessive disorder ataxia–telangiectasia (A-T), A-T cells are defected for DNA repair, hypersensitive to radiation, and show increased chromosomal instability.

3.1.2 PDBs Signaling

3.1.2.1 Cell Signaling Following Topoisomerases I Poison

CPT induces ATM-Chk2 and ATR-Chk1 activation. Since the cytotoxicity and the induced DSB by CTP are replication-dependent, ATR-Chk1 is the main pathway responsible for DDR activation in replicating cells. Depletion of ATR and CHK1, but not ATM, induces hypersensitivity to CPT [20, 21]. Besides its role in DNA repair, protein SUMOylation was found to be essential for DNA damage signaling, where ATRIP, ATR regulatory partner, SUMOylation is critical for ATRIP interaction with several components of ATR-Chk1 [22]. PIAS3 SUMO ligase is the only member of PIAS (protein inhibitor of activated STAT) family, known for its role in DNA repair, that was found to be playing many roles in ATR activation, and in the absence of PIAS3, ATR shows abnormal kinase activity. In CPT treated cells, PIAS3 aids to DSBs formation; where in hydroxyurea treated cells, PIAS3 is essential during early events of ATR activation, ATR autophosphorylation in particular [23]. Of notice, PIAS3 overexpression improves homologous recombination (HR) and NHEJ, the mechanisms behind this is still largely unknown [24].

Although ATM may not be primarily involved in DDR activation in response to CPT, ATM participates in many aspects of DNA repair in response to CPT: (1) ATM participates in HR repair [25, 26] (2) ATM, ATR and DNA-PK regulate the crosstalk between HR and NHEJ through the co-regulation of p53–RPA interaction.

Phosphorylation of p53 by ATM/ATR and RPA by DNA-PK leads to the dissociation of P53-RPA complex which is necessary to initiate HR [27]. (3) ATM/DNA-PK activates and recruits tyrosyl-DNA phosphodiesterase-1 (TDP1) to site of DSB [28, 29]. Recently, DNA-PKcs were found to regulate ATM negatively through phosphorylation, DNA-PKcs inhibition or deletion induces ATM hyperactivity and thus plays a role in determining PDBs repair pathway choice [30].

In contrast to cancer cells, ATM is mainly activated in post-mitotic cells by Top1 poison. In post-mitotic cells, CPT leads to transcription inhibition with R-loop formation and the formation of DSBs which activate ATM [31]. Activated ATM will activate the DNA-PK which in turn, triggers histone ubiquitination and Top1 ubiquitination leading to enhancement of Top1 proteolysis as well as to full ATM activity at DSB sites [32]. In addition, ATM depletion in neuronal cells leads to Top1cc accumulation due to elevated levels of reactive oxygen species [33].

3.1.2.2 Cell Signaling Following Topoisomerases II Poison

The activation of cell signaling pathways after Top2 poisons is drug-dependent. The cytotoxic mechanisms induced by many Top2 poisons are not exclusive to only targeting Top2, so it is difficult to elucidate the cell signaling pathway induced by each mechanism separately. Anthracyclines-Top2-poisoning effect induces ATM activation, but not ATR activation [34]. Depletion of ATM leads to slight enhancement in sensitivity in response to anthracycline Top2 poisoning effect [35, 36]. Anthracyclin-DNA adducts, induced by formaldehyde, require the activity of ATM and ATR for checkpoint activation, where ATR is required for G2/M checkpoint activation and ATM is required for G1 checkpoint activation [35].

Etopsoide induces ATR-Chk1 and ATM-Chk2 activation, but similar to CPT, in S-phase ATR-Chk1 is responsible for inhibiting DNA replication, and the role of ATM is dispensable [37]. Interestingly, the role of ATM in the repair of etoposide-induced DSB during G1-phase was found to also be dispensable, and the MRN complex was shown to be required for the etoposide-induced breaks repair by NHEJ-independent of ATM [38]. ATM depletion was shown to be dispensable for etopsoide-induced DSB repair, but it affects the repair of blocked DSBs by Top2 in the absence of TDP2 (see below) [39]. On the other hand, ATM is mainly activated in nonreplicating cells in response to etoposide treatment, and the inhibition of ATM in these cells is antiapoptotic [40].

In the light of the fact that topoisomerases poisons induce DSBs, one would expect an ATM dependent DDR activation. However, in response to either Top1 or Top2 poisons treatment, the cell cycle arrests in an ATR dependent manner [21, 41–44]. Three main conclusions could be made from this finding; (1) topoisomerases poisons induce cytotoxicity through interfering with major nuclear processes, mainly replication, rather than direct generation of DSBs (2) Topoisomerase poisons-induced DSBs might be produced in the course of replication restart, and not due to Topcc disruption (3) Topcc-induced DSBs termini are usually associated with proteins, because of this they are not acknowledged as original breaks, that can be recognized by ATM. In the latter regard, some NHEJ proteins, such as Ku and DNA-PKcs, bind to Top2 cleaved complexes only after its termini-bounded proteins are removed [45].

3.2 PDBs Repair

PDBs can be repaired by TDPs enzymes which precisely hydrolyze the bond between the trapped topoisomerases and the DNA, and nonspecifically by the nucleases which remove the Tops and cut part of the DNA. It is not fully clear how the cell decides on specific repair pathway, as the same type of DNA damage can be processed by several repair pathways. Some studies have shown that Poly (ADP-ribose) polymerase (PARP) is involved in favoring non-nucleolytic repair pathway for Top1 induced PDBs [33, 46]. Several PARP inhibitors are known to synergize CPT cytotoxicity; recently Top1-PARylation was found to counteract CPT mediated-Top1cc [47].

3.2.1 Protein Linked DNA Break Repair by Precision Scissors

Precision scissors are proteins that are capable of liberating the trapped topoisomerase from DNA termini without the need to cleave DNA. Topcc is maintained by a phosphotyrosyl bond between the DNA terminus and the topoisomerase. TDP1 is the first discovered 'scissor' that can counteract PDBs by releasing trapped topoisomerases. TDP1 mainly releases 3′-terminus-stalled Top1cc. Nevertheless, it has also been shown to release 5′-Top2cc, though only in yeast so far. The catalysis of Top1cc by TDP1 is structurally and mechanistically conserved from humans to yeast and depends on the formation of a DNA-TDP1 intermediate. Briefly, TDP1 breaks the 3′-phosphotyrosyl bond linking DNA with Top1 in a two-step cycle that incorporates two catalytic histidines. In the first step, the nucleophilic histidine (Hisnuc) attacks the 3′-phosphate to form a TDP1cc intermediate. This leads to the release of the Top1 from DNA. In the second step, the other histidine acts as a general acid/base (Hisgab) activating water to hydrolyze the 3′-phospho-histidyl bond made in step one, resulting in dissociation of TDP1 from DNA [48]. Importantly, the excision of Top1cc by TDP1 requires prior enzymatic degradation of Top1 by the ubiquitin/proteasome system to expose the Top1–3′-DNA phosphotyrosyl bond which facilitates its attacking by TDP1. DNA-PK mediates ubiquitination of Top1 which is a prerequisite for its subsequent proteolysis. The excision of Top1cc by TDP1 leaves a 3′-phosphate end that, before being processed by DNA polymerases and ligases, must first be dephosphorylated by polynucleotide kinase phosphatase (PNKP) and this makes PNKP a key protein with great importance in repairing damage caused by Top1cc.

Importantly, spinocerebellar ataxia with axonal neuropathy (SCAN1), a neurodegenerative disease, was found to arise due to a naturally occurring mutation that leads to conversion of the Hisgab to arginine [49]. This mutation was found to cause a delay in the hydrolysis of the 3′-phosphohistidyl bond (second step) [50] and thus enhances the stability of the TDP1cc covalent intermediate which results in sensitization to DNA damaging agents such as irradiation and CPT leading to high genomic instability [51]. This finding can be of great significance in cancer therapy as it paves the way toward developing TDP1 poisons that can stabilize the wild type TDP1 at DNA 3′-termini as in the case of Topoisomerases' poisons.

Posttranslational modifications are known to take a part in TDP1 recruitment, modulation of enzymatic activity and stability. TDP1 is PARylated by the Poly(ADP-ribose) polymerases 1 (PARP1) [46]. TDP1 PARylation, together with SUMOylation at K111, increases the accumulation of TDP1 at Top1cc sites [52]. The interaction between TDP1 and PARP1 recruits XRCC1 which acts as a scaffold for many repair proteins. TDP1 was also found to be phosphorylated at S81 by ATM and DNA-PK which increases TDP1 enrichment and stability at DNA damage sites and helps recruiting XRCC1 and ligase IIIα.

In fact, further mechanistic studies have shown that TDP1 can resolve a broad range of 3′-end blocking adducts such as 3′-phosphoglycolate induced by radiotherapy [53], apurinic or apyrimidinic sites caused by alkylating agents such as temozolomide [54] and chain-terminating nucleoside analogues [51]. This, in addition to its Top1cc resolving activity, suggests TDP1 as a promising target for cancer treatment. The crystal structure of TDP1 has been solved [55] which paved the way to developing effective TDP1 inhibitors to be used as novel chemotherapeutic agents, possibly combined with Top1 poisons. The nature of the catalytic cycle of TDP1 gave rise to two possible strategies to for targeting [56]. The first strategy depends on the inhibition of the first step of the two-step catalytic cycle by using TDP1 inhibitors that are capable of preventing the formation of the TDP1–DNA intermediate. While the second strategy depends on targeting the TDP1–DNA covalent complex, and thus trapping and stabilizing the toxic TDP1-DNA adduct just like the way Top1 poisons stabilize Top1-DNA adducts.

TDP2 is the first discovered 5′-tyrosyl DNA phosphodiesterase with a Top2-induced DSBs repair activity. The role of TDP2, originally known as TTRAP, in the DSBs repair was discovered in an attempt to find new human proteins that can resolve tyrosyl-linked protein adducts. For this purpose, a screen was made to identify candidates that can compensate for the function of TDP1 in TDP1Δrad1Δ double-mutant yeast cells. The screen found TTRAP to confer CPT resistance to the double-mutant cells. Further assays proved TTRAP to have a robust 5′-tyrosyl DNA phosphodiesterase activity that was metal dependent. Hence, TTRAP was designated as the novel protein TDP2 [57]. Further studies confirmed a specific role of TDP2 in resolving 5′-termini Top2cc and thus counteracting DSBs caused by Top2 poisons such as etoposide and doxorubicin. It is of great importance to note that unlike TDP1, the product of TDP2 catalysis is a phosphorylated 5′-terminus that is readily ligatable and thus is a substrate for NHEJ. It is therefore plausible that TDP2 is found to be epistatic with members of the NHEJ machinery such as KU70 and KU80 [58].

Originally, it was logical to suggest that TDP1 mainly repairs Top1cc and that TDP2 mainly repairs Top2cc. However, recent in vivo insights suggest that both proteins might have overlapping roles in DSB repair. TDP2 could actually play a role in Top1cc repair. Double knock-out murine and chicken cells overexpressing TDP2 showed increased rates of DNA breaks repair and cellular viability in response to Top1 poisons such as CPT. On the other hand, a contribution of TDP1 in repairing Top2 induced DNA damage is debatable [59].

Like TDP1, posttranslational modifications play a role in TDP2 activity as well. Extracellular signal regulated kinase 3 (ERK3) phosphorylates TDP2 at Ser60, and thus enhances its Phosphodiesterase activity in desensitizing cancer cells to DNA damage caused by Top2 poisons [60]. It is still unclear whether posttranslational modifications plays a role in TDP2 recruitment to DNA damaged sites or not. It is worth noting that TDP1 and TDP2 are structurally different, where Human TDP2 (362 amino acids) is smaller than TDP1 (608 amino acids) [61]. Although both proteins perform their functions as monomers and prefer substrates that are single stranded, they are still mechanistically different in that TDP2 uses Mg2+/Mn2+ coordination for the hydrolysis of 5′-phosphotyrosyl bonds in one step which is not the case with TDP1 whose action is a two-step, metal-independent process that requires the formation of a covalent intermediate [62].

Like Top1cc, the processing of Top2cc by TDP2 requires its previous proteolytic cleavage or heat denaturation [63]. Yet, the major distinction between the two enzymes is that the product of TDP1 catalysis, after 3′-DNA end dephosphorylation by PNKP, is consequently a substrate for SSBR while the product of TDP2 is a substrate for NHEJ. This goes along well with the finding that inducing Top1cc is most toxic when members of HR like Rad52, BRCA1 BRCA2 and MRE11 are mutated or chemically inhibited. On the other hand, TDP2 is epistatic with KU70, KU80 and DNA-PK which are core components of NHEJ [64].

Many attempts were made to discover potent TDP2 inhibitors. Isoeugenol was found to synergize cytotoxicity of the Top2 poison etoposide, but only in the absence of TDP1. This makes isoeugenol a promising lead compound for developing potent TDP2 inhibitors [65]. Certain Indenoisoquinoline compounds that were initially identified as Top1 and TDP1 inhibitors, were also found to be TDP2 inhibitors. This "triple inhibitor" opens the way for developing 'universal' drugs against important targets and thus are very attractive for further studying as chemotherapeutic anticancer agents [66].

3.2.2 Protein Linked DNA Break Repair by Nucleases

A building up evidences suggest that nucleases activity can remove topoisomerases from the DNA. Several groups of nucleases are suggested to carry out a redundant role in the removal of PDBs. Which nuclease is more representatives and what the regulations between these nucleases is still not clear. Recently, structure of DNA ends was found to be a determine factor for DNA repair pathway selection, where damaged ends requires Mre11 dependent resection, and CtIP was found essential for activating Mre11-dependent nuclease activity [67].

Work on *Xenopus laevis* egg clarified the importance of CtIP in repairing PDBs CtIP interaction with BRCA1 is necessary for repair of PDBs through HR, promoting cell survival against topoisomerase-poisons while resection of endonuclease-generated DSB ends is independent from this interaction [68]. CtIP show low expression levels in breast cancer patients, and its depletion enhance PARP inhibitors cytotoxicity in vivo and in vitro [69]. In addition to the specific role of CtIP in the removal of PDBS, CtIP and MRE11 nuclease activity is essential for HR repair of single ended breaks repair, by preventing Ku, from the NHEJ, binding to the broken DNA [70]. In contrast to the error-free repair mediated by TDPs (discussed above), CtIP mediates deletion of original sequences, error-prone repair, for rejoining distant broken DNA ends and single DNA strands generation by CtIP favors insertions of ectopic sequences through microhomology-mediated template switching, in depleted human 53BP1 cells [71]. HR proteins inhibition, such as BRCA2, BRCA1 and RPA, increases the rate of DNA breaks-induced mutation, and this action is dependent on the activity of CtIP and MRE11 [72]. CtIP was further defined as a cofactor of MRE11 activity, where MRE11, NSB1, RAD50 and CtIP cleave DNA near the break to resolve PDBs and initiate HR [73].

In budding yeast, MRE11 was shown to promote global sumoylation of repair proteins and allows initiation but, not processing of Spo11 during meiosis and its activity is independent from checkpoint phosphorylation [74]. Interestingly, NBS1 protects unmodified DNA ends and control exo and endo- nucletic activity of MRE11 and RAD50 in PDBs repair [75], which highlights a possible role of NBS1 (also called NBN) in human diseases. Moreover, EXD2 (EXDL2) was recently identified as a MRN/CtIP interactor that accelerate its 3′-5′ exonuclease activity required for the repair of CPT-induced PDBs via HR and promote genome stability in human cells [76]. More nucleases seem to be implicated in PDBs repair, yet it is still controversial whether they can actually remove topoisomerase or have a role in downstream repair events. Structure specific endonucleases complexes such as (Mus81–Mms4), (Slx1–Slx4) complex, and Yen1 process double holiday junctions to produce crossover and non-crossover products. Recently Mus81–Mms4 was suggested to take a critical part in repairing interhomolog joints [77].

SLX4, from Fanconi anemia pathway, is implicated in PDBs repair and is required for meiotic DSB formation [78]. SLX4 plays a role in coordinating the processing and repair of PDBs, where it is recruited near damaged DNA end through interaction with Rtt107 and Dpb11 [79]. SLX4 acts as a scaffold protein for MUS81, SLX1 and XPF complex. In addition, it controls function of several partner endonucleases as it show SUMO binding properties, that SUMOylates XPF-ERCC1 complex [80]. SLX4 interaction with XPF is dispensable for Top-1 induced PDBs repair while its interaction MUS81 is not. Earlier, studies showed a role for Mus81–Mms4, along with Rad1–Rad10, XPF, SLX4–SLX1 in repairing of Top1-induced PDBs. MUS81–EME1 acts to cleave the DNA at stalled replication sites [81] and the complex enzymatic activity is stimulated by Esc2, an adaptor protein with no enzymatic domains, which plays a role in resolving sister chromatid junctions [82]. Mus81 and XPF show a functional interplay in HR to resolve PDBs after Top1 removal. Mus81 plays an important role in resolving interhomology joint structures that promotes genetic instability [77]. XPF-ERCC1 complex participate in repairing Top1 PDBs by cleaving DNA upstream from the trapped Top1, XPF-ERCC1 was further promoted as an alternative repair pathway to CPT, in addition to the established PARP-TDP1 pathway [83]. A promising clinical outcome from combining PARP and Top1 inhibitors in XPF-ERCC1 deficient cancers was reported [84].

3.2.3 Protein Linked DNA Break Repair by Proteases

Proteases are conserved in all eukaryotes, where they function in DNA-protein cross links (DPCs) repair and are considered as guardians of the genome.

Early studies revealed a role for weak suppressor of smt3 (Wss1) in response genotoxic stress, and it was said to promote cell survival following top1 poison exposure, but the underlying mechanisms remained largely unknown [85, 86]. Deficient Wss1 yeast cells fail to repair DPCs and exhibit compromised genomic integrity [87]. It was not until recently, when Wss1 was reported as a DNA repair factor that resolve CPT induced DPCs in *Saccharomyces cerevisiae* [87]. Wss1 is now known to be activated against UV irradiation and Top1 positions treatment, and is essential for cell survival. In the absence of TDP1, resolving Top1-induced DPCs is Wss1 and SUMO dependent [88]. In consistence with this, DPC repair pathway analogue was identified in *Xenopus laevis* egg extract [89].

There are striking similarities between Wss1 and SprT-like domain-containing protein (SPRTN), which was considered to be Wss1 mammalian representative [87]. Later, SPRTN was identified as DPCs repair protease in higher eukaryotes and in *Xenopus laevis* egg extracts [90, 91]. SPRTN gene mutations result in Ruijs-Aalfs syndrome, characterized by premature aging, genomic instability and increased cancer predisposition. There biallelic SPRTN mutations were identified in patients exhibiting early onset of hepatocellular carcinoma, the authors suggested these mutations to cause slower replication fork progression [92]. SPRTN was further proposed as a specialized protein for the repair of PDBs generated during replication [93]. SPRTN deficient human cells show hypersensitivity to CPT and accumulate DPCs [87]. Cells with SPRTN deficiency/mutations sustain DPCs and are hypersensitive to DPCs inducing agents such as CPT and etoposide [90]. While SPRTN is an essential protein in mammalian cells, its nematode ortholog is unessential for worm viability [94], but worms lacking Dvc-1 are hypersensitive to formaldehyde and cisplatin, promoting SPRTN as a therapeutic target for improving cisplatin cancer treatment outcomes [90]. Finally, SPRTN role in DPC removal was confirmed *in vivo* recently [95].

3.2.4 DNA Helicases

Building up evidences suggest that Top1 poisons, CPT, slows the replication fork progression and reversal, which results from accumulation of positive supercoils, this was suggested to be controlled by PARP1 [96, 97].

RECQ1 helicase has an established role in promoting replication fork restart upon Top1 inhibition, and was also considered as a general mechanism against different replication challenges [98, 99]. PARP1 control RECQ1 helicase activity; the latter induce unscheduled fork restart, providing a link between fork restart, repair and PARP inactivation [98]. PARP inactivation, reduce reversed fork accumulation following DNA damage inducing agents treatment. The core HR protein, RAD51 is known to reside at replication forks [100, 101]; RAD51 was later identified as the first protein to promote fork reversal in vivo [99]. This highlights the involvement of other repair proteins in forming or processing of reversed forks, nucleases are known to participate in stalled forks processing in response to DNA damage [102, 103]. Indeed Several DNA resection factors, such as Mre11, NBSs and CtIP were reported to be involved in fork metabolism [104–107]. Another nuclease/helicase, the DNA2, was identified in DNA replication yeast mutants [108, 109]. DNA2 participate in DSB repair, DNA2 and EXO1 resect the 5′ end of DSB to initiate HR [110–112]. Later, DNA2 was found to work with BLM helicase to resect DSBs ends in human cells [113]. It was further suggested that DNA2 might play a similar role in repairing replication induced DSBs, through initiating HR repair or resecting structures that block replication fork [114]. Recently, a novel role for DNA2 was identified in mammalian cells, where DNA2 cooperates with (Werner protein) WRN to favor replication fork restart in mammalian cells and this process seems to be regulated by RECQ1 and RAD51 [115].

Another role for WRN was reported in vivo, where it shields the nascent strand from degradation by MRE11/EXO1 [116]. Furthermore, in Werner syndrome (WS), characterized by genomic instability and accelerated aging, WRN protein inhibits recruitment of CtIP and MRE11 to DSBs sites, preventing large deletions at 5′ end, WRN was also found to promote Classic (C-NHEJ) against (alternative) Alt-NHEJ for the repair of DSBs via helicase and exonuclease activity [117]. CPT was shown to alter the cellular localization of WRN helicase, inducing its degradation. Reversed fork restart by RECQL and stable WRN expression were presented as a PDBs repair pathways that mediates Top1 poisons resistance [118].

Recently a study has shown that BAZ1B-SMARCA5, chromatin remodeling complex, accumulates near replication forks and promotes topoisomerase I loading near forks in camptothecin treated cells. Suppression of the BAZ1B decrease the extent of CPT-mediated replication fork reversal and increase the cellular tolerance to CPT [119].

3.3 Topoisomerases to the Chromatin and Back

Topoisomerases relieves topological stress associated with DNA replication and transcription. These DNA associated processes are hindered by the chromosome compact structure by DNA wrapping around histone, forming nucleosomes, shielding DNA from topoisomerases activity. The interplay between topoisomerases and chromatin, in terms of assembly and disassembly mechanisms, is understudied. A recent series of studies highlight a role of histones epigenetics and chaperones, chromatin-remodelling complexes, and insulator proteins in topoisomerases recruitment to the chromatin, as well as repair of the trapped topoisomerases.

Topoisomerases activity must be tightly regulated to outside of nucleosome regions to maintain negative supercoiling that is essential for replication and transcription [120, 121]. Early studies have shown that DNA topoisomerases are required during nucleosome assembly to relief DNA tension generated by chromatin remodeler Snf2 activity [122]. In fission yeast, Snf2 and Chd1 homolog (Hrp1) interacts with the histone chaperone Nap1 to promote nucleosome disassembly [123]. A following study showed that Hrp1, Nap1 and topoisomerases have an overlapping genomic occupancy [124]. In budding yeast, two proteins were identified, Tof2 and Fob1, to have a role in Top1-chromatin recruitment during replication and transcription by forming a cleavage complex at ribosomal replication fork sites [125].

In addition, topoisomerases can be recruited to the chromatin through the chromatin remodelers such as SWI/SNF complex [126, 127]. The Top2α chromatin binding depends on the ATPase catalytic subunit of the SWI/SNF complexe (SMARCA4) and the ability of Top2α to suppress DNA entanglement during mitosis requires SWI/SNF complexes [126]. In addition, a recent study has shown that the SMARCA4 recruits Top1 to general chromatin to suppress the genomic instability and negative superhelicity, whereas the FACT complex, a histone chaperon, is required for Top1 binding to the transcriptionally active chromatin marker (H3K4me3), at non-canonical DNA structures for the site-specific cleavage [127].

Top3β is thought to be the new player in transcription and replication regulation. Top3β has recently been shown to possess an RNA activity. The depletion of TOP3β increases the risk of intellectual disability and schizophrenia [128, 129]. In addition, Top3β has been identified to inhibit R-loop formation in conjunction with Tudor domain–containing protein 3 (TDRD3). TDRD3 is a methylarginine effector molecule that recognizes methyl-histone marks and activates transcription. Also, TDRD3 acts as a bridge between Top3β and arginine-methylated histones and the Top3β-TDRD3 prevents R-loop accumulation and suppress the rate of c-Myc/Igh translocation [130]. TDRD3 also serves as a molecular bridge between Top3β and the translation regulator FMRP [131]. In addition to TDRD3 function of targeting Top3β to chromatin, a recent study has shown that TDRD3 enhances the biochemical activities of Top3β on both DNA and RNA substrates [132]. The BAZ1B-SMARCA5, a chromatin remodeling complex, was found to facilitate Top1 access to replication fork in CPT treated cells, BAZ1B was found to play a role in CPT sensitivity [119]. In addition, we have recently shown that perturbed histone H4K16 acetylation is responsible for irinotecan resistance in colorectal cancer cells [133]. These studies highlight the importance of chromatin regulation not only for topoisomeraseses recruitments but also for the repair of trapped topoisomerases.

3.4 Topoisomerases and Transcription Initiation

A canonical role of Topoisomerases in facilitating transcription has been agreed upon. Topoisomerases are essential for transcription elongation as well as Pol II pause release. The progressing Pol II generates supercoiling and torsion that need to be resolved by topoisomerases, otherwise the levels of such supercoils will be high enough to halt the transcription [134]. The important role of TopI and Top2B in facilitating transcription elongation is mostly pronounced in long genes, as confirmed by studies on both mouse and human cells. Chemical induction of Top1cc in cancer cells using CPT or topotecan causes a general inhibition of transcription elongation, but the efficiency of such inhibition was shown to increase as the genes are longer and including more introns [135]. Also, treating neuronal cells with topotecan was found to potently inhibit expression of long genes that are linked to autism [136]. And how do topoisomerases recognize actively transcribed genes? The chromatin of actively transcribed genes is marked by histone H3 Lys4 trimethylation (H3K4me3). These marks are recognized by the transcription elongation factor facilitates chromatin transcription (FACT) complex which recruits Topoisomerases to actively transcribed genes to release supercoils ahead of the progressing POL II [127]. Nevertheless, it would appear that topoisomerases have a noncanonical role in transcription initiation as well besides its already well-established role in facilitating transcription elongation.

In addition to the occasional DNA damage that takes place as a side effect of gene transcription, recent evidence show that cells are capable of utilizing "scheduled" and site-specific DNA damage events to trigger calculated transcription of specific genes.

Early insights in the role of DNA strand break in transcriptional initiation was provided by studies on yeast. The activities of Top1 or Top2 were shown to be required for transcription initiation of certain controlled genes (GAL and PHO) via facilitating the recruitment of RNA POL II to their promoters [137].

In 2006, a study by Rosenfeldand and colleagues confirmed that the same noncanonical topoisomerase function observed in yeast occurs in human cells, where they highlighted a role of Top2B in estrogen-induced transcription. This study showed that when breast cancer cells are estrogen-deprived, Top2B is associated with a repressor complex on the promoter of the pS2 gene whose expression is estrogen-dependent. Interestingly, treating these cells with estrogen lead to recruitment of estrogen receptor to the pS2 promoter. This lead to a series of events culminating eliminating nucleosomes from this promoter region and eviction of the repressor complex freeing Top2B. The now free Top2B, being in close proximity to the promoter region, catalyzes the production of DSB at the promoter. This transient lesion causes the suppressive linker histone H1 to be dissociated from the promoter and recruitment of histone acetylases. Furthermore, the DSB induced the activation and recruitment of NHEJ proteins such as XRCC5, DNA-PKc and Ku70 which seemed to be essential to avoid the undesired consequences of long-lasting unrepaired DNA damage [138]. Thus, this new role of topoisomerases created a new concept of "creative DNA damage" that lead to serious of studies following the same novel theme.

A very important study described a role of Top1 as a DNA break inducer that in essential for deriving cell-specific ligand-induced gene expression. Stimulating prostate cancer cells with DHT results in androgen receptor (AR) internalization and binding to certain gene enhancers. Top1 was shown to be recruited to enhancers bound by AR, catalyzing DNA breaks that induce transcription of eRNA and consequently affecting expression of many androgen-responsive genes. This is also followed by activation and recruitment of a set of DNA break repair genes including HR genes such as the MRN complex in addition to members of the base excision repair (BER) pathway, NHEJ genes like the heterodimer KU70–KU86 and DNA ligase IV to prevent persistence of DNA damage [139]. In another study, Top2B activity was shown to be important for inducing transcription of serum-inducible immediate genes such as Myc, Fos, Jun and EGR1. The transcription of such genes in response to serum supplementation was shown to be prevented by the Top2B inhibitor ICRF193. The DSB caused by Top2B in the promoters of the serum-inducible genes lead to enrichment of the noncanonical histone variant gamma-H2AX which facilitated initiation of transcription [140].

In the same context, it is of great importance to highlight that Top2B is of such significance in initiating transcription that even targeted artificial induction of DSB at promoters of the serum-inducible genes Fos and Npas4 was found lead to their transcription even in the absence of the inducing signal [141].

3.5 Topoismoerase1 Mutagenic Activity

Ribonucleotides may be misincorporated into the DNA by polymerases during replication [142]. Ribonucleotide excision repair (RER) pathway is responsible for ribonucleotide removal and RNase H2 is the initiator of RER [143]. Top1 is known to have a ribonuclease activity [144], and this activity increases mutations, chromosomal translocations and checkpoint activation at ribonucleotide sites [145–148]. Top1 deletion decreased all these signs of genomic instability. This mutagenic ribonucleotide activity of Top1 could be attributed to Top1 binding to ribonucleotides before RNase H2, which converts them to nicks when Top1 is removed [145, 149]. In addition, Top1cc formed at ribonucleotide sites allows nucleophilic attacks on the phosphotyrosyl linkages by the 2-hydroxyl on rNMPs (ribonucleotide monophosphates), producing to a 2,3-cyclic phosphate and liberating Top1 [145, 150]. These nicks hampers DNA elongations and ligation [145, 149, 150]. Loss of RNase H2 in yeast cells induces Top1 activity induce hyper-recombinations and chromosomal translocations and probably causing upregualtion of DSB repair genes [147, 151–153]. In absence of RNase H2, both Srs2 and Exo1 work together to repair Top1-induced nicks, also Sgs1 helicase, from the RecQ family, was shown to play a role in this process [154].

3.6 Protein Linked DNA Breaks in Cancer

Topcc have been implicated in several human cancers, neurodegenerative and autoimmune diseases. The role of Topcc in cancers started with therapy induced secondary leukemias in mixed lineage leukemia (MLL), where etoposide was found to trap Top2β which initiates chromosomal translocations [155–158]. TDP1, TDP2 mutations are already connected to neurological disorders [49, 58]. The presence of Top1 autoantibodies is associated with reduced survival in scleroderma patients [159]. As an example the role of Topcc induced breaks in prostate cancer is discussed in details below.

3.6.1 Protein Linked DNA Breaks and Prostate Cancer

Prostate cancer has been linked to topoisomerases-induced DSBs. Androgen receptor, the main player in prostate cancer, recruits Top2β to the promoters of hormone-dependent genes, resulting in chromosomal rearrangements such as those between transmembrane protease serine 2 (TMPRSS2) and ETS transcription factors coding regions, ERG and ETS variants (ETV) [160]. The resulting TMPRSS2-ERG fusion causes overexpression of oncogenic genes and is found in almost half of prostate cancer samples. More gene fusions have been subsequently revealed including TMPRSS2–ETV4, TMPRSS2-ETV5, KLK2–ETV4 and others [161–163]. TMPRSS2-ERG fusions is a distinctive feature of prostate cancer aggressiveness and poor prognosis, where absence of ERG fusions is considered as a good prognostic indicator [161, 164, 165].

Rate of TMPRSS2-ERG fusions depends on androgen treatment time where transient treatment TMPRSS2–ERG fusion in cancer cells, but not in normal cells [164]; while prolonged treatment induces this fusion in normal cells as well [166]. This highlights the presence of proficient Top2 induced PDBs repair mechanism that prevents translocations in normal cells, and this mechanism apparently inhibited, mutated or absent in prostate cancer cells. As TDP2 is responsible for repairing Top2 induced PDBs, one would expect it to have a role in Top2 initiated chromosomal translocations as well. Other DNA repair genes such as NKX3.1 acts as a suppressor for TMPRSS2-ERG rearrangement through accelerating DNA repair [167]. Also, NKX3.1 blocks the AR of ERG gene [130]. In this regard Reduced NKX3.1 levels is correlated with increased TMPRSS2-ERG recombination events in prostate cancer tissues [168]. Also, Nkx3.1 knockedout mice were shown to have a delayed DDR in response to etoposide treatment [169]. Chromosomal translocations could be induced by some inflammatory stimuli [170], suggesting a role of other repair proteins in gene fusions and translocations that still needs to be identified. Recently, the chromatin remodeler SMARCA4 was found responsible for recruiting Top1 to chromatin in B-cells and that SMARCA4 depletion induced Igh/c-Myc chromosomal translocations due to low TOP1 recruitment. Another protein from the Top1 complex, FACT was found to be Important for Top1 binding to H3K4me3 which is essential for DNA cleavage and AID-induced translocations [127].

3.6.2 Protein Linked DNA Breaks and Personalized Medicine

The identification of prostate cancer gene fusions had a significant clinical application in the era of personalized medicine, now researchers are able to detect the TMPRSS2–ERG fusion in blood and urine [171]. This non-invasive and easy detection mode of such an aggressive prostate cancer phenotypes, along with the elevated PSA levels, lead to a significant decrease in the need for invasive biopsies and an improvement in the overall patient survival rate [172]. In this regard, tumors with TMPRSS2–ERG fusions have a distinct DNA methylation profile than negative tumors, indicating that gene methylation profile could be playing a role in prostate cancer progression and tumorgenesis [173]. In addition to their role in cancer, it is notable that protein-linked DNA breaks are pathogenic in a number of neurological disorders, most recently in frontotemporal dementia and ALS, in a study came out this month in Nature Neuroscience (Ref: https://www.ncbi.nlm.nih.gov/pubmed/28714954). Thus, harnessing our knowledge on the homeostatic control of PDBs will open new frontiers in personalised medical decisions and approcahes that are not only useful in cancer but also in a number of neurological disorders [174].

3.7 Conclusion

Protein linked DNA breaks are the result of uncontrolled topoisomerases activity that usually end up with inducing cell death or chromosomal translocations. In fact topoisomerases are the targets for most of the current anticancer drugs. These drugs mode of action depends on trapping the enzyme covalently on the DNA to induce DNA damage in cancer cells. Topoisomerases based drugs selectivity replay on two observations, first cancer cells show high levels and activity of topoisomerases 1 and 2, second cancer cells are usually defective for one or more of the DNA repair pathways. Our understanding of the role of protein linked DNA breaks in cancer, and probably response to therapy, is hampered by our lack of knowledge on chromosomal translocations specificity and the role of gene-gene interaction in chromosomal translocations. Considering Top1 mutagenic activity in ribonucleotide repair, and the high abundance of ribonucleotides in the genome it seems plausible to think that it might contribute to cancer or response to topoisomerases targeted therapy or perhaps other topoisomerases may exhibit a similar activity. A growing number of studies report a strong line of evidence suggest a novel roles of other DNA repair proteins in PDBs initiation or repair or response to therapy. This urges the need for more comprehensive studies that considers the overlapping and contradicting roles of repair factors. Improving our understanding on PDBs induction and repair, will eventually lead to identification of individual variations that control cancer initiation, progression and improve response to cancer therapy.

References

1. Schilsky RL (1996) Methotrexate: an effective agent for treating cancer and building careers. The polyglutamate era. Stem Cells 14:29–32. doi:10.1002/stem.140029
2. Miura S, Yoshimura Y, Satoh H, Izuta S (2001) The antitumor mechanism of 1-(2-deoxy-2-fluoro-4--thio-beta-D-arabinofuranosyl)-cytosine: effects of its triphosphate on mammalian DNA polymerases. Jpn J Cancer Res 92:562–567
3. Povirk LF (1996) DNA damage and mutagenesis by radiomimetic DNA-cleaving agents: bleomycin, neocarzinostatin and other enediynes. Mutat Res 355:71–89
4. Zorbas H, Keppler BK (2005) Cisplatin damage: are DNA repair proteins saviors or traitors to the cell? Chembiochem 6:1157–1166. doi:10.1002/cbic.200400427
5. Chen T, Stephens PA, Middleton FK, Curtin NJ (2012) Targeting the S and G2 checkpoint to treat cancer. Drug Discov Today 17:194–202. doi:10.1016/j.drudis.2011.12.009
6. Biss M, Xiao W (2012) Selective tumor killing based on specific DNA-damage response deficiencies. Cancer Biol Ther 13:239–246. doi:10.4161/cbt.18921
7. Yang X, Wood PA, Hrushesky WJ (2010) Mammalian TIMELESS is required for ATM-dependent CHK2 activation and G2/M checkpoint control. J Biol Chem 285:3030–3034. doi:10.1074/jbc.M109.050237
8. Bakkenist CJ, Kastan MB (2003) DNA damage activates ATM through intermolecular autophosphorylation and dimer dissociation. Nature 421:499–506. doi:10.1038/nature01368
9. Lee JH, Paull TT (2007) Activation and regulation of ATM kinase activity in response to DNA double-strand breaks. Oncogene 26:7741–7748. doi:10.1038/sj.onc.1210872
10. Buscemi G et al (2001) Chk2 activation dependence on Nbs1 after DNA damage. Mol Cell Biol 21:5214–5222. doi:10.1128/MCB.21.15.5214-5222.2001
11. Nakanishi K et al (2002) Interaction of FANCD2 and NBS1 in the DNA damage response. Nat Cell Biol 4:913–920. doi:10.1038/ncb879
12. Uziel T et al (2003) Requirement of the MRN complex for ATM activation by DNA damage. EMBO J 22:5612–5621. doi:10.1093/emboj/cdg541
13. Lee JH, Paull TT (2005) ATM activation by DNA double-strand breaks through the Mre11-Rad50-Nbs1 complex. Science 308:551–554. doi:10.1126/science.1108297
14. Woods D, Turchi JJ (2013) Chemotherapy induced DNA damage response: convergence of drugs and pathways. Cancer Biol Ther 14:379–389. doi:10.4161/cbt.23761
15. Liu X et al (2012) Overlapping functions between XLF repair protein and 53BP1 DNA damage response factor in end joining and lymphocyte development. Proc Natl Acad Sci U S A 109:3903–3908. doi:10.1073/pnas.1120160109
16. McGowan CH, Russell P (2004) The DNA damage response: sensing and signaling. Curr Opin Cell Biol 16:629–633. doi:10.1016/j.ceb.2004.09.005
17. Harrison JC, Haber JE (2006) Surviving the breakup: the DNA damage checkpoint. Annu Rev Genet 40:209–235. doi:10.1146/annurev.genet.40.051206.105231
18. Stewart L, Redinbo MR, Qiu X, Hol WG, Champoux JJ (1998) A model for the mechanism of human topoisomerase I. Science 279:1534–1541
19. Staker BL et al (2002) The mechanism of topoisomerase I poisoning by a camptothecin analog. Proc Natl Acad Sci U S A 99:15387–15392. doi:10.1073/pnas.242259599
20. Wang JC (2002) Cellular roles of DNA topoisomerases: a molecular perspective. Nat Rev Mol Cell Biol 3:430–440. doi:10.1038/nrm831
21. Flatten K et al (2005) The role of checkpoint kinase 1 in sensitivity to topoisomerase I poisons. J Biol Chem 280:14349–14355. doi:10.1074/jbc.M411890200
22. Wu CS et al (2014) SUMOylation of ATRIP potentiates DNA damage signaling by boosting multiple protein interactions in the ATR pathway. Genes Dev 28:1472–1484. doi:10.1101/gad.238535.114
23. Wu CS, Zou L (2016) The SUMO (Small Ubiquitin-like Modifier) ligase PIAS3 primes ATR for checkpoint activation. J Biol Chem 291:279–290. doi:10.1074/jbc.M115.691170

24. Liu S et al (2013) PIAS3 promotes homology-directed repair and distal non-homologous end joining. Oncol Lett 6:1045–1048. doi:10.3892/ol.2013.1472
25. Sakasai R, Teraoka H, Tibbetts RS (2010) Proteasome inhibition suppresses DNA-dependent protein kinase activation caused by camptothecin. DNA Repair (Amst) 9:76–82. doi:10.1016/j.dnarep.2009.10.008
26. Kocher S, Spies-Naumann A, Kriegs M, Dahm-Daphi J, Dornreiter I (2013) ATM is required for the repair of Topotecan-induced replication-associated double-strand breaks. Radiother Oncol 108:409–414. doi:10.1016/j.radonc.2013.06.024
27. Serrano MA et al (2013) DNA-PK, ATM and ATR collaboratively regulate p53-RPA interaction to facilitate homologous recombination DNA repair. Oncogene 32:2452–2462. doi:10.1038/onc.2012.257
28. Das BB et al (2009) Optimal function of the DNA repair enzyme TDP1 requires its phosphorylation by ATM and/or DNA-PK. EMBO J 28:3667–3680. doi:10.1038/emboj.2009.302
29. Chiang SC, Carroll J, El-Khamisy SF (2010) TDP1 serine 81 promotes interaction with DNA ligase IIIalpha and facilitates cell survival following DNA damage. Cell Cycle 9:588–595. doi:10.4161/cc.9.3.10598
30. Zhou Y et al (2017) Regulation of the DNA damage response by DNA-PKcs inhibitory phosphorylation of ATM. Mol Cell 65:91–104. doi:10.1016/j.molcel.2016.11.004
31. Sordet O et al (2009) Ataxia telangiectasia mutated activation by transcription- and topoisomerase I-induced DNA double-strand breaks. EMBO Rep 10:887–893. doi:10.1038/embor.2009.97
32. Cristini A et al (2016) DNA-PK triggers histone ubiquitination and signaling in response to DNA double-strand breaks produced during the repair of transcription-blocking topoisomerase I lesions. Nucleic Acids Res 44:1161–1178. doi:10.1093/nar/gkv1196
33. Alagoz M, Chiang SC, Sharma A, El-Khamisy SF (2013) ATM deficiency results in accumulation of DNA-topoisomerase I covalent intermediates in neural cells. PLoS One 8:e58239. doi:10.1371/journal.pone.0058239
34. Huelsenbeck SC et al (2012) Rac1 protein signaling is required for DNA damage response stimulated by topoisomerase II poisons. J Biol Chem 287:38590–38599. doi:10.1074/jbc.M112.377903
35. Forrest RA et al (2012) Activation of DNA damage response pathways as a consequence of anthracycline-DNA adduct formation. Biochem Pharmacol 83:1602–1612. doi:10.1016/j.bcp.2012.02.026
36. Maede Y et al (2014) Differential and common DNA repair pathways for topoisomerase I- and II-targeted drugs in a genetic DT40 repair cell screen panel. Mol Cancer Ther 13:214–220. doi:10.1158/1535-7163.MCT-13-0551
37. Rossi R, Lidonnici MR, Soza S, Biamonti G, Montecucco A (2006) The dispersal of replication proteins after Etoposide treatment requires the cooperation of Nbs1 with the ataxia telangiectasia Rad3-related/Chk1 pathway. Cancer Res 66:1675–1683. doi:10.1158/0008-5472.CAN-05-2741
38. Quennet V, Beucher A, Barton O, Takeda S, Lobrich M (2011) CtIP and MRN promote non-homologous end-joining of etoposide-induced DNA double-strand breaks in G1. Nucleic Acids Res 39:2144–2152. doi:10.1093/nar/gkq1175
39. Alvarez-Quilon A et al (2014) ATM specifically mediates repair of double-strand breaks with blocked DNA ends. Nat Commun 5:3347. doi:10.1038/ncomms4347
40. Korwek Z et al (2012) Inhibition of ATM blocks the etoposide-induced DNA damage response and apoptosis of resting human T cells. DNA Repair (Amst) 11:864–873. doi:10.1016/j.dnarep.2012.08.006
41. Cliby WA, Lewis KA, Lilly KK, Kaufmann SH (2002) S phase and G2 arrests induced by topoisomerase I poisons are dependent on ATR kinase function. J Biol Chem 277:1599–1606. doi:10.1074/jbc.M106287200
42. Costanzo V et al (2003) An ATR- and Cdc7-dependent DNA damage checkpoint that inhibits initiation of DNA replication. Mol Cell 11:203–213
43. Siu WY et al (2004) Topoisomerase poisons differentially activate DNA damage checkpoints through ataxia-telangiectasia mutated-dependent and -independent mechanisms. Mol Cancer Ther 3:621–632
44. Ho CC et al (2005) The relative contribution of CHK1 and CHK2 to Adriamycin-induced checkpoint. Exp Cell Res 304:1–15. doi:10.1016/j.yexcr.2004.10.016
45. Martensson S, Nygren J, Osheroff N, Hammarsten O (2003) Activation of the DNA-dependent protein kinase by drug-induced and radiation-induced DNA strand breaks. Radiat Res 160:291–301
46. Das BB et al (2014) PARP1-TDP1 coupling for the repair of topoisomerase I-induced DNA damage. Nucleic Acids Res 42:4435–4449. doi:10.1093/nar/gku088
47. Das SK et al (2016) Poly(ADP-ribose) polymers regulate DNA topoisomerase I (Top1) nuclear dynamics and camptothecin sensitivity in living cells. Nucleic Acids Res 44:8363–8375. doi:10.1093/nar/gkw665
48. Cuya SM, Comeaux EQ, Wanzeck K, Yoon KJ, van Waardenburg RC (2016) Dysregulated human Tyrosyl-DNA phosphodiesterase I acts as cellular toxin. Oncotarget 7:86660–86674. doi:10.18632/oncotarget.13528
49. Takashima H et al (2002) Mutation of TDP1, encoding a topoisomerase I-dependent DNA damage repair enzyme, in spinocerebellar ataxia with axonal neuropathy. Nat Genet 32:267–272. doi:10.1038/ng987
50. He X et al (2007) Mutation of a conserved active site residue converts tyrosyl-DNA phosphodiesterase I into a DNA topoisomerase I-dependent poison. J Mol Biol 372:1070–1081. doi:10.1016/j.jmb.2007.07.055
51. Huang SY et al (2013) TDP1 repairs nuclear and mitochondrial DNA damage induced by

chain-terminating anticancer and antiviral nucleoside analogs. Nucleic Acids Res 41:7793–7803. doi:10.1093/nar/gkt483
52. Hudson JJ, Chiang SC, Wells OS, Rookyard C, El-Khamisy SF (2012) SUMO modification of the neuroprotective protein TDP1 facilitates chromosomal single-strand break repair. Nat Commun 3:733. doi:10.1038/ncomms1739
53. El-Khamisy SF, Hartsuiker E, Caldecott KW (2007) TDP1 facilitates repair of ionizing radiation-induced DNA single-strand breaks. DNA Repair 6:1485–1495. doi:10.1016/j.dnarep.2007.04.015
54. Alagoz M, Wells OS, El-Khamisy SF (2014) TDP1 deficiency sensitizes human cells to base damage via distinct topoisomerase I and PARP mechanisms with potential applications for cancer therapy. Nucleic Acids Res 42:3089–3103. doi:10.1093/nar/gkt1260
55. Davies DR, Interthal H, Champoux JJ, Hol WG (2002) The crystal structure of human tyrosyl-DNA phosphodiesterase, Tdp1. Structure 10:237–248
56. Comeaux EQ, van Waardenburg RC (2014) Tyrosyl-DNA phosphodiesterase I resolves both naturally and chemically induced DNA adducts and its potential as a therapeutic target. Drug Metab Rev 46:494–507. doi:10.3109/03602532.2014.971957
57. Malik M, Nitiss KC, Enriquez-Rios V, Nitiss JL (2006) Roles of nonhomologous end-joining pathways in surviving topoisomerase II-mediated DNA damage. Mol Cancer Ther 5:1405–1414. doi:10.1158/1535-7163.MCT-05-0263
58. Gomez-Herreros F et al (2013) TDP2-dependent non-homologous end-joining protects against topoisomerase II-induced DNA breaks and genome instability in cells and in vivo. PLoS Genet 9:e1003226. doi:10.1371/journal.pgen.1003226
59. Zeng Z et al (2012) TDP2 promotes repair of topoisomerase I-mediated DNA damage in the absence of TDP1. Nucleic Acids Res 40:8371–8380. doi:10.1093/nar/gks622
60. Bian K et al (2016) ERK3 regulates TDP2-mediated DNA damage response and chemoresistance in lung cancer cells. Oncotarget 7:6665–6675. doi:10.18632/oncotarget.6682
61. Pommier Y et al (2014) Tyrosyl-DNA-phosphodiesterases (TDP1 and TDP2). DNA Repair 19:114–129. doi:10.1016/j.dnarep.2014.03.020
62. Gao R, Huang SY, Marchand C, Pommier Y (2012) Biochemical characterization of human tyrosyl-DNA phosphodiesterase 2 (TDP2/TTRAP): a Mg(2+)/Mn(2+)-dependent phosphodiesterase specific for the repair of topoisomerase cleavage complexes. J Biol Chem 287:30842–30852. doi:10.1074/jbc.M112.393983
63. Gao R et al (2014) Proteolytic degradation of topoisomerase II (Top2) enables the processing of Top2. DNA and Top2.RNA covalent complexes by tyrosyl-DNA-phosphodiesterase 2 (TDP2). J Biol Chem 289:17960–17969. doi:10.1074/jbc.M114.565374
64. Heo J et al (2015) TDP1 promotes assembly of non-homologous end joining protein complexes on DNA. DNA Repair 30:28–37. doi:10.1016/j.dnarep.2015.03.003
65. Elsayed W, El-Shafie L, Hassan MK, Farag MA, El-Khamisy SF (2016) Isoeugenol is a selective potentiator of camptothecin cytotoxicity in vertebrate cells lacking TDP1. Sci Rep 6:26626. doi:10.1038/srep26626
66. Beck DE et al (2016) Synthesis and biological evaluation of new fluorinated and chlorinated indenoisoquinoline topoisomerase I poisons. Bioorg Med Chem 24:1469–1479. doi:10.1016/j.bmc.2016.02.015
67. Liao S, Tammaro M, Yan H (2016) The structure of ends determines the pathway choice and Mre11 nuclease dependency of DNA double-strand break repair. Nucleic Acids Res 44:5689–5701. doi:10.1093/nar/gkw274
68. Aparicio T, Baer R, Gottesman M, Gautier J (2016) MRN, CtIP, and BRCA1 mediate repair of topoisomerase II-DNA adducts. J Cell Biol 212:399–408. doi:10.1083/jcb.201504005
69. Wang J et al (2016) Loss of CtIP disturbs homologous recombination repair and sensitizes breast cancer cells to PARP inhibitors. Oncotarget 7:7701–7714. doi:10.18632/oncotarget.6715
70. Chanut P, Britton S, Coates J, Jackson SP, Calsou P (2016) Coordinated nuclease activities counteract Ku at single-ended DNA double-strand breaks. Nat Commun 7:12889. doi:10.1038/ncomms12889
71. Guirouilh-Barbat J et al (2016) 53BP1 protects against CtIP-dependent capture of ectopic chromosomal sequences at the junction of distant double-strand breaks. PLoS Genet 12:e1006230. doi:10.1371/journal.pgen.1006230
72. Ahrabi S et al (2016) A role for human homologous recombination factors in suppressing microhomology-mediated end joining. Nucleic Acids Res 44:5743–5757. doi:10.1093/nar/gkw326
73. Anand R, Ranjha L, Cannavo E, Cejka P (2016) Phosphorylated CtIP functions as a co-factor of the MRE11-RAD50-NBS1 endonuclease in DNA end resection. Mol Cell 64:940–950. doi:10.1016/j.molcel.2016.10.017
74. Chen YJ et al (2016) S. cerevisiae Mre11 recruits conjugated SUMO moieties to facilitate the assembly and function of the Mre11-Rad50-Xrs2 complex. Nucleic Acids Res 44:2199–2213. doi:10.1093/nar/gkv1523
75. Deshpande RA, Lee JH, Arora S, Paull TT (2016) Nbs1 converts the human Mre11/Rad50 nuclease complex into an endo/exonuclease machine specific for protein-DNA adducts. Mol Cell 64:593–606. doi:10.1016/j.molcel.2016.10.010
76. Broderick R et al (2016) EXD2 promotes homologous recombination by facilitating DNA end resection. Nat Cell Biol 18:271–280. doi:10.1038/ncb3303
77. Keyamura K, Arai K, Hishida T (2016) Srs2 and Mus81-Mms4 prevent accumulation of toxic inter-homolog recombination intermediates. PLoS Genet 12:e1006136. doi:10.1371/journal.pgen.1006136

78. Higashide M, Shinohara M (2016) Budding yeast SLX4 contributes to the appropriate distribution of crossovers and meiotic double-strand break formation on bivalents during meiosis. G3 (Bethesda) 6:2033–2042. doi:10.1534/g3.116.029488
79. Dibitetto D et al (2016) Slx4 and Rtt107 control checkpoint signalling and DNA resection at double-strand breaks. Nucleic Acids Res 44:669–682. doi:10.1093/nar/gkv1080
80. Guervilly JH, Gaillard PH (2016) SLX4 gains weight with SUMO in genome maintenance. Mol Cell Oncol 3:e1008297. doi:10.1080/23723556.2015.1008297
81. Regairaz M et al (2011) Mus81-mediated DNA cleavage resolves replication forks stalled by topoisomerase I-DNA complexes. J Cell Biol 195:739–749. doi:10.1083/jcb.201104003
82. Sebesta M et al (2017) Esc2 promotes Mus81 complex-activity via its SUMO-like and DNA binding domains. Nucleic Acids Res 45:215–230. doi:10.1093/nar/gkw882
83. Zhang YW et al (2011) Poly(ADP-ribose) polymerase and XPF-ERCC1 participate in distinct pathways for the repair of topoisomerase I-induced DNA damage in mammalian cells. Nucleic Acids Res 39:3607–3620. doi:10.1093/nar/gkq1304
84. LoRusso PM et al (2016) Phase I safety, pharmacokinetic, and pharmacodynamic study of the poly(ADP-ribose) polymerase (PARP) inhibitor veliparib (ABT-888) in combination with irinotecan in patients with advanced solid tumors. Clin Cancer Res 22:3227–3237. doi:10.1158/1078-0432.CCR-15-0652
85. Mullen JR, Chen CF, Brill SJ (2010) Wss1 is a SUMO-dependent isopeptidase that interacts genetically with the Slx5-Slx8 SUMO-targeted ubiquitin ligase. Mol Cell Biol 30:3737–3748. doi:10.1128/MCB.01649-09
86. O'Neill BM, Hanway D, Winzeler EA, Romesberg FE (2004) Coordinated functions of WSS1, PSY2 and TOF1 in the DNA damage response. Nucleic Acids Res 32:6519–6530. doi:10.1093/nar/gkh994
87. Stingele J, Schwarz MS, Bloemeke N, Wolf PG, Jentsch S (2014) A DNA-dependent protease involved in DNA-protein crosslink repair. Cell 158:327–338. doi:10.1016/j.cell.2014.04.053
88. Balakirev MY et al (2015) Wss1 metalloprotease partners with Cdc48/Doa1 in processing genotoxic SUMO conjugates. Elife 4. doi:10.7554/eLife.06763
89. Duxin JP, Dewar JM, Yardimci H, Walter JC (2014) Repair of a DNA-protein crosslink by replication-coupled proteolysis. Cell 159:346–357. doi:10.1016/j.cell.2014.09.024
90. Stingele J et al (2016) Mechanism and regulation of DNA-protein crosslink repair by the DNA-dependent metalloprotease SPRTN. Mol Cell 64:688–703. doi:10.1016/j.molcel.2016.09.031
91. Lopez-Mosqueda J et al (2016) SPRTN is a mammalian DNA-binding metalloprotease that resolves DNA-protein crosslinks. Elife 5. doi:10.7554/eLife.21491
92. Lessel D et al (2014) Mutations in SPRTN cause early onset hepatocellular carcinoma, genomic instability and progeroid features. Nat Genet 46:1239–1244. doi:10.1038/ng.3103
93. Vaz B et al (2016) Metalloprotease SPRTN/DVC1 orchestrates replication-coupled DNA-protein crosslink repair. Mol Cell 64:704–719. doi:10.1016/j.molcel.2016.09.032
94. Mosbech A et al (2012) DVC1 (C1orf124) is a DNA damage-targeting p97 adaptor that promotes ubiquitin-dependent responses to replication blocks. Nat Struct Mol Biol 19:1084–1092. doi:10.1038/nsmb.2395
95. Morocz M et al (2017) DNA-dependent protease activity of human Spartan facilitates replication of DNA-protein crosslink-containing DNA. Nucleic Acids Res. doi:10.1093/nar/gkw1315
96. Ray Chaudhuri A et al (2012) Topoisomerase I poisoning results in PARP-mediated replication fork reversal. Nat Struct Mol Biol 19:417–423. doi:10.1038/nsmb.2258
97. Solier S et al (2013) Transcription poisoning by Topoisomerase I is controlled by gene length, splice sites, and miR-142-3p. Cancer Res 73:4830–4839. doi:10.1158/0008-5472.CAN-12-3504
98. Berti M et al (2013) Human RECQ1 promotes restart of replication forks reversed by DNA topoisomerase I inhibition. Nat Struct Mol Biol 20:347–354. doi:10.1038/nsmb.2501
99. Zellweger R et al (2015) Rad51-mediated replication fork reversal is a global response to genotoxic treatments in human cells. J Cell Biol 208:563–579. doi:10.1083/jcb.201406099
100. Hashimoto Y, Puddu F, Costanzo V (2011) RAD51- and MRE11-dependent reassembly of uncoupled CMG helicase complex at collapsed replication forks. Nat Struct Mol Biol 19:17–24. doi:10.1038/nsmb.2177
101. Petermann E, Orta ML, Issaeva N, Schultz N, Helleday T (2010) Hydroxyurea-stalled replication forks become progressively inactivated and require two different RAD51-mediated pathways for restart and repair. Mol Cell 37:492–502. doi:10.1016/j.molcel.2010.01.021
102. Hu J et al (2012) The intra-S phase checkpoint targets Dna2 to prevent stalled replication forks from reversing. Cell 149:1221–1232. doi:10.1016/j.cell.2012.04.030
103. Ying S, Hamdy FC, Helleday T (2012) Mre11-dependent degradation of stalled DNA replication forks is prevented by BRCA2 and PARP1. Cancer Res 72:2814–2821. doi:10.1158/0008-5472.CAN-11-3417
104. Schlacher K et al (2011) Double-strand break repair-independent role for BRCA2 in blocking stalled replication fork degradation by MRE11. Cell 145:529–542. doi:10.1016/j.cell.2011.03.041
105. Shiotani B et al (2013) Two distinct modes of ATR activation orchestrated by Rad17 and Nbs1. Cell Rep 3:1651–1662. doi:10.1016/j.celrep.2013.04.018

106. Murina O et al (2014) FANCD2 and CtIP cooperate to repair DNA interstrand crosslinks. Cell Rep 7:1030–1038. doi:10.1016/j.celrep.2014.03.069
107. Yeo JE, Lee EH, Hendrickson EA, Sobeck A (2014) CtIP mediates replication fork recovery in a FANCD2-regulated manner. Hum Mol Genet 23:3695–3705. doi:10.1093/hmg/ddu078
108. Kuo C, Nuang H, Campbell JL (1983) Isolation of yeast DNA replication mutants in permeabilized cells. Proc Natl Acad Sci U S A 80:6465–6469
109. Budd ME, Campbell JL (1995) A yeast gene required for DNA replication encodes a protein with homology to DNA helicases. Proc Natl Acad Sci U S A 92:7642–7646
110. Gravel S, Chapman JR, Magill C, Jackson SP (2008) DNA helicases Sgs1 and BLM promote DNA double-strand break resection. Genes Dev 22:2767–2772. doi:10.1101/gad.503108
111. Zhu Z, Chung WH, Shim EY, Lee SE, Ira G (2008) Sgs1 helicase and two nucleases Dna2 and Exo1 resect DNA double-strand break ends. Cell 134:981–994. doi:10.1016/j.cell.2008.08.037
112. Nicolette ML et al (2010) Mre11-Rad50-Xrs2 and Sae2 promote 5′ strand resection of DNA double-strand breaks. Nat Struct Mol Biol 17:1478–1485. doi:10.1038/nsmb.1957
113. Nimonkar AV et al (2011) BLM-DNA2-RPA-MRN and EXO1-BLM-RPA-MRN constitute two DNA end resection machineries for human DNA break repair. Genes Dev 25:350–362. doi:10.1101/gad.2003811
114. Peng G et al (2012) Human nuclease/helicase DNA2 alleviates replication stress by promoting DNA end resection. Cancer Res 72:2802–2813. doi:10.1158/0008-5472.CAN-11-3152
115. Thangavel S et al (2015) DNA2 drives processing and restart of reversed replication forks in human cells. J Cell Biol 208:545–562. doi:10.1083/jcb.201406100
116. Iannascoli C, Palermo V, Murfuni I, Franchitto A, Pichierri P (2015) The WRN exonuclease domain protects nascent strands from pathological MRE11/EXO1-dependent degradation. Nucleic Acids Res 43:9788–9803. doi:10.1093/nar/gkv836
117. Shamanna RA et al (2016) WRN regulates pathway choice between classical and alternative non-homologous end joining. Nat Commun 7:13785. doi:10.1038/ncomms13785
118. Shamanna RA et al. (2016) Camptothecin targets WRN protein: mechanism and relevance in clinical breast cancer. Oncotarget 7:13269–13284. doi:10.18632/oncotarget.7906
119. Ribeyre C et al (2016) Nascent DNA proteomics reveals a chromatin remodeler required for topoisomerase I loading at replication forks. Cell Rep 15:300–309. doi:10.1016/j.celrep.2016.03.027
120. Pommier Y, Kohlhagen G, Wu C, Simmons DT (1998) Mammalian DNA topoisomerase I activity and poisoning by camptothecin are inhibited by simian virus 40 large T antigen. Biochemistry 37:3818–3823. doi:10.1021/bi972067d
121. Seinsoth S, Uhlmann-Schiffler H, Stahl H (2003) Bidirectional DNA unwinding by a ternary complex of T antigen, nucleolin and topoisomerase I. EMBO Rep 4:263–268. doi:10.1038/sj.embor.embor770
122. Gavin I, Horn PJ, Peterson CL (2001) SWI/SNF chromatin remodeling requires changes in DNA topology. Mol Cell 7:97–104
123. Walfridsson J, Khorosjutina O, Matikainen P, Gustafsson CM, Ekwall K (2007) A genome-wide role for CHD remodelling factors and Nap1 in nucleosome disassembly. EMBO J 26:2868–2879. doi:10.1038/sj.emboj.7601728
124. Durand-Dubief M, Svensson JP, Persson J, Ekwall K (2011) Topoisomerases, chromatin and transcription termination. Transcription 2:66–70. doi:10.4161/trns.2.2.14411
125. Krawczyk C, Dion V, Schar P, Fritsch O (2014) Reversible Top1 cleavage complexes are stabilized strand-specifically at the ribosomal replication fork barrier and contribute to ribosomal DNA stability. Nucleic Acids Res 42:4985–4995. doi:10.1093/nar/gku148
126. Dykhuizen EC et al (2013) BAF complexes facilitate decatenation of DNA by topoisomerase IIalpha. Nature 497:624–627. doi:10.1038/nature12146
127. Husain A et al (2016) Chromatin remodeller SMARCA4 recruits topoisomerase 1 and suppresses transcription-associated genomic instability. Nat Commun 7:10549. doi:10.1038/ncomms10549
128. Stoll G et al (2013) Deletion of TOP3beta, a component of FMRP-containing mRNPs, contributes to neurodevelopmental disorders. Nat Neurosci 16:1228–1237. doi:10.1038/nn.3484
129. Xu D et al (2013) Top3beta is an RNA topoisomerase that works with fragile X syndrome protein to promote synapse formation. Nat Neurosci 16:1238–1247. doi:10.1038/nn.3479
130. Yang Y et al (2014) Arginine methylation facilitates the recruitment of TOP3B to chromatin to prevent R loop accumulation. Mol Cell 53:484–497. doi:10.1016/j.molcel.2014.01.011
131. Ahmad M et al (2016) RNA topoisomerase is prevalent in all domains of life and associates with polyribosomes in animals. Nucleic Acids Res 44:6335–6349. doi:10.1093/nar/gkw508
132. Siaw GE, Liu IF, Lin PY, Been MD, Hsieh TS (2016) DNA and RNA topoisomerase activities of Top3beta are promoted by mediator protein Tudor domain-containing protein 3. Proc Natl Acad Sci U S A 113:E5544–E5551. doi:10.1073/pnas.1605517113
133. Meisenberg C et al. (2016) Epigenetic changes in histone acetylation underpin resistance to the topoisomerase I inhibitor irinotecan. Nucleic Acids Res. doi:10.1093/nar/gkw1026
134. Maxwell A, Costenaro L, Mitelheiser S, Bates AD (2005) Coupling ATP hydrolysis to DNA strand passage in type IIA DNA topoisomerases.

Biochem Soc Trans 33:1460–1464. doi:10.1042/BST20051460
135. Joshi RS, Pina B, Roca J (2012) Topoisomerase II is required for the production of long Pol II gene transcripts in yeast. Nucleic Acids Res 40:7907–7915. doi:10.1093/nar/gks626
136. King IF et al (2013) Topoisomerases facilitate transcription of long genes linked to autism. Nature 501:58–62. doi:10.1038/nature12504
137. Roedgaard M, Fredsoe J, Pedersen JM, Bjergbaek L, Andersen AH (2015) DNA topoisomerases are required for preinitiation complex assembly during GAL gene activation. PLoS One 10:e0132739. doi:10.1371/journal.pone.0132739
138. Ju BG et al (2006) A topoisomerase IIbeta-mediated dsDNA break required for regulated transcription. Science 312:1798–1802. doi:10.1126/science.1127196
139. Puc J et al (2015) Ligand-dependent enhancer activation regulated by topoisomerase-I activity. Cell 160:367–380. doi:10.1016/j.cell.2014.12.023
140. Bunch H et al (2015) Transcriptional elongation requires DNA break-induced signalling. Nat Commun 6:10191. doi:10.1038/ncomms10191
141. Madabhushi R et al (2015) Activity-induced DNA breaks govern the expression of neuronal early-response genes. Cell 161:1592–1605. doi:10.1016/j.cell.2015.05.032
142. Williams JS, Lujan SA, Kunkel TA (2016) Processing ribonucleotides incorporated during eukaryotic DNA replication. Nat Rev Mol Cell Biol 17:350–363. doi:10.1038/nrm.2016.37
143. Williams JS et al (2013) Topoisomerase 1-mediated removal of ribonucleotides from nascent leading-strand DNA. Mol Cell 49:1010–1015. doi:10.1016/j.molcel.2012.12.021
144. Sparks JL, Burgers PM (2015) Error-free and mutagenic processing of topoisomerase 1-provoked damage at genomic ribonucleotides. EMBO J 34:1259–1269. doi:10.15252/embj.201490868
145. Kim N et al (2011) Mutagenic processing of ribonucleotides in DNA by yeast topoisomerase I. Science 332:1561–1564. doi:10.1126/science.1205016
146. Williams JS, Kunkel TA (2014) Ribonucleotides in DNA: origins, repair and consequences. DNA Repair (Amst) 19:27–37. doi:10.1016/j.dnarep.2014.03.029
147. Potenski CJ, Niu H, Sung P, Klein HL (2014) Avoidance of ribonucleotide-induced mutations by RNase H2 and Srs2-Exo1 mechanisms. Nature 511:251–254. doi:10.1038/nature13292
148. Lazzaro F et al (2012) RNase H and postreplication repair protect cells from ribonucleotides incorporated in DNA. Mol Cell 45:99–110. doi:10.1016/j.molcel.2011.12.019
149. Sekiguchi J, Shuman S (1997) Site-specific ribonuclease activity of eukaryotic DNA topoisomerase I. Mol Cell 1:89–97
150. Huang SY, Ghosh S, Pommier Y (2015) Topoisomerase I alone is sufficient to produce short DNA deletions and can also reverse nicks at ribonucleotide sites. J Biol Chem 290:14068–14076. doi:10.1074/jbc.M115.653345
151. Arana ME et al (2012) Transcriptional responses to loss of RNase H2 in Saccharomyces cerevisiae. DNA Repair (Amst) 11:933–941. doi:10.1016/j.dnarep.2012.09.006
152. Conover HN et al (2015) Stimulation of chromosomal rearrangements by ribonucleotides. Genetics 201:951–961. doi:10.1534/genetics.115.181149
153. Epshtein A, Potenski CJ, Klein HL (2016) Increased spontaneous recombination in RNase H2-deficient cells arises from multiple contiguous rNMPs and not from single rNMP residues incorporated by DNA polymerase epsilon. Microb Cell 3:248–254. doi:10.15698/mic2016.06.506
154. Niu H, Potenski CJ, Epshtein A, Sung P, Klein HL (2016) Roles of DNA helicases and Exo1 in the avoidance of mutations induced by Top1-mediated cleavage at ribonucleotides in DNA. Cell Cycle 15:331–336. doi:10.1080/15384101.2015.1128594
155. Pendleton M, Lindsey RH Jr, Felix CA, Grimwade D, Osheroff N (2014) Topoisomerase II and leukemia. Ann N Y Acad Sci 1310:98–110. doi:10.1111/nyas.12358
156. Cowell IG et al (2012) Model for MLL translocations in therapy-related leukemia involving topoisomerase IIbeta-mediated DNA strand breaks and gene proximity. Proc Natl Acad Sci U S A 109:8989–8994. doi:10.1073/pnas.1204406109
157. Azarova AM et al (2007) Roles of DNA topoisomerase II isozymes in chemotherapy and secondary malignancies. Proc Natl Acad Sci U S A 104:11014–11019. doi:10.1073/pnas.0704002104
158. Lovett BD et al (2001) Near-precise interchromosomal recombination and functional DNA topoisomerase II cleavage sites at MLL and AF-4 genomic breakpoints in treatment-related acute lymphoblastic leukemia with t(4;11) translocation. Proc Natl Acad Sci U S A 98:9802–9807. doi:10.1073/pnas.171309898
159. Mahler M, Silverman ED, Schulte-Pelkum J, Fritzler MJ (2010) Anti-Scl-70 (topo-I) antibodies in SLE: myth or reality? Autoimmun Rev 9:756–760. doi:10.1016/j.autrev.2010.06.005
160. Haffner MC et al (2010) Androgen-induced TOP2B-mediated double-strand breaks and prostate cancer gene rearrangements. Nat Genet 42:668–675. doi:10.1038/ng.613
161. Tomlins SA et al (2005) Recurrent fusion of TMPRSS2 and ETS transcription factor genes in prostate cancer. Science 310:644–648. doi:10.1126/science.1117679
162. Helgeson BE et al (2008) Characterization of TMPRSS2:ETV5 and SLC45A3:ETV5 gene fusions in prostate cancer. Cancer Res 68:73–80. doi:10.1158/0008-5472.CAN-07-5352
163. Hermans KG et al (2008) Truncated ETV1, fused to novel tissue-specific genes, and full-length ETV1 in prostate cancer. Cancer Res 68:7541–7549. doi:10.1158/0008-5472.CAN-07-5930
164. Lin C et al (2009) Nuclear receptor-induced chromosomal proximity and DNA breaks underlie spe-

cific translocations in cancer. Cell 139:1069–1083. doi:10.1016/j.cell.2009.11.030
165. Kumar-Sinha C, Tomlins SA, Chinnaiyan AM (2008) Recurrent gene fusions in prostate cancer. Nat Rev Cancer 8:497–511. doi:10.1038/nrc2402
166. Bastus NC et al (2010) Androgen-induced TMPRSS2:ERG fusion in nonmalignant prostate epithelial cells. Cancer Res 70:9544–9548. doi:10.1158/0008-5472.CAN-10-1638
167. Bowen C, Gelmann E (2010) P. NKX3.1 activates cellular response to DNA damage. Cancer Res 70:3089–3097. doi:10.1158/0008-5472.CAN-09-3138
168. Bowen C, Zheng T, Gelmann EP (2015) NKX3.1 suppresses TMPRSS2-ERG gene rearrangement and mediates repair of androgen receptor-induced DNA damage. Cancer Res 75:2686–2698. doi:10.1158/0008-5472.CAN-14-3387
169. Zhang H, Zheng T, Chua CW, Shen M, Gelmann EP (2016) Nkx3.1 controls the DNA repair response in the mouse prostate. Prostate 76:402–408. doi:10.1002/pros.23131
170. Mani RS et al (2016) Inflammation-induced oxidative stress mediates gene fusion formation in prostate cancer. Cell Rep 17:2620–2631. doi:10.1016/j.celrep.2016.11.019
171. Laxman B et al (2006) Noninvasive detection of TMPRSS2:ERG fusion transcripts in the urine of men with prostate cancer. Neoplasia 8:885–888. doi:10.1593/neo.06625
172. Merdan S et al (2015) Assessment of long-term outcomes associated with urinary prostate cancer antigen 3 and TMPRSS2:ERG gene fusion at repeat biopsy. Cancer 121:4071–4079. doi:10.1002/cncr.29611
173. Geybels MS et al (2015) Epigenomic profiling of prostate cancer identifies differentially methylated genes in TMPRSS2:ERG fusion-positive versus fusion-negative tumors. Clin Epigenetics 7:128. doi:10.1186/s13148-015-0161-6
174. Walker C, Herranz-Martin S, Karyka E, Liao C, Lewis K, Elsayed W, Lukashchuk V, Chiang SC, Ray S, Mulcahy PJ, Jurga M, Tsagakis I, Iannitti T, Chandran J, Coldicott I, De Vos KJ, Hassan MK, Higginbottom A, Shaw PJ, Hautbergue GM, Azzouz M, El-Khamisy SF (2017, July) C9orf72 expansion disrupts ATM-mediated chromosomal break repair. Nat Neurosci. doi:10.1038/nn.4604. [Epub ahead of print]

The Emerging Role of Proteomics in Precision Medicine: Applications in Neurodegenerative Diseases and Neurotrauma

4

Rana Alaaeddine, Mira Fayad, Eliana Nehme, Hisham F. Bahmad, and Firas Kobeissy

Abstract

Inter-individual variability in response to pharmacotherapy has provoked a higher demand to personalize medical decisions. As the field of pharmacogenomics has served to translate personalized medicine from concept to practice, the contribution of the "omics" disciplines to the era of precision medicine seems to be vital in improving therapeutic outcomes. Although we have observed significant advances in the field of genomics towards personalized medicine, the field of proteomics-with all its capabilities- is still in its infancy towards the area of personalized precision medicine. Neurodegenerative diseases and neurotrauma are among the areas where the implementation of neuroproteomics approaches has enabled neuroscientists to broaden their understanding of neural disease mechanisms and characteristics. It has been shown that the influence of epigenetics, genetics and environmental factors were among the recognized factors contributing to the diverse presentation of a single disease as well as its treatment establishing the factor–disease interaction. Thus, management of these variable single disease presentation/outcome necessitated the need for factoring the influence of epigenetics, genetics, epigenetics, and other factors on disease progression to create a custom treatment plan unique to each individual. In fact, neuroproteomics with its high ability to decipher protein alterations along with their post translational modifications (PTMs) can be an ideal tool for personalized medicine goals includ-

R. Alaaeddine
Department of Pharmacology and Therapeutics, Faculty of Medicine, American University of Beirut, Beirut, Lebanon

M. Fayad
Biomedical Engineering Program, Faculty of Engineering and Architecture and Faculty of Medicine, American University of Beirut, Beirut, Lebanon

E. Nehme • F. Kobeissy (✉)
Department of Biochemistry and Molecular Genetics, Faculty of Medicine, American University of Beirut, Beirut, Lebanon
e-mail: firasko@gmail.com

H.F. Bahmad (✉)
Department of Anatomy, Cell Biology and Physiological Sciences, Faculty of Medicine, American University of Beirut, Beirut, Lebanon
e-mail: hfbahmad@gmail.com

S. El-Khamisy (ed.), *Personalised Medicine*, Advances in Experimental Medicine and Biology 1007,
DOI 10.1007/978-3-319-60733-7_4

ing: discovery of molecular mechanisms underlying disease pathobiology, development of novel diagnostics, enhancement of pharmacological neurotherapeutic approaches and finally, providing a "proteome identity" for patients with certain disorders and diseases. So far, neuroproteomics approaches have excelled in the areas of biomarker discovery arena where several diagnostic, prognostic and injury markers have been identified with a direct impact on the neurodegenerative diseases and neurotrauma. However, other applications in proteomics such as "individual" proteome sequencing with its signature PTMs, have not been fully investigated as compared to the achievements in the genomics discipline This infers that proteomics research work has promising potential, yet to be discovered, in the precision medicine and comprises a major component of the personalized medicine infrastructure as it allows individual characterization of disease at the protein level. To conclude, the field of proteomics-based personalized medicine is still in its infancy compared to genomics field due to several technical and instrumentation-based obstacles; however, we anticipate to have this initiative leading in the coming future. This chapter will discuss briefly how neuroproteomics can impact personalized medicine in the fields of neurodegenerative disorders particularly in Alzheimer's disease and brain injury.

Keywords

Post-translational modifications • Neurodegenerative diseases • Brain injury • Neurotrauma • Personalized medicine • Alzheimer's disease • proteomics

4.1 Introduction

The continuing progression of disease complexities introduced an incentive to revolutionize how medical field looks at diseases [1]. Currently, medicine's universal treatment approach has shown several shortcomings in delivering suitable treatment response for patients with the same disease, as these treatment methodologies are based on an average person response. Nevertheless, patients respond to treatment differently due to several factors including their specific genetic and proteomic profile [2]. Fittingly, the human genome was sequenced in 2003, and since then, advances in next generation sequencing (NGS) facilitated the discovery of several genetically based diseases such as the *BRCA* gene in breast cancer [2]. Identification of genetic diseases was the first step into what is called "*personalized medicine*" [3]. The latter term refers to a unique therapeutic treatment intended for individuals based on their genetic makeup [3]. The more recently used term in scientific articles is "precision medicine", which conveys targeted medicine aimed for subgroups of patients with similar genomic profile and not specifically based on disease afflicted individuals [3]. Precision medicine could be used to treat genetic mutation-based diseases (such as cystic fibrosis), and could be applied in the field of oncology to target solid tumors. Moreover, it could be used in pharmacogenesis area to adjust drug dosages based on the individual's genetic information; and recently, it has been applied in assessing neurodegenerative diseases such as Alzheimer's disease (AD) and brain injury (BI) [3]. AD is a neurodegenerative disease that impairs memory and motor function [4]. It affects about 44 million people globally [5]. In 2014, AD was found to be the sixth leading cause of death in the United States, making it a major burden on the health care system worldwide [6]. Studies have shown that AD has a long incubation period. This indicated that early onset interventions could be preventative and could possibly reduce the severity of AD and its treatment. As such, AD as a neurodegenerative disorder would be a perfect candidate for precision medicine which can be applied at different stages of AD characterization and assessment.

These include: (1) identifying the underlying factors using comprehensive risk assessment to understand the source of disease risk, whether it is due to genetic causes, a mutation or environmental factors [7]; (2) utilizing tools for preclinical detection since treatment is rarely applied based on risk, instead it is processed based on detection of latent pathophysiological processes [7]; and (3) tailoring molecular-based platforms as an important stage in precision medicine for targeted treatment aiming to slow or reverse the latent pathophysiological processes [7]. Moreover, clinical precision medicine approaches have proven that it can benefit from biomarkers research as it can stratify individuals with preclinical condition of AD for treatment response [4]. The three aforementioned stages allow for effective and promising precision medicine approaches to treat AD and other neurodegenerative diseases.

Neurotrauma is known to increase the risk of developing AD [8, 9]. Approximately 1% of the populations in developing countries have sustained BI [10]. The severity of (BI) and its long term implications on neurodegenerative diseases alerted the medical societies on the importance of utilizing targeted treatment and preventative therapy [8]. Accordingly, precision medicine in the area of BI aims at categorizing BI patients based on mechanistically homogeneous endotypes such as traumatic axonal injury or contusions, each of which responds to targeted therapy differently; regardless of the trauma severity [8]. For the past 42 years, Glasgow Coma Scale (GCS) has been the basic tool used to assess the neurological state of patients after sustaining BI [8]. However, GCS alone does not account for other confounding factors such as genetic heterogeneity which implicates the use of precision medicine [8]. This gap raised a new concern as to whether GCS is still the best approach to assess and detect BI severity, and whether alternative tools need to be implemented to achieve the aims of precision medicine [8]. Among the proposed approaches are to focus on biofluids analysis such as cerebrospinal fluid (CSF) in conjunction with neuroimaging biomarkers of BI, which were found to be promising in terms of diagnosis, prediction and monitoring of neuropathological progression as well as in AD risk prediction [10]. CSF biomarkers are useful injury indicators as they are in close proximity to the brain injured tissue which reflects biochemical changes in the brain, and can predict more precisely molecular and cellular changes in the brain post injury [10]. Axonal proteins and tau are one of the most promising CSF biomarkers reflecting the extent of axonal damage after acute BI [10]. In terms of neuroimaging, tau pathology relationship to BI severity could also be validated using corresponding imaging signals [10].

Collectively, if implemented on large scale, precision medicine could prove to be a promising approach for better assessment, diagnosis and treatment of BI patients. This could be achieved by comprehensively studying proteome makeup along with protein changes in individual patients to advise therapy and treatment. Such quest is best achieved by utilizing several neuroproteomics platforms [10].

4.2 Capabilities of Neuroproteomics in Precision Medicine

Most neurodegenerative diseases are characterized by neural dysfunction and injury, but they differ in terms of genetics, pathologies, phenotypes as well as treatments. Proteomics is the study of global protein (proteome) expressed at a specific condition [11]. Neuroproteomics specializes in the study of proteins that are part of the nervous system [10]. While precision medicine can be easily adapted to genomic medicine, proteomics precision medicine is far more complicated than that of genetic medicine due to the complex nature of the proteome make up [12]. The human proteome is characterized by its dynamic components involving protein-protein interaction, PTMs as well as its tissue, cellular and organelle specific-expression. Personalized proteomics is also dynamic; the expressed proteome profile at the steady control state is completely different compared to those expressed post disease state influenced by several factors which is highly complicated in neurodegenerative diseases due to the critical role of brain proteome in regulating the central nervous system (CNS) functions [13, 14].

Among the major neurodegenerative diseases with complex pathophysiology is AD. AD pathophysiology has complicated the progress in drug developments for cure or treatment [15]. This complexity arises from the fact that AD progresses from a latency phase where no signs or symptoms are observed even though pathophysiological processes are ongoing, to a prodromal phase with mild cognitive impairment (MCI), and eventually to dementia [15]. Identifying the latency and the prodromal phase windows is among the most successful approach for studying AD [15]. Thus, identifying predictive biomarkers at these stages is a key step for individualized medicine to diagnose patients who are advancing from prodromal phase with MCI to early and late AD stages [11]. This entails characterizing each patient proteome profile prior and during AD development to indicate for any protein changes associated with the critical stages of pre-AD development.

Different approaches have been considered in neuroproteomics platforms, one of which is the analysis of biomarkers in the CSF due to the continuous diffusion of proteins from the CNS to the CSF [11]. Another approach is to analyze biochemical changes that occur in patients sustaining advanced AD to compare their "altered" molecular and cellular proteomic profiles associated with dementia or memory loss [11].

4.3 Implications of Neuroproteomics in Traumatic Brain Injury and Alzheimer's Disease

4.3.1 Implications of Neuroproteomics in Traumatic Brain Injury

Traumatic brain injury (TBI) is an injury that occurs to the brain, brought about by external mechanical impact [16]. TBI interferes with normal brain function affecting memory, behavior and neuropsychological status of TBI patients. TBI is categorized into mild, moderate and severe injury; where mild injury being the most common among TBI comprising 70% of all TBI incidence [16]. Upon initiation, TBI occurs via two phases; the primary and secondary phase. The former starts at the moment of injury and comprises axonal shearing and hemorrhage followed by the secondary injury. Several consequences result from secondary injury phase, such as the disruption of the blood brain barrier (BBB) and the overproduction of reactive species that cause oxidative stress, neural cell death and altered proteome profile affecting the general protein functions [16]. Neuroproteomic techniques applied to the central nervous system injury have risen as a promising field for assessing novel pathways and mechanisms applicable to TBI pathophysiology, identifying key proteins as potential biomarkers and potential restorative medication targets as will be discussed later [17].

Among the leading studies in the areas of TBI biomarker research, Xu et al. applied proteomic and bioinformatics techniques to examine variation in protein expression levels in human brains post severe TBI conducted on Chinese TBI cohort [18]. Around 4031 proteins were identified using tandem mass tags (TMT) labeling followed by LC-MS/MS; 160 proteins were overexpressed and 5 proteins were downregulated in the injured compared to the control group. Among the overexpressed proteins, myelin basic protein (MBP), and myelin proteolipid protein (MYPR), that are involved in glial cell differentiation pathway. Moreover, matrix metallopeptidase 9 (MMP9) and s100 calcium binding protein A8 (S100A8) were found in elevated levels in the severe TBI brain tissue and these are associated with inflammatory pathways [18]. Several of these proteins were added to the databases of proteins associated with severe forms of brain injury.

In a recent study conducted by Thelin et al., protein profile in serum post-TBI was evaluated [19]. In their study, antibody bead suspension array was utilized to study serum proteins in a rat model of severe TBI. A total of 68 sera were analyzed leading to the identification of 143 different proteins. The levels of these proteins were compared between the injured and uninjured groups as well as in different oxygen status. Several of the identified proteins were implicated in injury mechanisms; it was shown that that the complement factor 9 (C9) and complement factor B (CFB) that are implicated in the innate complement system were identified during the first days post injury [19]. Similarly, aldolase c (ALDOC) was increased in the early stage after injury. Conversely, hypoxia inducing factor (HIF)1α, amyloid precursor protein (APP) and Williams-Beuren syndrome chromosome region 17 (WBSCR17) protein that has cerebral specificity were shown to be increased weeks following TBI [19]. Taken together, these serum protein profiles could be categorized according to disease staging and can reflect on the injury modulating factors (oxygenation levels) to help in TBI mechanisms assessment; however, such studies lack patient specificity as they rely more on pooling without associating with specific patients characteristics such as genetic profile, global proteomic makeup, epigenetic conditions, as well as PTMs alterations that can lead to precision evaluation.

Of interest, one study stands up discussing genotype-disease interaction [20]. Crawford et al. used apolipoprotein E (APOE)3 and APOE4 transgenic mice to study the effect of brain injury interaction in these two transgenic mice, which exhibited favorable and unfavorable outcomes respectively, following experimental TBI. Using a quantitative proteomics platform, altered regulated proteins were characterized as a function of disease-genotype (TBI*APOE genotype) interaction [20]. This important study clearly demonstrated that plasma protein changes are not only injury related but also genetic- make up dependent. The translatability of this work is of extreme importance as it can potentially extend to combat veterans receiving rehabilitation assessment exhibiting different genetic make-up and demonstrating different neurorehabilitative response to treatment.

4.3.2 Implications of Neuroproteomics in Alzheimer's Disease

Alzheimer's disease is defined as a chronic neurodegenerative disease that is manifested gradually that starts slowly and exacerbates over time. It is the most common type of dementia that causes injuries in the brain regions that are involved in memory [21]. In its initial stages, memory impairment is mild, yet at later stages, AD patients lose the capacity to bear on a discussion and react to their surroundings. In addition, more symptoms, such as mood swings and altered personality, become prevalent as the disease progresses. This staggering illness causes extraordinary suffering over patients and relatives. People over the age of 65 are at an increased risk of developing AD than younger people. The pervasiveness of AD in the overall public increments ranges around 1% in people at ages less than 65 years to around 40% in nonagenarians [22].

Alzheimer's disease is characterized by neuropathological features such as cerebral atrophy, extracellular senile plaques and intracellular neurofibrillary tangles (NFTs) [23]. The senile plaques consist of amyloid beta-peptide (Aβ) and the NFTs consist of the hyperphosphorylated microtubule-associated protein tau [24]. Albeit current Alzheimer's medications cannot prevent AD from advancing, these medications can incidentally moderate the compounding of dementia manifestations and enhance personal satisfaction for those with Alzheimer's and their caretakers. In addition, AD has a complex pathogenesis due to the fact that mitochondrial dysfunction, inflammatory mechanisms and oxidative stress play a role in the production and development of the disease [25]. Because of this complex origination and development, proteomics techniques have immediately developed as high-throughput methodologies for the identification of illness particular proteins [24].

Gozal et al. designed a study that aimed to analyze protein specific changes in neurodegenerative diseases using a proteomic approach [24]. Utilizing high performance liquid chromatography combined with tandem mass spectrometry (LC-MS/MS), they examined detergent-insoluble frontal cortex lysates from AD and unaffected control cases. In addition, they investigated specimens from frontotemporal lobar degeneration (FTLD) cases to recognize AD-particular changes not present in other neurodegenerative illnesses. Shotgun sequencing as well as label-free quantification procedure based on extracted ion current (XIC) were performed. Out of the 1045 identified proteins, 512 were clustered into the same group depending on similar peptides. Furthermore, quantitation analysis showed huge changes in 81 AD-particular proteins. Eleven proteins were acknowledged with high certainty as expanded in AD contrasted with control and FTLD brains, including β-amyloid, tau and apolipoprotein E, which were AD related proteins. Finally, Gozal et al. distinguished and approved the existence of serine protease 15, ankyrin B, and 14-3-3η in the detergent-insoluble part [24].

In another study, Musunuri et al. aimed to quantify and compare various proteins in the post mortem brain tissue from AD patients and control subjects (non-AD individuals) to better understand the mechanisms underlying the changes occurring in AD patient brains [25]. This was conducted in human subjects by utilizing shotgun mass spectrometry utilizing a steady isotope dimethyl labeling technique. A total of 827 proteins were quantitated. Of these, 227 proteins were found in no less than nine out of ten AD patient pairs. A sum of 69 proteins (37 upregulated and 32 downregulated) in the AD compared to the non-AD subjects were identified. Among the increased proteins, glial fibrillary acidic protein (GFAP), α-enolase (ENOA) and ferritin light chain (FRIL), were identified; whereas, tubulin β-3 chain (TBB3), involved in axon guidance and maintenance, was shown to be downregulated [25]. In addition, twenty-three novel proteins that have not been previously identified in AD were characterized. These involved: neuronal-particular septin-3 (SEPT 3), septin-2 (SEPT 2), septin-5 (SEPT 5), dihydropteridine reductase (DHPR), and clathrin heavy chain 1 (CHC1). Altered proteins were associated with a wide assortment of biological pathways related to disease pathogenesis, including glycolysis, oxidative anxiety, apoptosis, flag transduction, and synaptic function proposing new candidates for AD specific biomarker candidates [25].

4.4 Functional Neuroproteomics: Synapse Proteomics, Protein Interaction Networks, and Post-Translational Modifications

Functional proteomics constitutes another area of investigation in the proteomics field whose methodologies are inclined towards two noteworthy focuses: the explanation of the biological function of obscure altered proteins and deciphering cell mechanisms. On the other hand, brain functional proteomics allows to assess the metabolic changes occurring inside neuronal cells and brain tissue that may infer some pathophysiological adjustments [26]. Functional neuroproteomics led the way to the study of synapse proteomics and protein interaction networks as well as analysis of post-translational modifications (PTMs) of proteins as discussed later. A synapse is a small gap found at the end of a neuron that functions as a bridge to transmit information or signal from one cell to another. Each synapse comprises a neurotransmitter, integrating and discharging mechanical assembly, the presynapse, and a transmitter receiving component, the postsynapse [27]. To understand the underlying mechanisms of the synapse abnormalities we have to comprehend the atypical protein expression and protein–protein interaction, that are known to occur in different disorders such as psychiatric diseases [27]. Post-translational modification (PTM) refers to the enzyme catalyzed changes that occur to the protein after being translated by ribosomes. There are various forms of these PTMs including phosphorylation, carbonylation and acetylation that can be detected by several techniques like mass spectrometry and western blotting. These modifications play vital distinctive roles in physiological as well as pathological conditions.

Ansari et al. conducted a study where young male rats were subjected to a one-sided direct cortical injury to assess oxidation redox in TBI [28]. Given that oxidative stress in TBI results from the disruption of the balance between oxidants and antioxidants, altered proteomic data identified a number of antioxidants like glutathione [GSH], glutathione peroxidase [GPx], and glutathione reductase [GR]. Synaptic markers such as synapsin-I, post-synaptic density protein 95 (PSD-95), synapse-associated protein 97 (SAP-97), and GAP-43 were validated by Western blot. All action levels were contrasted with sham-injured animals. Changes in pre-and post-synaptic proteins (Synapsin-I and PSD-95) occurred mid (24 h), while SAP-97 levels showed an extended decrease. These results indicated that disruption in the antioxidants affects the synaptic proteins and consequently their functions [28].

In another study, Yu et al. utilized a bioinformatics systems biology strategy based on assessing four distinct high-throughput gene expression studies of experimental TBI to elucidate molecular pathological pathways underlying the progression of TBI mechanisms [29]. For this aim, canonical pathways as well as protein-interaction network were exploited as a scaffold to predict protein markers and identify novel molecular mechanisms involved in TBI. Of interest, systems biology results indicated that 24 h post-injury, the essentially actuated molecular marks were nonspecific to TBI, while the fundamentally smothered molecular marks were components of the nervous system and associated with synaptic function. A suppressed subnetwork comprising of 58 proteins related to synaptic capacity were identified. Among these, three proteins were selected including: postsynaptic density protein 95 (PSD 95), nitric oxide synthase 1 (NOS 1), and disrupted in schizophrenia 1 (DISC 1), that were validated using penetrating ballistic-like brain injury rat model validating the bioinformatics predictive model of protein interaction [29].

The analysis of synaptic proteome wasn't solely applied to TBI. Among the various disorders or conditions that this analysis is applied to is Alzheimer's disease. In 2012, Chang et al. focused on distinguishing synaptosomal proteins that contrast in expression between subjects with and without AD in two brain regions (the hippocampus and the temporal cortex) that are influenced in AD by utilizing an enhancement method combined with proteomics and mass spectrometry (MS) [30]. Twenty-six proteins indicated more than 20% contrast in expression. Of these, 10 related with vesicular trafficking (septin-11, septin-8, a-tubulin, b-actin, and annexin A5). Others are associated with signal transduction, energy metabolism and antioxidant activity [30].

Additionally, in a recently published article by Zali et al. protein-protein interaction prediction (PIP) analysis of the hippocampus proteins between AD patients and non-AD patients was investigated [31]. Out of the 245 modified proteins that were identified, 105 were observed to be solely communicated in AD while 140 proteins were identified in decreased levels. The differentially expressed proteins and related systems were investigated utilizing cytoscape and the PIP examination techniques: MCODE and CluGO. The network analysis outlines 22 clusters with different seed genes. The CluGO method exhibited expanding in apoptosis, immune system processes, and glutathione transferase activity. However, GTPase activity and glucose metabolism were down-regulated [32].

Of interest, not many studies have investigated the role of protein carbonylation on different neural cell types and brain regions post TBI [33]. In one study, Lazarus et al. aimed to determine the regions in the brain that are susceptible to carbonylation as well as the neural cell types affected [33]. Immunostaining was utilized to assess carbonylated proteins and cell-specific markers in the brains of male and female rats that were subjected to experimental brain injury of controlled cortical impact (CCI). Results demonstrated that the highest levels of protein carbonylation occurred in the immediate area of the injury lesion site specifically in the astrocytes, along with the ependymal cells lining the dorsal third ventricle, and the floor of the third ventricle above the median eminence. Furthermore, protein carbonylation was shown to be much greater in male rats at sites distant from the lesion. This finding proposes that hormonal systems may serve a defensive part against oxidative stress. In addition, proteomic investigation verified that glial fibrillary acidic protein (GFAP), dihydropyrimidase-related protein 2, fructose-bisphosphate aldolase C (ALDOC), and fructose bisphosphate aldolase A (ALDOA) were the most influenced proteins via carbonylation in response to TBI. However, protein carbonylation was not detected in different neural cell types such as oligodendrocytes, microglia, and macrophages. These results signify that protein carbonylation post-TBI occurs in a regional as well as protein specific manner [33].

Another investigated PTM process was S-nitrosation where cysteine (Cys) thiol is converted to nitrosothiol (RSNO). This type of PTM is altered in physiological as well as pathological conditions [34]. Senevirante et al. used a CK-p25–inducible mouse model of Alzheimer's disease-like neurodegeneration and applied the SNOTRAP (SNO trapping by triaryl phosphine) approach in order to tag the targeted cysteine residues in the proteins of the brain [34]. SNO-proteins were detected using liquid chromatography-mass spectrometry. They were able to detect 313 nitrosated protein sites in 251 proteins in the mouse brain, where 135 SNO-proteins were detected only during neurodegeneration. Moreover, this study demonstrated an increase in the S-nitrosation of proteins during early neurodegeneration which were shown to be critical for metabolism, synapse function and AD pathology [34].

4.5 Clinical Neuroproteomics

The compelling capabilities of proteomics methodologies in analyzing proteins implicated in physiological or pathophysiological pathways have paved the way to a better understanding of diseases, particularly neurological ones. This is due to the fact that neuroproteomics analysis techniques have been highly implemented to fill the gaps of neuropathology research. Knowing that the cellular mechanisms of most neurological disorders are still vague, the investment of neuroproteomics along with neuropathology in the field of personalized medicine is highly appreciated [35].

Advanced neuroproteomics analysis platform has proven itself to be greatly efficient in the discovery of novel proteins. High throughput proteomics tools have allowed researchers to profile the human proteome and identify protein dysfunctions in terms of quantity and quality. Since neurodegenerative diseases and neurotrauma are contributed to protein dysfunction, clinical neuroproteomics is expected to make a leap in diagnosis, treatment, early detection, as well as delaying progression of such diseases, taking into account individual variations. Nevertheless, it is important to notify that other diseases -such as drug addiction, epilepsy, or multiple sclerosis- are also active areas in clinical neuroproteomics [35].

This section summarizes the most important clinical and research findings related to neurodegenerative diseases and neurotrauma. Moreover, the link between these diseases and pharmacological therapies is also highlighted. Most importantly, the implication of proteomics in biomarker discovery is later discussed in this section.

4.5.1 Neurodegenerative Disease

Neuroproteomics has a remarkable contribution in the advancement of the understanding of neurodegenerative diseases (NDD), such as

Alzheimer's disease (AD), Parkinson's disease (PD), and Huntington's disease (HD). Although these diseases differ in their clinical manifestations, they all have the same mechanistic background, in terms of protein aggregation, oxidative damage, and neuronal apoptosis, that lead to neuron degeneration [36]. Being one of the most prevalent forms of dementia [37], AD has been a subject of interest of neuroproteomics research. Given that amyloid plaques and neurofibrillary tangles are two characteristics of AD, a number of studies have been conducted to elucidate the protein components and PTMs occurring at the molecular level. Various studies have confirmed the presence of new protein constituents within amyloid plaques [38, 39]. In addition, there are phosphorylation sites in tau protein, that are modified in AD [38]. Most of the literature's focus has been on the phosphorylation PTM, yet it is crucial to point out that many other PTMs of tau protein take place. A study carried out by Thomas et al. in 2012 have stated that lysine methylation is another form of PTM of tau proteins in the neurofibrillary tangles [40].

The research work conducted by Troncone et al. in 2016 provides evidence that the pathology of AD is not restricted to brain tissues only, yet it may involve other vital organs [41]. The findings of this research prove that Aβ-amyloid residues also exist in myocardial tissues. Therefore, it's very reasonable to regard AD as a metastatic disease that causes organ failure, particularly heart failure. Owing to the coexistence of AD and HF among many patients, these results will lead the advancement of novel clinical approaches to treat HF in AD.

Given that patients with TBI are at a higher risk of developing certain NDDs, advanced proteomic platforms have been implemented in the investigation of the pathophysiological mechanisms mutual between TBI and the corresponding NDDs [9]. The findings have shown that numerous PTMs occurring in TBI are exclusively shared with AD, yet not PD [9]. Furthermore, oligomers of tau, well-known to aggregate in neurofibrillary tangles in AD, may likewise be causing the toxicity in TBI [42]. Other studies have also proved the existence of amyloid plaques not only in AD, yet in TBI as well as illustrated in a number of clinical TBI studies [43–46].

Redox proteomics is an arising branch of proteomics that studies PTMs of proteins occurring under oxidative stress or in redox signaling [47]. Thus, redox proteomics aims at studying oxidative stress-based changes occurring at the proteome level which has implications on drug administration and drug design and testing [48, 49]. Apparently, reactive oxygen/nitrogen species trigger an alteration in the PTM of various proteins, where the resulting oxidized proteins are thought to be involved in the progression of numerous diseases, such as cardiovascular diseases, diabetes mellitus type 2, cancer, and many others [47]. It has been identified that oxidative stress and the corresponding oxidized species are underlying the pathophysiology and worsening of NDDs in specific [35, 50]. Redox proteomics has aided in spotting proteins that are associated with the dysfunction of AD, thus implicating oxidative damage [38]. Interestingly, these protein alterations are found at an early onset of the disease which highlights the role of oxidation in the early processes of AD [38, 51]. On the other hand, neuroproteomics with the discipline of redox proteomics has contributed to the advancement of drug discovery since this field permits the identification of various target proteins that are target for oxidative modifications prior to or upon drug administration contributing to drug testing and evaluation [36]. In this regard, there is an immense need to design biomarker panels for the assessment of biological and metabolic oxidative stress brought about by administration or treatment of pharmaceutical drugs [52]. The work of Domenico et al. in 2016 has demonstrated that oxidized proteins in the CSF exist in states of mild cognitive impairment, prior to the development of AD, thus may serve as a biomarker for early detection of AD [53]. Apolipoprotein A-I [54] and 24S-Hydroxycholesterol [38] are two examples of potential biomarkers that can be detected by redox neuroproteomics. So far, the investment of neuroproteomics in pharmacological clinical research and drug development is still in its infancy and only preliminary research has been performed; nevertheless, neuroproteomics will have a major role in evaluating the effect of neuropharmacological therapies on neurodegenerative diseases.

4.5.2 Biomarker Discovery

Biomarker discovery is one of the most important fields where neuroproteomics has been implemented. It engages the detection of protein alterations in the human plasma or CSF, that indicates the presence or progression of diseases [35]. Proteomics-related biomarkers have facilitated the diagnosis of neurodegenerative diseases and provided an insight of disease condition [38]. However, as the field of neuroproteomics gets more integrated in clinical aspects, it's urged to utilize modern tools to achieve diagnostic precision. Furthermore, it is crucial to standardize laboratory protocols in order to narrow variations in laboratory results [35]. These variations may be a result of either utilizing more than one method in each laboratory or testing a heterogeneous tissue sample.

Biomarkers can be detected in both plasma and CSF; however, screening of the CSF is preferred over plasma screening considering that the sooner occurs within close proximity with the CNS and is somewhat easy to be collected as well [35]. Nonetheless, plasma is still obtained from control healthy individuals for its ease of collection and enrichment in higher quantities of protein biomarkers· [55]. In addition, the characteristics of an ideal biomarker encompass having remarkable sensitivity and specificity, indicating early disease stages, and being insensitive to handling of samples [55]. New biomarkers, in both blood and CSF, has not only been implicated for the detection of Alzheimer's disease, yet it has also been used to determine the stage of AD in patients [37]. Recent data from a study carried out by Kitamura et al. has revealed three downregulated proteins and two upregulated ones in early AD, thus aiding in the early detection of AD [37]. In another study, Jauch et al. concluded that the S100β protein and myelin basic protein were elevated in blood of patients 24 h after brain injury [56]. It is important to note that the use of neuroproteomics *in clinica* faces similar challenges observed in basic research [57] attributed to the failure of biomarker identification and translation to a large population. This fact of lack of translatability may require stringent standards for discovery/identification coupled with more validated platforms for biomarker validation [58, 59].

4.6 Conclusion and Future Directions

As discussed, the different neuroproteomics tools and platforms represent a promising target for personalized medicine as it can segregate patients proteome based on different factors such as epigenetics, environmental as well as genetic makeup [35]. The application of proteomic research on clinical studies would benefit the medical field as it eliminates treatment response variability, and provides a more targeted approach therapy. The ultimate aim of precision medicine is to match specifically patient response with the best course of treatment to obtain the optimal outcomes [57]. However, a major challenge in the area of proteomics compared to the genomics field is the high cost and instrument robustness. In addition, most biofluids proteomics studies rely on sample pooling rather than running individual sample assessment where the results are validation step relies on random selected individual samples.

However, with the recent advances in the area of mass spectrometry and proteomics platforms in general, it is expected that such steps would advance our knowledge proteome dynamics [38] where the analysis outcomes rely on the accuracy and sensitivity of mass spectrometry. As a result, such advances will guide researchers to overcome the failure of translation of research innovations into drug discovery [60]. Taken together, the application of proteomics into the field of precision medicine is still in infancy compared to other omics fields; due to several challenges pertaining to cost, instrumentation, and sample characteristics. However, we anticipate that we would observe a huge leap in the area of proteomics-based precision medicine as we are observing advances in the areas of proteomics.

References

1. Collins FS, McKusick VA (2001) Implications of the human genome project for medical science. JAMA 285(5):540–544
2. Juengst E, McGowan ML, Fishman JR, Settersten RA Jr (2016) From "Personalized" to "Precision" medicine: the ethical and social implications of rhetorical reform in genomic medicine. Hast Cent Rep 46(5):21–33
3. Ashley EA (2016) Towards precision medicine. Nat Rev Genet 17(9):507–522
4. Schelke MW et al (2016) Nutritional interventions for Alzheimer's prevention: a clinical precision medicine approach. Ann N Y Acad Sci 1367(1):50–56
5. Prince M, Comas-Herrera A, Knapp M, Guerchet M, Karagiannidou M (2016) World Alzheimer report 2016: improving healthcare for people living with dementia: coverage, quality and costs now and in the future. Alzheimer's Disease International, London
6. Heron M, Anderson RN (2016) Changes in the leading cause of death: recent patterns in heart disease and cancer mortality. Cancer 400(500000):600000
7. Montine TJ, Montine KS (2015) Precision medicine: clarity for the clinical and biological complexity of Alzheimer's and Parkinson's diseases. J Exp Med 212(5):601–605
8. Menon DK, Maas AI (2015) Traumatic brain injury in 2014. Progress, failures and new approaches for TBI research. Nat Rev Neurol 11(2):71–72
9. Abou-Abbass H et al (2016) Glycosylation and other PTMs alterations in neurodegenerative diseases: current status and future role in neurotrauma. Electrophoresis 37(11):1549–1561
10. DeKosky ST, Blennow K, Ikonomovic MD, Gandy S (2013) Acute and chronic traumatic encephalopathies: pathogenesis and biomarkers. Nat Rev Neurol 9(4):192–200
11. Moya-Alvarado G, Gershoni-Emek N, Perlson E, Bronfman FC (2016) Neurodegeneration and Alzheimer's disease (AD). What can proteomics tell us about the Alzheimer's brain? Mol Cell Proteomics 15(2):409–425
12. Roberts S, Julius M (2016) Precision medicine: now, not when. Healthc Manag Forum 29(4):158–161
13. Ozdemir V et al (2017) Personalized medicine beyond genomics: alternative futures in big data-proteomics, environtome and the social proteome. J Neural Transm 124(1):25–32
14. Colinge J, Rix U, Bennett KL, Superti-Furga G (2012) Systems biology analysis of protein-drug interactions. Proteomics Clin Appl 6(1–2):102–116
15. Veenstra TD (2016) Neuroproteomic tools for battling Alzheimer's disease. Proteomics 16(22):2847–2853
16. Henderson M et al (2016) Neuroproteomic study of nitrated proteins in moderate traumatic brain injured rats treated with gamma glutamyl cysteine ethyl ester administration post injury: Insight into the role of glutathione elevation in nitrosative stress. PROTEOMICS – Clin Appl 10(12):1218–1224
17. Kobeissy FH et al (2016) Neuroproteomics and systems biology approach to identify temporal biomarker changes post experimental traumatic brain injury in rats. Front Neurol 7
18. Xu B et al (2016) Protein profile changes in the frontotemporal lobes in human severe traumatic brain injury. Brain Res 1642:344–352
19. Thelin EP et al. (2016) Protein profiling in serum after traumatic brain injury in rats reveals potential injury markers. Behav Brain Res.
20. Crawford F et al (2012) Identification of plasma biomarkers of TBI outcome using proteomic approaches in an APOE mouse model. J Neurotrauma 29(2):246–260
21. Kovacech B, Zilka N, Novak M (2009) New age of neuroproteomics in Alzheimer's disease research. Cell Mol Neurobiol 29(6–7):799–805
22. Jaber Z et al (2016) Role of systems biology in brain injury biomarker discovery: neuroproteomics application. Methods Mol Biol 1462:157–174
23. Brinkmalm A et al (2015) Explorative and targeted neuroproteomics in Alzheimer's disease. Biochim Biophys Acta 1854(7):769–778
24. Gozal YM et al (2009) Proteomics analysis reveals novel components in the detergent-insoluble subproteome in Alzheimer's disease. J Proteome Res 8(11):5069–5079
25. Musunuri S et al (2014) Quantification of the brain proteome in Alzheimer's disease using multiplexed mass spectrometry. J Proteome Res 13(4):2056–2068
26. Federico VR, Federica F (2016) Functional proteomics as marker for neurological and psychiatric disorders: the first application to dementia for an immediate future. J Neurol Neurosci 7:S2
27. Li KW, Klemmer P, Smit AB (2010) Interaction proteomics of synapse protein complexes. Anal Bioanal Chem 397(8):3195–3202
28. Ansari MA, Roberts KN, Scheff SW (2008) A time course of contusion-induced oxidative stress and synaptic proteins in cortex in a rat model of TBI. J Neurotrauma 25(5):513–526
29. Yu C et al (2015) A systems biology strategy to identify molecular mechanisms of action and protein indicators of traumatic brain injury. J Neurosci Res 93(2):199–214
30. Chang RY, Nouwens AS, Dodd PR, Etheridge N (2013) The synaptic proteome in Alzheimer's disease. Alzheimer's Dement J Alzheimer's Assoc 9(5):499–511
31. Zali H, Tavirani MR, Jalilian FA, Khodarahmi R (2013) Proteins expression clustering of Alzheimer disease in rat hippocampus proteome. J Paramedical Sci 4(3):111–118

32. Butterfield DA, Reed TT (2016) Lipid peroxidation and tyrosine nitration in traumatic brain injury: insights into secondary injury from redox proteomics. Proteomics Clin Appl 10(12):1191–1204
33. Lazarus RC, Buonora JE, Jacobowitz DM, Mueller GP (2015) Protein carbonylation after traumatic brain injury: cell specificity, regional susceptibility, and gender differences. Free Radic Biol Med 78: 89–100
34. Seneviratne U et al (2016) S-nitrosation of proteins relevant to Alzheimer's disease during early stages of neurodegeneration. Proc Natl Acad Sci U S A 113(15):4152–4157
35. Bayes A, Grant SG (2009) Neuroproteomics: understanding the molecular organization and complexity of the brain. Nat Rev Neurosci 10(9):635–646
36. D'Alessandro A, Rinalducci S, Zolla L (2011) Redox proteomics and drug development. J Proteome 74(12):2575–2595
37. Kitamura Y et al (2017) Plasma protein profiling for potential biomarkers in the early diagnosis of Alzheimer's disease. Neurol Res 39(3):231–238
38. Lovestone S et al (2007) Proteomics of Alzheimer's disease: understanding mechanisms and seeking biomarkers. Expert Rev Proteomics 4(2):227–238
39. Liao L et al (2004) Proteomic characterization of postmortem amyloid plaques isolated by laser capture microdissection. J Biol Chem 279(35): 37061–37068
40. Thomas SN et al (2012) Dual modification of Alzheimer's disease PHF-tau protein by lysine methylation and ubiquitylation: a mass spectrometry approach. Acta Neuropathol 123(1):105–117
41. Troncone L et al (2016) Abeta amyloid pathology affects the hearts of patients with Alzheimer's disease: mind the heart. J Am Coll Cardiol 68(22):2395–2407
42. Gerson J et al (2016) Tau oligomers derived from traumatic brain injury cause cognitive impairment and accelerate onset of pathology in Htau mice. J Neurotrauma 33(22):2034–2043
43. Johnson VE, Stewart W, Smith DH (2010) Traumatic brain injury and amyloid-beta pathology: a link to Alzheimer's disease? Nat Rev Neurosci 11(5):361–370
44. Roberts GW, Gentleman SM, Lynch A, Graham DI (1991) beta A4 amyloid protein deposition in brain after head trauma. Lancet 338(8780):1422–1423
45. Roberts GW et al (1994) Beta amyloid protein deposition in the brain after severe head injury: implications for the pathogenesis of Alzheimer's disease. J Neurol Neurosurg Psychiatry 57(4):419–425
46. Raby CA et al (1998) Traumatic brain injury increases beta-amyloid peptide 1-42 in cerebrospinal fluid. J Neurochem 71(6):2505–2509
47. Butterfield DA, Dalle-Donne I (2012) Redox proteomics. Antioxid Redox Signal 17(11):1487–1489
48. Sheehan D, McDonagh B, Barcena JA (2010) Redox proteomics. Expert Rev Proteomics 7(1):1–4
49. McDonagh B, Sheehan D (2008) Effects of oxidative stress on protein thiols and disulphides in *Mytilus edulis* revealed by proteomics: actin and protein disulphide isomerase are redox targets. Mar Environ Res 66(1):193–195
50. Butterfield DA, Sultana R (2008) Redox proteomics: understanding oxidative stress in the progression of age-related neurodegenerative disorders. Expert Rev Proteomics 5(2):157–160
51. Keller JN et al (2005) Evidence of increased oxidative damage in subjects with mild cognitive impairment. Neurology 64(7):1152–1156
52. Beretta G, Facino RM (2010) Recent advances in the assessment of the antioxidant capacity of pharmaceutical drugs: from in vitro to in vivo evidence. Anal Bioanal Chem 398(1):67–75
53. Di Domenico F et al (2016) Oxidative signature of cerebrospinal fluid from mild cognitive impairment and Alzheimer disease patients. Free Radic Biol Med 91:1–9
54. Keeney JT et al (2013) Apolipoprotein A-I: insights from redox proteomics for its role in neurodegeneration. Proteomics Clin Appl 7(1–2):109–122
55. Shoemaker LD, Achrol AS, Sethu P, Steinberg GK, Chang SD (2012) Clinical neuroproteomics and biomarkers: from basic research to clinical decision making. Neurosurgery 70(3):518–525
56. Jauch EC et al (2006) Association of serial biochemical markers with acute ischemic stroke: the National Institute of Neurological Disorders and Stroke recombinant tissue plasminogen activator stroke study. Stroke 37(10):2508–2513
57. Duarte TT, Spencer CT (2016) Personalized proteomics: the future of precision medicine. Proteomes 4(4)
58. Scherl A (2015) Clinical protein mass spectrometry. Methods 81:3–14
59. Lehmann S, et al. (2016) Clinical mass spectrometry proteomics (cMSP) for medical laboratory: what does the future hold? Clin Chim Acta; Int J Clin Chem
60. Guest FL, Guest PC, Martins-de-Souza D (2016) The emergence of point-of-care blood-based biomarker testing for psychiatric disorders: enabling personalized medicine. Biomark Med 10(4):431–443

The Role of Nitric Oxide from Neurological Disease to Cancer

5

Ahmed Maher, Mohamed F. Abdel Rahman, and Mohamed Z. Gad

Abstract

Until the beginning of the 1980s, nitric oxide (NO) was just a toxic molecule of a lengthy list of environmental pollutants such as cigarette smoke and smog. In fact, NO had a very bad reputation of being destroyer of ozone, suspected carcinogen and precursor of acid rain. However, by the early 1990s it was well recognized by the medical research community. Over the last two decades, the picture has been totally changed. Diverse lines of evidence have converged to show that this sometime poison is a fundamental player in the everyday business of the human body. NO activity was probed in the brain, arteries, immune system, liver, pancreas, uterus, peripheral nerves, lungs, and almost every system in the human body. NO is a major player in the cardiovascular system as it is involved in regulating blood pressure. In the CNS, it is involved in memory formation and the regulation of cerebral blood flow to ensure adequate supply of blood to the brain. Because NO is involved in many pathways, it has a role in several diseases related to modern life as hypertension, coronary heart diseases, Alzheimer's Disease, stroke and cancer. This chapter focuses on the discussion of the role of NO in neurological diseases and cancer and how can this Janus-faced molecule play a role in the pathology and personalized treatment of these diseases.

A. Maher • M.F. Abdel Rahman
Biochemistry Department, Faculty of Pharmacy, October University for Modern Sciences and Arts (MSA), Cairo, Egypt

M.Z. Gad (✉)
Clinical Biochemistry Unit, Faculty of Pharmacy & Biotechnology, German University in Cairo (GUC), Cairo, Egypt
e-mail: mohamed.gad@guc.edu.eg

S. El-Khamisy (ed.), *Personalised Medicine*, Advances in Experimental Medicine and Biology 1007,
DOI 10.1007/978-3-319-60733-7_5

Keywords
Nitric oxide (NO) • NO signal transduction • CNS • Neurodegeneration disorders • Cancer • NOS expression • NO-targeted therapy

5.1 Introduction

In 1978, Murad hypothesized that endogenous factors such as hormones may influence smooth muscles via nitric oxide (NO). In 1980, Furchgott and his group discovered that an unknown substance was formed in the endothelium that could relax the smooth muscle cells in blood vessels. He named the substance EDRF, Endothelium Derived Relaxing Factor [1]. Nine years later, Ignarro reached the conclusion that EDRF was identical to NO [2].

In 1998, the three American professors Robert Furchgott, Ferid Murad and Louis Ignarro were awarded Nobel Prize for their eminent contribution in the discovery of NO role in the cardiovascular system.

NO is an unusual gaseous messenger. It is a free radical that can react with thiol groups on proteins to form new complexes. In contrast to other second messengers, NO does not require energy to transport itself in and out the cell, it acts as a second messenger in a paracrine and autocrine manner. NO travels in the bloodstream by forming complexes with glutathione, hemoglobin and other proteins. Upon dissociation from these complexes, NO can affect some distant cells which qualifies NO to be classified as a hormone [3].

NO biological targets include transition metals as well as free radicals. The NO/metal reactions mainly involve ferrous iron and to a lesser extent copper. NO reacts with free radicals because they possess unpaired electrons. NO reacts with superoxide anion (O_2^-) to give peroxynitrite ($ONOO^-$) whose formation has been implicated in the pathology of several conditions involving oxidative stress such as atherosclerosis. The most significant effect of $ONOO^-$ may be attributed to the scavenging of NO and O_2^-, thereby diminishing their signaling capabilities [4].

5.1.1 NO Synthesis

Intracellular NO synthesis is catalyzed by three isoforms of nitric oxide synthase (NOS, EC1.14.13.39) which use L-arginine and molecular oxygen as substrates to produce NO and the amino acid L-citrulline. The three identified isoforms of NOS are constitutive neuronal NOS (nNOS, NOS-1) found in neuronal tissue, inducible NOS (iNOS, NOS-2) inducible in a wide range of cells and tissues and endothelial NOS (eNOS, NOS-3) found in vascular endothelial cells [5]. These forms are products of different genes, with different localization, regulation, catalytic properties and inhibitor sensitivity, and with 51–57% homology between the human isoforms [6].

5.1.2 NO Signal Transduction

5.1.2.1 NO/cGMP-Dependent Signaling

Many of the NO actions are done through the soluble guanylyl cyclase (sGC). sGC is a heterodimer consisting of alpha and beta subunits. There can be two different alpha subunits, α1 and α2, and two different beta subunits, β1 and β2. Most tissues possess the α1β1 heterodimer which was also found to be the receptor for NO. NO binds to a heme group liganded to His_{105} of the β-subunit. The binding of NO to sGC increases its V_{max} 200–400-fold and decreases the K_m [7]. sGC converts guanosine triphosphate (GTP) into guanosine 3′,5′-cyclic monophosphate (cGMP) which triggers

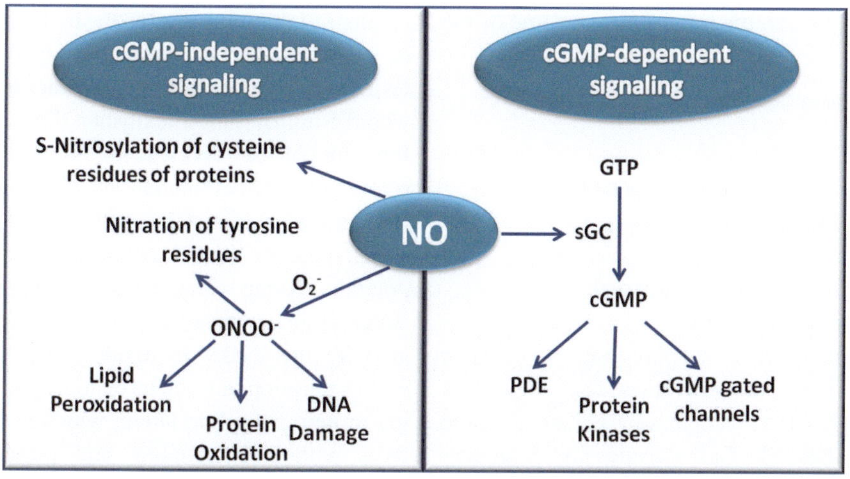

Fig. 5.1 cGMP signal transduction pathways

several downstream signaling events, including activation of cGMP-dependent protein kinases, cGMP-gated channels and cGMP-regulated phosphodiesterases (PDE) [8] (Fig. 5.1).

5.1.2.2 NO/cGMP-Independent Signaling

Modifications done by NO and its derivatives in important target molecules including thiols, lipids and aromatic amino acids are important for normal physiology. However, high levels of NO lead to cytotoxicity and nitrosative stress [9].

Protein S-nitrosylation reaction between NO derived species and the reduced thiol of a cysteine residue is an important posttranslational modification that regulates protein stability and functions and thus, is implicated in normal physiology as well as in various diseases. Tyrosine nitration is another modification induced by NO derived species. NO reacts with superoxide in a diffusion-limited manner to generate peroxynitrite which causes tissue damage by inducing protein oxidation, lipid peroxidation and DNA damage [8] (Fig. 5.1).

5.2 Nitric Oxide in Neurological Disorders

The impact of neurological disorders on the international society is high and in continuous increase where the World Health Organization (WHO) is estimating that the percentage of disability-adjusted life years (DALYs) due to neurological disorders will increase by 12% by the year 2030 and by 66% for specific diseases such as Alzheimer's Disease (AD) [10]. Also diseases such as dementia, epilepsy, migraine and stroke are among the top 50 causes of DALY [11].

According to the WHO, one DALY can be thought of as one lost year of "healthy" life. The sum of these DALYs across the population, or the burden of disease, can be thought of as a measurement of the gap between current health status and an ideal health situation where the entire population lives to an advanced age, free of disease and disability [10].

NO is a regulatory cellular messenger in the nervous system; it plays a role in the cerebral endothelium-dependent vasodilatation [12], synaptic plasticity and behavior being a modulator of several neurotransmitters [13], sleep cycle regulator and a component in the CNS defense mechanism being produced by astrocytes and microglial cells [14].

In this chapter, the role of NO in some of the common neurological disorders will be discussed.

5.2.1 Physiological Role of NO in CNS

5.2.1.1 Role of NO in Memory and Cognition

As mentioned earlier, NO plays a role in synaptic plasticity. Upon the activation of N-methyl-D-aspartate (NMDA) receptors by glutamate, there is a Ca^{2+} influx. The Ca^{2+} activates nNOS producing NO that acts on the sGC producing cGMP. The gaseous nature of NO allows it to diffuse into the presynapse where it stimulates the release of glutamate thus, increases synaptic plasticity as well as the production of presynaptic cGMP which in turn, enhances the regeneration of the glutamate vesicles [15, 16]. Post-synaptically, NO/cGMP potentiates neurotransmission and its role in long-term potentiation (LTP) is mediated by cGMP-dependent activation of the transcription factor cAMP response element-binding protein (CREB) [15]. Animal studies showed that blocking nNOS by different inhibitors impedes memory and learning, an effect that was reversed by NO-donors [17].

5.2.1.2 Neuroprotective Role of NO

The NO-activated CREB was found to inhibit apoptosis and so does the nitrosylated caspase-3 [14]. Nitrosylation also inhibits apoptosis through the inhibition of protein kinase Cε (PKCε) [18] and through the inhibition of NMDA receptors thus decreasing Ca^{2+} influx and preventing excitotoxicity [19]. NO guards against oxidative stress through the activation of the transcription factor Nrf2 [20].

5.2.2 Neurotoxicity of NO

NO can react with sulphur residues causing S-nitrosylation. This S-nitrosylation can affect several proteins such as Glyceraldehyde-3-phosphate dehydrogenase (GAPDH) which results in inhibition of glycolysis, peroxiredoxin II, an antioxidant expressed mainly in neurons, Hsp90 and protein-disulphide isomerase proteins where S-nitrosylation abolishes their chaperone function [21, 22]. NO was incriminated to play a role in the demyelination of oligodendrocytes [23] as well as interacting with the cyclooxygenase enzyme (COX) thus enhancing its neurotoxic potential. Along with the depletion of glutathione stores, high concentration of NO, mainly generated by the iNOS, is highly neurotoxic as it causes nitration of tyrosine residues thus preventing protein phosphorylation, which in turn interferes with cell signaling and protein-protein interaction [24].

5.2.2.1 NO Role in Alzheimer's Disease and Other Neurodegenerative Disorders

By the end of 2015 there were 46.8 million people living with dementia worldwide and the number is projected to increase by the year 2050 to reach 131.5 million [25]. AD accounts for 70% of dementia among elderly people [26].

The hallmarks of AD are the presence of amyloid beta protein Aβ and neurofibrillary tangles. Aβ is a product of the pathogenic processing of amyloid precursor protein (APP) by β-secretases – rather than α-secretases – followed by γ-secretases [27]. The deposition of Aβ triggers inflammatory responses and causes increased oxidative stress within the cell thus, disrupting its normal signaling pathways [28]. Tau is the major neuronal microtubule-associated protein where it interacts with tubulin and promotes its assembly into microtubules that stabilize neuronal structure. Hyperphosphorylation of the tau protein results in the disruption of microtubules and the formation of neurofibrillary tangles [29].

Only 1% of AD cases have been attributed to hereditary causes. Numerous factors are considered predisposing factors for AD, starting from genetic variations in the presenilins and apoE genes [30] to systemic inflammation [31]. Oxidative and nitrosative stress play a major role in AD. They are found before Aβ plaques and may exacerbate and even induce the formation of Aβ and the hyperphosphorylation of tau, as well as causing mitochondrial dysfunction, disrupting calcium signaling and activating microglia resulting in neuroinflammation [32].

NO effect on the brain can be converged in three main cellular effects, the effect on sGC and cGMP level, the effect on tyrosine nitration, and S-nitrosylation. Activating the sGC and increasing the level of cAMP is considered protective as it causes vasodilatation thus reduces cerebral oxidative stress and enhances the production of brain-derived neurotrophic factor (BDNF) through the CREB/BDNF pathway which has a neuroprotective effect [33]. It also reduces intracellular Ca^{2+} thus prevents excitotoxicity [19].

Increased concentration of NO has been directly correlated with neurodegeneration and AD. High NO concentration results in the nitration of the tyrosine residue in the Hsp90 protein resulting in decrease in mitochondrial activity and neuronal death [34]. Nitrotyrosination of Aβ has been reported to stabilize the more toxic Aβ oligomers and prevent its polymerizations to the less toxic fibrils [35]. In addition, high concentrations of nitrotyrosine were found in the spinal cord neurons of amyotrophic lateral sclerosis (ALS) patients and mice [21].

Finally, aberrant S-nitrosylation (SNO-) results in the malfunction of several proteins. These can be categorized into three categories; those affecting protein misfolding, those affecting mitochondrial dysfunction and those regulating cell death pathway:

Protein misfolding

(a) **Parkin**: a ligase and a transcriptional p-53 repressor, upon nitrosylation both functions are lost leading to the accumulation of misfolded proteins, aggregated Lewy bodies and neuronal death in Parkinson's disease (PD) [36, 37].
(b) **Protein disulfide isomerase (PDI)**: is a chaperone enzyme that is active during protein synthesis and activation. Nitrosylation of PDI results in the accumulation of misfolded proteins and neuronal death in various neurodegenerative diseases where its concentration increases significantly in patients with AD and PD [38, 39]. Studies also correlate between the loss of PDI function and the oligomerization of α-synuclein. α-synuclein aggregates are primary components of Lewy bodies, the defining pathological feature of PD [40]. In addition, SNO-PDI cannot guard the neuronal cells against the aggregation of misfolded superoxide dismutase 1 (SOD1), a common component in ALS [37].

Mitochondrial dysfunction

(a) **Dynamin-related protein 1 (Drp1)**: is a GTPase essential for mitochondrial fission. Nitrosylating Drp1 increases its GTPase activity leading to the formation of pathologically small, fragmented mitochondria with a compromised function. It was found that Aβ and mutant Huntington-induced nitrosative stress cause aberrant *S*-nitrosylation of Drp1 in models of AD and Huntington disease (HD) respectively. This was further confirmed by the high concentrations of SNO-Drp1 found in the postmortem brains of AD and HD patients [37, 41, 42].
(b) **Cyclin-dependent kinase 5 (Cdk5)**: is a serine/threonine kinase highly present in neurons. Upon activation, it phosphorylates a number of proteins related to neurodegenerative diseases such as tau, MEF2 and Drp1. Cdk5 forms a complex with nNOS which facilitates the formation of the hyperactive SNO-Cdk5 under Aβ-induced nitrosative stress conditions. This explains the neuronal damage occurring in AD as a result of hyperphosphorylation of the tau protein due to the loss of the cytoskeleton and the presence of high concentrations of SNO-Cdk5 in postmortem brains of AD patients [43]. SNO-Cdk5 also acts as an *S*-nitrosylase for Drp1, transnitrosylating an adducted NO group from Cdk5 to Drp1, to form the hyperactive SNO-Drp1 [44].

Cell death regulating pathway

(a) **Glyceraldehyde-3-phosphate dehydrogenase (GAPDH)**: a unique enzyme with a role in glycolysis and nuclear signaling of apoptosis. Upon nitrosylation, GAPDH not only loses its function in the glycolytic pathway resulting in a decrease in the ATP production, it also binds to an E3 ubiquitin ligase enzyme named SIAH1. The GAPDH/SIAH1 complex allows the GAPDH into the nucleus where it stabilizes the SIAH1 allowing it to degrade nuclear proteins and initiate an apoptotic cascade that may contribute to the pathology of neurodegenerative diseases [37, 45]. The GAPDH/SIAH1 complex facilitates the translocation of the mutant Huntington protein (mtHtt) into the nucleus suggesting a possible role in HD [45]. Also deprenyl, a drug preventing the S-nitrosylation of GAPDH and thus the binding to SIAH1 showed anti PD activity [21].

(b) **Caspases and X-linked inhibitor of apoptosis protein (XIAP)**: Caspases are a family of cysteine proteases that consist of 14 isoforms, which play an essential role in the apoptotic signal cascade. Caspases are formed constitutively in an inactive form which is activated in the presence of a proapoptotic signal by proteolytic cleavage by initiator caspases including caspase-8, -9 and -10 [46]. XIAP is a protein that directly binds to caspase-3, -7 and -9 inhibiting their activity and targeting them for ubiquitination and degradation thus, accounting for its antiapoptotic role and neuroprotective effect [37]. S-nitrosylation ceases this inhibition resulting in apoptosis and neuronal death. There is also evidence that nitrosylated caspases act as transnitrosylases to S-nitrosylate XIAP thus inhibiting the XIAP and activating themselves. Increased levels of SNO-XIAP have been found in brain samples from human patients with HD, PD and AD [47–49] which supports the notion that SNO-XIAP contributes to the pathogenesis of several neurodegenerative diseases.

(c) **Myocyte enhancer factor 2 (MEF2)**: is a transcription factor regulating neuronal survival in different regions in the brain as well as controlling synapse formation and dendritic remodeling. This is associated with neuronal plasticity, memory and learning [36]. S-nitrosylation prevents MEF2 from binding to the promoter region of downstream effector genes, thus inhibiting transcriptional activity and contributing to both, impaired neurogenesis and neuronal death. Also, high levels of SNO-MEF2 were found in the brains of transgenic AD mice models and in AD patients [50].

5.2.3 Role of NO in Regulating Cerebral Blood Flow

NO plays a role in the regulation of cerebral blood flow via the additive effects of eNOS and nNOS. The eNOS-derived NO results in the relaxation of vascular smooth muscles and thus ensures an adequate blood flow to the brain despite of changing blood pressure [51].

Cerebral hyperaemia or neurovascular coupling is the process of linking the cerebral blood flow to the neuronal activity to ensure an adequate blood supply to the brain. The excitatory neurotransmitter glutamate acts on NMDA receptors resulting in the production of NO. The release of NO causes vasodilatation of cerebral blood vessels directly and through the production of the vasodilatory epoxyeicosatrienoic acids. Conversely, the depletion of NO decreases the production of epoxyeicosatrienoic acids and favors the synthesis of the vasoconstrictor 20-hydroxyeicosatetraenoic acid [52].

5.2.4 Role of NO in Stroke

Stroke is defined by the WHO as the rapid onset of cerebral deficit lasting for more than 24 h, with no apparent cause other than a vascular one. It is considered the third leading cause of death after coronary heart disease and cancer [10]. Broadly it can be divided into ischemic strokes and hemorrhagic strokes.

According to the WHO 2006 report, cerebrovascular diseases represent 55% of DALYs of neurological diseases and represent more than 10% of the deaths worldwide [10].

NO plays a dual pivotal role in the pathology of strokes on the vascular and cellular levels being both neuroprotective and neurotoxic.

5.2.4.1 Vascular Level

After cerebral insults, decreased consciousness is common, leading to hypoventilation and both hypoxia and hypercapnia. Depletion of NO will result in the loss of physiological response to the changes in oxygen and carbon dioxide, further exacerbating neuronal damage.

P-selectin is an endothelial cell adhesion molecule that promotes platelet aggregation and fibrin deposition. An association was found between the decrease in the level of NO and the expression of p-selectin, therefore NO depletion favors the formation of microthrombi and microinfarctions characteristic of hemorrhagic strokes as well as increasing the probability of ischemic strokes [53, 54].

Cortical spreading depression is a wave of abrupt and sustained mass depolarization in the cortical surface and promotes neuronal death in energy compromised tissues [55]. It plays a role in early brain injury, delayed ischemia after hemorrhagic strokes, traumatic brain injuries [51, 55] as well as migraine episodes [55]. Cerebral ischemia is an inducer of spreading depression and thus, NO depletion may be a predisposing factor for cortical spreading depression. Also, spreading depression is accompanied by severe vasoconstriction resulting in further ischemia, a process that is reversed by NO-donors as *S*-nitroso-*N*-acetylpenicillamine [55].

5.2.4.2 Cellular Level

Ischemia-reperfusion is accompanied by the production of large concentrations of reactive oxygen species (ROS). iNOS is believed to be overexpressed in the neutrophils migrating to the brain as a consequence of the stroke. Unlike the protective role of eNOS-NO, high concentrations of iNOS-NO within these cells was found to be neurotoxic as it reacts with the ROS produced during the ischemia-reperfusion forming another neurotoxic compound, peroxynitrite [56, 57]. Experiments showed that inhibiting iNOS or deleting the iNOS gene reduced the infarct size in mice by approximately 30% [57] (Fig. 5.2).

5.3 NO in Cancer

Due to the wide range of functions of NO in the body, its role in cancer is still controversial as several studies reported that NO has tumoricidal effects while others reported that it has tumor promoting properties. The dual role of NO in cancer and several diseases might be explained by concentration dependence [58, 59].

In 2012, WHO estimated that there were 14 million new cases of cancer per year with a projection for this figure to rise to 22 million annually within the next two decades. WHO cancer deaths are predicted to rise from an estimated 8.2 million annually to 13 million per year. Globally, in 2012 the cancer types with the highest prevalence were lung, breast, and large bowel [141]. According to WHO, An estimated 169.3 million years of healthy life (DALYs) were lost globally because of cancer in 2008 [142].

A concentration of NO less than 100 nM acts as an antiapoptotic and thereby favors tumor formation and progression [60, 61] while, higher concentration of NO (more than 500 nM) is cytotoxic and proapoptotic thereby has an antitumor activity [62]. Macrophages, neutrophils, endothelial cells, hepatocytes, cardiac myocytes and chondrocytes might produce high concentrations of NO capable of inducing cytotoxicity [63].

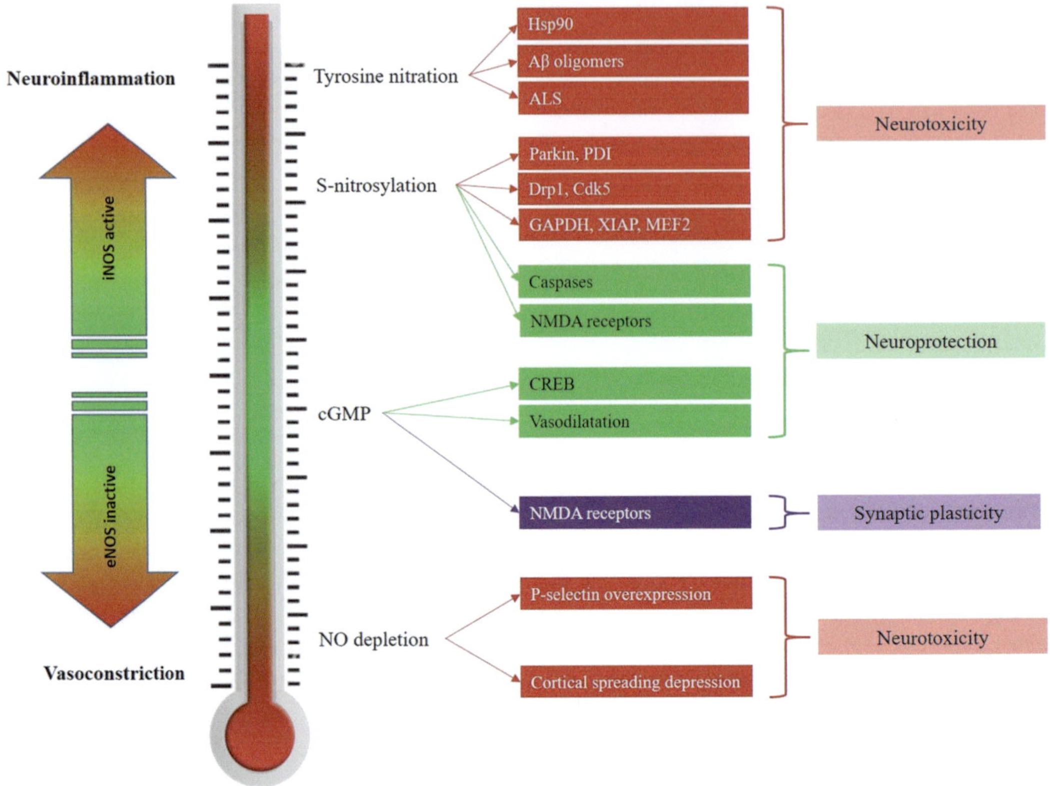

Fig. 5.2 The Janus-face of NO in the CNS demonstrating its role in neuroprotection and neurotoxicity

However, the concentration of NO is not the only factor, as the cellular response of cancer cells are complicated by several factors including the cell or tumor type, duration of exposure, NO flux, and immune and vascular cells. Hence, the overall outcome of NO results from the interplay between NO itself and the tumor cell [63].

5.3.1 NO Tumoricidal Effects

5.3.1.1 cGMP Signaling Pathway

In the 1970s Criss et al. reported that sGC levels were low in the tissue extracts in the proliferating tissues. Furthermore, NO failed to increase cGMP levels in these tissues or activate sGC in the homogenates [64]. Recently, the same research group found that sGC α1 and β1 subunits expression is significantly lower in glioma preparations and cell lines. Furthermore, they revealed that restoring sGC function either by blocking PDE or the expression of the constitutively active mutant sGCβ1Cys$_{105}$ (instead of the wild type sGCβ1His$_{105}$) correlated inversely with glioma cells growth [65]. This finding suggests that NO can prevent tumorigenesis, given that tumorigenesis and organogenesis possess common aspects [66].

5.3.1.2 NO Proapoptotic Effects

In 1993, Albina et al. reported that NO can induce apoptosis in macrophages [67]. Since then, several studies have shown that several cells including macrophages, pancreatic islets, thymocytes, and certain neuron types undergo apoptosis in response to NO by p53-dependent and p53-independent apoptosis [68].

p53-dependent apoptosis: p53 is a tumor suppressor gene whose expression leads to apoptosis caused by most of the DNA-damaging agents. The nuclear phosphoprotein p53 acts as a checkpoint control in the cell cycle. p53 activation blocks G_1/S and induces apoptosis in the case of severe DNA damage [68]. Several mechanisms have been suggested for p53 proapoptotic action. Direct translocation of the p53 protein to the mitochondria activates pro-apoptotic Bcl-2 family members [69, 70]. A recent study suggests that p53 activation can also induce caspase-independent programmed cell death [71]. p53 eliminates tumor cells through the induction of senescence mediated by the cell cycle inhibitor p21 leading to tumor cells engulfment by macrophages [72]. NO induces p53 up-regulation and activates wild-type p53 by inducing its phosphorylation [68].

p53-independent apoptosis: NO initiated apoptosis in $p53^{-/-}$ mice [73] and p53-negative cell lines such as HL-60 and U937 [74]. A proposed mechanism is through the nitrosylation of PKC [18].

5.3.2 NO Tumor Promoting Effects

5.3.2.1 NO Direct Genotoxicity

Under oxidative stress NO generates peroxynitrite and N_2O_3. Peroxynitrite can oxidize and nitrate DNA. It also attacks the sugar-phosphate backbone and may potentially cause single-strand DNA breaks. N_2O_3 is capable of nitrosating amines then alkylating DNA. Nitrosation of DNA bases leads to the formation of diazonium ions and subsequent deamination forming DNA-crosslinks [75].

Additionally, cytokine-mediated induction of iNOS was reported to diminish DNA repair capacity in carcinoma cell lines [76]. NO can also inactivate several DNA repair enzymes such as DNA alkyl-transferase, xeroderma pigmentosum-A protein and 8-oxoguanine glycosylase-1 by S-nitrosylation of the cysteine residue in their active sites [77].

5.3.2.2 NOS Expression

Increased iNOS expression was observed in cancer both on the mRNA and protein levels. Thomsen et al. reported that iNOS activity was higher in less differentiated tumors in human breast cancer [78]. Other studies confirmed that iNOS is expressed by breast carcinoma cells and correlates with tumor stage and microvessel density [79–81].

Similarly, iNOS is markedly expressed in approximately 60% of human colon adenomas and in 20–25% of colon carcinomas, while the expression is either low or absent in the surrounding normal tissues. Head and neck, esophageal, lung, prostate, bladder and pancreatic carcinomas, brain tumors, Kaposi's sarcoma, mesothelioma, and hematological malignancies were all associated with high iNOS expression [77].

Increased expression of the other two isoforms of NOS was reported by several studies. High expression of nNOS and eNOS was detected in astrocytic tumors with the highest levels of expression found in higher grade tumors [82]. Another interesting finding was the presence of a strong positive correlation between eNOS and iNOS in breast carcinoma patients [81].

Lim et al. showed that eNOS induces Ras proteins nitrosylation and activation in tumorigenesis. They suggested that the wild type Ras activates PI3K-AKT-eNOS-wild type Ras pathway in cancer cells [83].

5.3.2.3 Caveolae Signaling

Caveolae are 50–100 nm invaginations of the plasma membrane. They serve as sites for the sequestration of signaling proteins and are characterized by the presence of caveolin [84]. Caveolin1 (CAV1) binds eNOS and inhibits NO generation. When CAV1 is absent overproduction of NO takes place [85]. Overproduction of NO leads to mitochondrial dysfunction due to disruption of electron transport. NO reacts with superoxide to form peroxynitrite which inhibits complex I. NO also competes with oxygen and inhibits complex IV [86].

Many aggressive cancers are characterized by the underexpression of CAV1 cancer-associated fibroblasts. CAV1 underexpression is mediated by oxidative stress which leads to CAV1 degradation by autophagy. This aggravates oxidative stress which will lead to more decrease in CAV1 via a feed-forward manner [87]. Absence of CAV1 was linked to poor cancer prognosis. Several studies reported the association of poor clinical outcomes including early tumor recurrence, lymph node metastasis and resistance to tamoxifen to absence of CAV1 in breast cancer stroma [88, 89]. In contrast, a study showed that high CAV1 expression in breast cancer stroma was correlated with low survival [90].

Low CAV1 was also correlated to poor clinical outcomes in other types of cancer including prostate [91] and gastric cancer [92].

5.3.2.4 NO Antiapoptotic Effects

In addition to its actions as a proapoptotic agent, NO mediates several antiapoptotic effects. The accumulated data indicate that physiological levels of NO contribute to the balance between the antiapoptotic and proapoptotic forces within a cell by suppressing the apoptotic pathway at multiple levels and by several mechanisms. Through the activation of sGC, NO can increase cGMP levels, this interrupts apoptotic signaling in some cell types, including hepatocytes and splenocytes [93].

The cGMP-dependent antiapototic effects of NO include the suppression of mitochondrial cytochrome c release, ceramide generation, and caspase activation [94]. NO/cGMP induced the expression level of Bcl-2 in splenic B lymphocytes [95]. Li et al. pointed to the involvement of Akt/PKB activation in NO/cGMP-mediated antiapoptosis [96] which induces phosphorylation of Bcl-2-associated death promoter (BAD) and procaspase-9 and cytoprotective gene expression through NF-κB activation [94].

A second mechanism of antiapoptosis is the inhibition of caspase activity directly by S-nitrosylation [93] and indirectly by the activation of XIAP [49]. NO-mediated S-nitrosylation of the cysteine in caspase active site has been reported to inhibit apoptosis in hepatocytes [97, 98], endothelial cells [99] and other tumor cell lines [100]. XIAP overexpression was considered a poor prognostic sign in breast cancer [101]. XIAP is a novel target for new anticancer agents [102, 103].

The release of cytochrome c is a key component in the activation of caspase cascade and apoptosis [104]. NO inhibits cytochrome c release through the inhibition of caspase-8 [105]. The inhibition of caspase-8 inhibits the proteolytic cleavage and activation of Bid (BH3-interacting domain death agonist), a pro-apoptotic member of the Bcl-2 family. Cleavage and activation of Bid is an important step for its translocation to the mitochondria and induction of the cytochrome c release, which leads to the activation of downstream caspases and apoptosis [106].

NO was found also to regulate the expression of several proteins that take part in the apoptotic cascade. NO potentially induces cytoprotective proteins including Hsp70 and Hsp32, which protect hepatocytes from apoptosis induced by TNFα and oxidative or nitrosative stress [107, 108]. The iNOS activating cytokines prevents apoptosis of wild type mice beta cells through the induction of Hsp70, the same cytokines failed to prevent apoptosis in iNOS-/- beta-cells [109]. NO also upregulates Bcl-2 [95] and COX [94] and downregulates MAP kinase phosphatise-3 [110] which prevents apoptosis.

NO produced from iNOS contributes directly in GC to AT mutations in p53 which leads to loss of its repressor activity [111].

5.3.2.5 Cancer Metastasis

NO facilitates the blood flow to the tumor by vasodilation and inhibition of leukocyte adhesion and increase in vascular permeability [112]. In addition, it promotes metastasis through inducing angiogenesis. When iNOS was transfected into colon adenocarcinoma line it produced tumors that grew more rapidly and more vascularized than wild type cells [113]. Excessive production of NO sustained tumor growth, which was correlated with invasive ability of tumor cells in vitro and induced tumor angiogenesis in vivo. Blocking of iNOS activity retarded the growth of xenografted tumors [114].

> Cancer Metastasis is a multistage process that causes the spread and growth of tumor cells through angiogenesis, invasion, colonization, and ultimately proliferation from the original neoplasm to other organs [143]. Angiogenesis is the process by which blood vessels are formed [144].

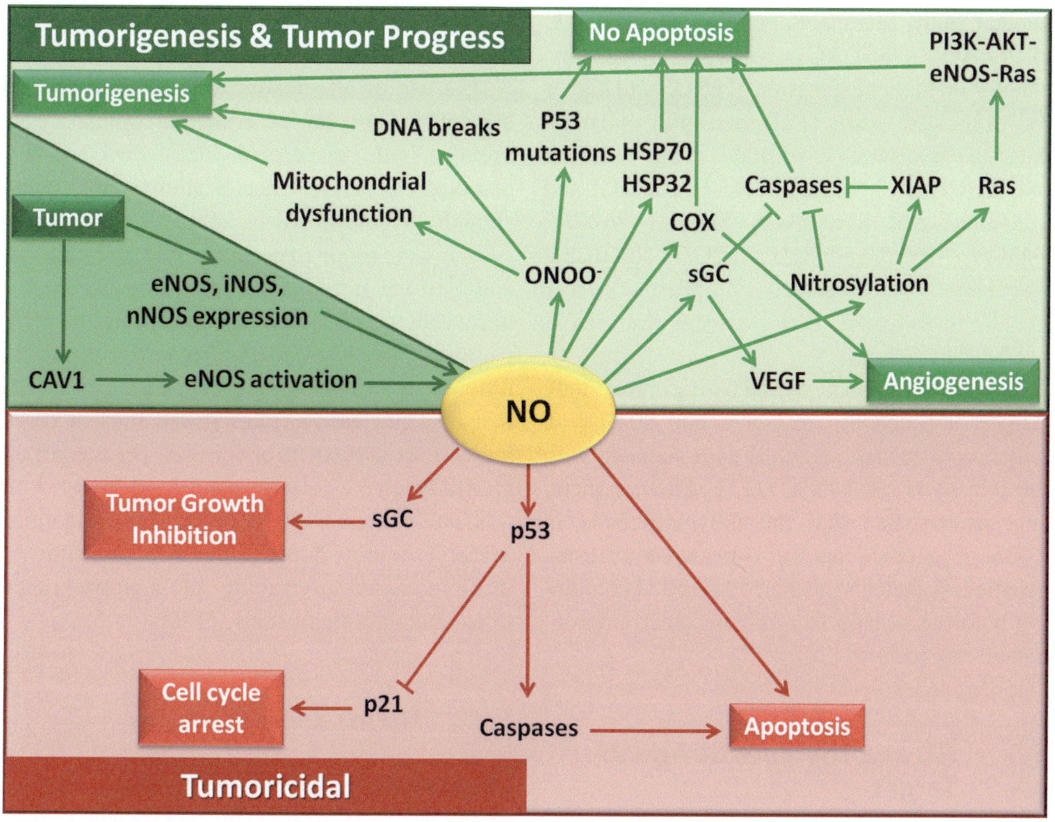

Fig. 5.3 NO tumor promoting versus tumoricidal actions

Clinical studies also confirmed the positive correlation between iNOS activity and tumor vascularization in human head and neck cancer specimens [115, 116].

Vascular endothelial growth factor (VEGF) is an important proangiogenic factor which potentiates microvascular hyperpermeability [117]. Purified VEGF as well as VEGF produced by tumor cells require functional NO/cGMP pathway to promote neovascular growth via stimulation of NO synthesis [118].

NO also activates COX-2 which has two important effects on tumor progression. It stimulates the production of proangiogenic factors and prostaglandins and concomitantly inhibits apoptosis [112]. Sappayatosok et al. showed that iNOS, VEGF and COX-2 are expressed in oral squamous cell carcinoma and reported that VEGF correlates with tumor grading, tumor staging and angiogenesis while COX-2 correlates with cervical lymph node metastasis [119] (Fig. 5.3).

5.3.3 NOS Gene Polymorphisms and Cancer Risk

Several studies aimed at assessing the association between genetic polymorphism and the risk of cancer development, tumor aggressiveness and prognosis [120–122].

Medeiros et al. reported that the a-allele of eNOS 4a/b is associated with prostate cancer risk with a higher prevalence among patients with high-grade prostate cancer. On the other hand they found no significant difference in allele and genotype frequencies of Glu-Asp298 between prostate cancer patients and controls [120]. In another study, Marangoni et al. identified that C allele eNOS −786T > C polymorphism was associated with higher expression of eNOS and higher risk of prostate cancer [123]. In a study that evaluated the association of prostate cancer with four iNOS SNPs (−2892T/C, +14C/T, +88T/G, and +524G/A) and five eNOS SNPs (−762C/T, −43C/T, −26A/G, −63G/T, −62G/T) significant associations were observed with prostate cancer in all investigated SNPs except for iNOS −2892T/C [124].

A recent meta-analysis and case–control study suggest that eNOS -786T > C and 894G > T polymorphisms are significantly associated with the risk of breast cancer [125]. Another meta-analysis revealed that the polymorphisms in iNOS gene could not be considered a strong genetic risk factor. It also recommended combining both the genetic factors with other environmental risk factors [126].

5.4 NO as a Therapeutic Agent/Target

Due to its vital role in some of the most common neurological diseases and cancer, NO has been studied as a potential therapeutic agent/target.

5.4.1 In Neurodegenerative Diseases

Although nNOS and iNOS are responsible for the production of NO in the brain, iNOS is a more suitable target as it is directly related to inflammation and is responsible for the production of copious NO levels. Several iNOS inhibitors have been reported to have neuroprotective effects in Parkinson's disease and showed an improvement in the models being studied [127].

5.4.2 In Stroke

In stroke NO is essential for vasodilatation thus improving cerebral blood flow and preventing ischemia and spreading depression as well as migraine episodes. The use of NO-donors as potential treatments for different types of strokes is currently under study.

The use of NO-donors was found to reduce the infarct size in experimental animals and improve both the cerebral blood flow and the neurological performance if administered early enough [55, 128]. Also, some of these compounds were found to decrease lipid peroxidation and tyrosine nitration by inhibiting nNOS via nitrosylation and iNOS via suppressing the JNK pathway. The NO produced from these donors is different from that produced endogenously in that it is not easily released and thus, it can't increase to the extent of forming peroxynitrites [128, 129].

Large clinical trials on the use of transdermal glyceryl trinitrate directly after the stroke showed that it increased survivability and improved functional outcome significantly [130].

5.4.3 NO in Cancer Medicine

The dual role of NO as tumoricidal and tumor promoting mediator had attracted the researchers to investigate both NOS inhibitors and NO-donating compounds as potential anti-cancer agents [131].

NO-mediated anticancer drugs act either by direct killing or chemosensitization. Direct killing of cancer cells can be achieved with high concentration of micromolar to millimolar concentrations of NO [132]. The use of NO-donors in direct killing is limited due to poor bioavailability and instability during storage and systemic circulation [133].

Combinations of the NO-donating with an existing anticancer drug were prepared to increase its efficacy. From these combinations the compound PABA/NO had been effective against human leukemia cell [134] and the NO-releasing prodrug JS-K could inhibit tumor growth in multiple myeloma cells [135]. A recent study revealed that JS-K stimulated caspase-3, caspase-9, Bax, TNFα, and IL-1b leading to apoptosis in Hep3B cells [136]. JS-K has been also shown to upregulate the expression of anti-angiogenesis genes thrombospodin-1 and its receptor CD36 in HL-60 cells [137].

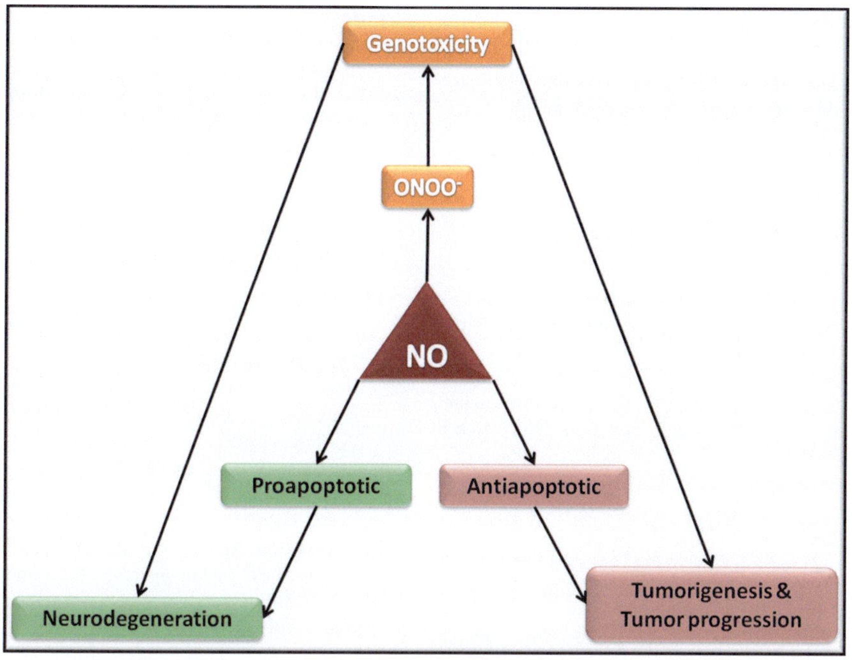

Fig. 5.4 The link between NO roles in neurodegenerative diseases and cancer

GT-094 was the first promising nitrate for colorectal cancer chemoprevention due to its anti-inflammatory and cytoprotective activity [138]. Another study demonstrated that NO-releasing aspirin NO-ASA has 1000-fold antiproliferative effects compared to aspirin in human colon cancer models [139].

NO can be used to overcome the multidrug resistance of cancer cells by reducing DNA repair and detoxification capacity, enhancing nuclear transport of drug, inhibiting HIF and NF-κB, and/or inactivating drug efflux proteins [133].

5.5 Conclusion

NO is a central molecule in many signaling cascades in various organs. This accounts for its dual role and sometimes the contradictory effects of NO, physiologically and pathologically.

NO concentration is one important factor in determining how NO acts. In CNS, physiological concentrations of NO play a role in memory formation and regulation of cerebral blood flow thus, acting as a neuroprotective factor. High NO concentrations mediate neurotoxicity leading to neurodegenerative diseases and stroke. In cancer, low concentrations of NO favor tumor formation while high concentrations have tumoricidal effects. However, the concentration is not the only factor that controls NO actions as other factors including cell type and duration of exposure to NO also play a considerable role in the determination of NO outcome [62].

The NO-mediated neurodegenerative diseases and cancer share many common aspects as oxidative stress and DNA damage. High concentrations of NO, secreted mainly by iNOS, react with free radicals including superoxide to produce reactive nitrogen species (RNS) such as peroxynitrite that has a direct genotoxic effect by inducing DNA alkylation and DNA breaks. The use of antioxidants is believed to reduce the incidence of both diseases [140].

In contrast, the dual role of NO in apoptosis plays a role in the reciprocal regulation of both diseases. The proapoptotic effect of NO induces neurodegenerative diseases and inhibits tumorigenesis and tumor progression while the antiapoptotic effect of NO is neuroprotective but tumor promoting (Fig. 5.4).

References

1. Moncada S, Palmer RM, Higgs EA (1988) The discovery of nitric oxide as the endogenous nitrovasodilator. Hypertension 12:365–372
2. Ignarro LJ (1989) Endothelium-derived nitric oxide: actions and properties. FASEB J 3:31–36
3. Murad F (2011) Nitric oxide: the coming of the second messenger. Rambam Maimonides Med J 2:e0038
4. Thomas DD (2015) Breathing new life into nitric oxide signaling: a brief overview of the interplay between oxygen and nitric oxide. Redox Biol 5:225–233
5. Forstermann U, Sessa WC (2012) Nitric oxide synthases: regulation and function. Eur Heart J 33:829–837
6. Alderton WK, Cooper CE, Knowles RG (2001) Nitric oxide synthases: structure, function and inhibition. Biochem J 357:593–615
7. Bian K, Murad F (2014) What is next in nitric oxide research? From cardiovascular system to cancer biology. Nitric Oxide 43:3–7
8. El-Sehemy A, Postovit L-M, Fu Y (2016) Nitric oxide signaling in human ovarian cancer: a potential therapeutic target. Nitric Oxide Biol Chem 54:30–37
9. Adams L, Franco MC, Estevez AG (2015) Reactive nitrogen species in cellular signaling. Exp Biol Med (Maywood) 240:711–717
10. WHO (2006) Public health challenges WHO Library Cataloguing-in-Publication Data. World Health Organization
11. Thakur KT et al (2016) Chapter 5 Neurological disorders. Ment Neurol Subst Use Disord Dis Control Priorities, Third Ed 4:265
12. Jiang Z et al (2014) Role of nitric oxide synthases in early blood-brain barrier disruption following transient focal cerebral ischemia. PLoS One 9:e93134
13. Kudlow P, Cha DS, Carvalho AF, McIntyre RS (2016) Nitric oxide and major depressive disorder: pathophysiology and treatment implications. Curr Mol Med 16:206–215
14. Calabrese V et al (2007) Nitric oxide in the central nervous system: neuroprotection versus neurotoxicity. Nat Rev Neurosci 8:766–775
15. Benarroch EE (2011) Nitric oxide: a pleiotropic signal in the nervous system. Neurology 77:1568–1576
16. Pierrefiche O, Naassila M (2014) Endogenous nitric oxide but not exogenous no-donor S-nitroprussiate facilitates NMDA excitation in spontaneous rhythmic neonatal rat brainstem slice. Brain Res 1543:9–16
17. Prast H, Philippu A (2001) Nitric oxide as modulator of neuronal function. Prog Neurobiol 64:51–68
18. Dash PR et al (2007) Fas ligand-induced apoptosis is regulated by nitric oxide through the inhibition of fas receptor clustering and the nitrosylation of protein kinase Cε. Exp Cell Res 313:3421–3431
19. Benarroch EE (2011) NMDA receptors: recent insights and clinical correlations. Neurology 76:1750–1757
20. Um H-C, Jang J-H, Kim D-H, Lee C, Surh Y-J (2011) Nitric oxide activates Nrf2 through S-nitrosylation of Keap1 in PC12 cells. Nitric Oxide 25:161–168
21. Knott AB, Bossy-Wetzel E (2009) Nitric oxide in halth and disease of the nervous system. Antioxid Redox Signal 11:541–553
22. Nakamura T, Lipton SA (2011) Redox modulation by S-nitrosylation contributes to protein misfolding, mitochondrial dynamics, and neuronal synaptic damage in neurodegenerative diseases. Cell Death Differ 18:1478–1486
23. Linares D et al (2006) Neuronal nitric oxide synthase plays a key role in CNS demyelination. J Neurosci 26:12672–12681
24. Calabrese V et al (2009) Nitric oxide in cell survival: a janus molecule. Antioxid Redox Signal 11:2717–2739
25. Alzheimer's Association (2016) 2016 Alzheimer's disease facts and figures. Alzheimers Dement 12:459–509
26. Rivera DS, Inestrosa NC, Bozinovic F (2016) On cognitive ecology and the environmental factors that promote Alzheimer disease: lessons from *Octodon degus* (Rodentia: Octodontidae). Biol Res 49:10
27. Querfurth HW, LaFerla FM (2010) Alzheimer's Disease. N Engl J Med 362:329–344
28. Berridge MJ (2014) Calcium regulation of neural rhythms, memory and Alzheimer's disease. J Physiol 592:281–293
29. Iqbal K, Liu F, Gong C-X (2014) Alzheimer disease therapeutics: focus on the disease and not just plaques and tangles. Biochem Pharmacol 88:631–639
30. Bird TD (2008) Genetic aspects of Alzheimer disease. Genet Med 10:231–239
31. Holmes C et al (2009) Systemic inflammation and disease progression in Alzheimer disease. Neurology 73:768–774
32. Balez R, Ooi L (2016) Getting to NO Alzheimer's disease: neuroprotection versus neurotoxicity mediated by nitric oxide. Oxidative Med Cell Longev 2016:3806157
33. Guo H et al (2017) FFPM, a PDE4 inhibitor, reverses learning and memory deficits in APP/PS1 transgenic mice via cAMP/PKA/CREB signaling and anti-inflammatory effects. Neuropharmacology 116:260–269
34. Franco MC et al (2015) Nitration of Hsp90 on tyrosine 33 regulates mitochondrial metabolism. J Biol Chem 290:19055–19066
35. Guivernau B et al (2016) Amyloid-peptide nitrotyrosination stabilizes oligomers and enhances NMDAR-mediated toxicity. J Neurosci 36:11693–11703
36. Ryan SD et al (2013) Isogenic human iPSC parkinson's model shows nitrosative stress-induced dysfunction in MEF2-PGC1α transcription. Cell 155:1351–1364

37. Nakamura T et al (2015) Aberrant protein S-nitrosylation contributes to the pathophysiology of neurodegenerative diseases. Neurobiol Dis 84:99–108
38. Xu B et al (2014) Alpha-synuclein oligomerization in manganese-induced nerve cell injury in brain slices: a role of NO-mediated S-nitrosylation of protein disulfide isomerase. Mol Neurobiol 50:1098–1110
39. Uehara T et al (2006) S-nitrosylated protein-disulphide isomerase links protein misfolding to neurodegeneration. Nature 441:513–517
40. Benskey MJ, Perez RG, Manfredsson FP (2016) The contribution of alpha synuclein to neuronal survival and function – implications for Parkinson's disease. J Neurochem 137:331–359
41. Cho D-H, Nakamura T, Lipton SA (2010) Mitochondrial dynamics in cell death and neurodegeneration. Cell Mol Life Sci 67:3435–3447
42. Haun F et al (2013) S-nitrosylation of dynamin-related protein 1 mediates mutant huntingtin-induced mitochondrial fragmentation and neuronal injury in huntington's disease. Antioxid Redox Signal 19:1173–1184
43. Qu J et al (2011) S-nitrosylation activates Cdk5 and contributes to synaptic spine loss induced by -amyloid peptide. Proc Natl Acad Sci 108:14330–14335
44. Nakamura T, Cho D-H, Lipton SA (2012) Redox regulation of protein misfolding, mitochondrial dysfunction, synaptic damage, and cell death in neurodegenerative diseases. Exp Neurol 238:12–21
45. Bae B-I et al (2006) Mutant huntingtin: nuclear translocation and cytotoxicity mediated by GAPDH. Proc Natl Acad Sci 103:3405–3409
46. Wu H et al (2014) Caspases: a molecular switch node in the crosstalk between autophagy and apoptosis. Int J Biol Sci 10:1072–1083
47. Tsang AHK et al (2009) S-nitrosylation of XIAP compromises neuronal survival in Parkinson's disease. Proc Natl Acad Sci U S A 106:4900–4905
48. Nakamura T et al (2010) Transnitrosylation of XIAP regulates caspase-dependent neuronal cell death. Mol Cell 39:184–195
49. Nakamura T, Lipton SA (2016) Protein S-nitrosylation as a therapeutic target for neurodegenerative diseases. Trends Pharmacol Sci 37:73–84
50. Okamoto S, Lipton SA (2015) S-nitrosylation in neurogenesis and neuronal development. Biochim Biophys Acta 1850:1588–1593
51. Garry PS, Ezra M, Rowland MJ, Westbrook J, Pattinson KTS (2015) The role of the nitric oxide pathway in brain injury and its treatment – from bench to bedside. Exp Neurol 263:235–243
52. Attwell D et al (2010) Glial and neuronal control of brain blood flow. Nature 468:232–243
53. Minamino T et al (1998) Increased expression of P-selectin on platelets is a risk factor for silent cerebral infarction in patients with atrial fibrillation: role of nitric oxide. Circulation 98:1721–1727
54. Sabri M et al (2012) Mechanisms of microthrombi formation after experimental subarachnoid hemorrhage. Neuroscience 224:26–37
55. Dreier JP, Reiffurth C (2015) The stroke-migraine depolarization continuum. Neuron 86:902–922
56. Kim JY, Park J, Chang JY, Kim S-H, Lee JE (2016) Inflammation after ischemic stroke: the role of leukocytes and glial cells. Exp Neurobiol 25:241–251
57. Garcia-Bonilla L et al (2014) Inducible nitric oxide synthase in neutrophils and endothelium contributes to ischemic brain injury in mice. J Immunol 193:2531–2537
58. Ridnour LA et al (2006) The biphasic nature of nitric oxide responses in tumor biology. Antioxid Redox Signal 8:1329–1337
59. Martínez MC, Andriantsitohaina R (2009) Reactive nitrogen species: molecular mechanisms and potential significance in health and disease. Antioxid Redox Signal 11:669–702
60. Oronsky B, Fanger GR, Oronsky N, Knox S, Scicinski J (2014) The implications of hyponitroxia in cancer. Transl Oncol 7:167–173
61. Lechner M, Lirk P, Rieder J (2005) Inducible nitric oxide synthase (iNOS) in tumor biology: the two sides of the same coin. Semin Cancer Biol 15:277–289
62. Ridnour LA et al (2008) Molecular mechanisms for discrete nitric oxide levels in cancer. Nitric Oxide 19:73–76
63. Vannini F, Kashfi K, Nath N (2015) The dual role of iNOS in cancer. Redox Biol 6:334–343
64. Criss WE, Murad F, Kimura H, Morris HP (1976) Properties of guanylate cyclase in adult rat liver and several Morris hepatomas. Biochim Biophys Acta Enzymol 445:500–508
65. Zhu H et al (2011) Restoring soluble guanylyl cyclase expression and function blocks the aggressive course of glioma. Mol Pharmacol 80:1076
66. Singh SK et al (2004) Identification of human brain tumour initiating cells. Nature 432:396–401
67. Albina JE, Cui S, Mateo RB, Reichner JS (1993) Nitric oxide-mediated apoptosis in murine peritoneal macrophages. J Immunol 150:5080–5085
68. Messmer UK, Brüne B (1996) Nitric oxide-induced apoptosis: p53-dependent and p53-independent signalling pathways. Biochem J 319:299–305
69. Chipuk JE et al (2004) Direct activation of bax by p53 mediates mitochondrial membrane permeabilization and apoptosis. Science (80-.) 303:1010–1014
70. Mihara M et al (2003) p53 has a direct apoptogenic role at the mitochondria. Mol Cell 11:577–590
71. Tovar C et al (2013) MDM2 small-molecule antagonist RG7112 activates p53 signaling and regresses human tumors in preclinical cancer models. Cancer Res 73:2587–2597
72. Lujambio A et al (2013) Non-cell-autonomous tumor suppression by p53. Cell 153:449–460
73. Strasser A, Harris AW, Jacks T, Cory S (1994) DNA damage can induce apoptosis in proliferat-

ing lymphoid cells via p53-independent mechanisms inhibitable by Bcl-2. Cell 79:329–339
74. Bicknell GR, Snowden RT, Cohen GM (1994) Formation of high molecular mass DNA fragments is a marker of apoptosis in the human leukaemic cell line, U937. J Cell Sci 107:2483
75. Xu W, Lliu LZ, Loizidou M, Ahmed M, Charles IG (2002) The role of nitric oxide in cancer. Cell Res 12:311–320
76. Jaiswal M, LaRusso N, Burgart L, Gores G (2000) Inflammatory cytokines induce DNA damage and inhibit DNA repair in cholangiocarcinoma cells by a nitric oxide-dependent mechanism. Cancer Res 60(1):184–190
77. Mocellin S, Bronte V, Nitti D (2007) Nitric oxide, a double edged sword in cancer biology: searching for therapeutic opportunities. Med Res Rev 27:317–352
78. Thomsen LL et al (1995) Nitric oxide synthase activity in human breast cancer. Br J Cancer 72:41–44
79. Reveneau S et al (1999) Nitric oxide synthase in human breast cancer is associated with tumor grade, proliferation rate, and expression of progesterone receptors. Lab Investig 79:1215–1225
80. Vakkala M et al (2000) Inducible nitric oxide synthase expression, apoptosis, and angiogenesis in in situ and invasive breast carcinomas. Clin Cancer Res 6:2408–2416
81. Loibl S et al (2002) Expression of endothelial and inducible nitric oxide synthase in benign and malignant lesions of the breast and measurement of nitric oxide using electron paramagnetic resonance spectroscopy. Cancer 95:1191–1198
82. Nathan C, Xie QW (1994) Nitric oxide synthases: roles, tolls, and controls. Cell 78:915–918
83. Lim K-H, Ancrile BB, Kashatus DF, Counter CM (2008) Tumour maintenance is mediated by eNOS. Nature 452:646–649
84. Martinez-Outschoorn UE, Sotgia F, Lisanti MP (2015) Caveolae and signalling in cancer. Nat Rev Cancer 15:225–237
85. Feron O, Saldana F, Michel JB, Michel T (1998) The endothelial nitric-oxide synthase-caveolin regulatory cycle. J Biol Chem 273:3125–3128
86. Cleeter MWJ, Cooper JM, Darley-Usmar VM, Moncada S, Schapira AHV (1994) Reversible inhibition of cytochrome c oxidase, the terminal enzyme of the mitochondrial respiratory chain, by nitric oxide. FEBS Lett 345:50–54
87. Martinez-Outschoorn UE, Lisanti MP, Sotgia F (2014) Catabolic cancer-associated fibroblasts transfer energy and biomass to anabolic cancer cells, fueling tumor growth. Semin Cancer Biol 25:47–60
88. Witkiewicz AK et al (2009) An absence of stromal caveolin-1 expression predicts early tumor recurrence and poor clinical outcome in human breast cancers. Am J Pathol 174:2023–2034
89. Sloan EK et al (2009) Stromal cell expression of caveolin-1 predicts outcome in breast cancer. Am J Pathol 174:2035–2043
90. Goetz JG et al (2011) Biomechanical remodeling of the microenvironment by stromal caveolin-1 favors tumor invasion and metastasis. Cell 146:148–163
91. Ayala G et al (2013) Loss of caveolin-1 in prostate cancer stroma correlates with reduced relapse-free survival and is functionally relevant to tumour progression. J Pathol 231:77–87
92. Zhao X et al (2013) Caveolin-1 expression level in cancer associated fibroblasts predicts outcome in gastric cancer. PLoS One 8:e59102
93. Kim YM, Bombeck CA, Billiar TR (1999) Nitric oxide as a bifunctional regulator of apoptosis. Circ Res 84:253–256
94. Choi B-M, Pae H-O, Jang SII, Kim Y-M, Chung H-T (2002) Nitric oxide as a pro-apoptotic as well as anti-apoptotic modulator endogenous NO production and NO donors. J Biochem Mol Biol 35:116–126
95. Genaro AM, Hortelano S, Alvarez A, Martínez C, Boscá L (1995) Splenic B lymphocyte programmed cell death is prevented by nitric oxide release through mechanisms involving sustained Bcl-2 levels. J Clin Invest 95:1884–1890
96. Li J, Yang S, Billiar TR (2000) Cyclic nucleotides suppress tumor necrosis factor alpha-mediated apoptosis by inhibiting caspase activation and cytochrome c release in primary hepatocytes via a mechanism independent of Akt activation. J Biol Chem 275:13026–13034
97. Kim Y et al (2000) Nitric oxide prevents tumor necrosis factor α–induced rat hepatocyte apoptosis by the interruption of mitochondrial apoptotic signaling through S-nitrosylation of caspase-8. Hepatology 32:770–778
98. Kim YM, Talanian RV, Billiar TR (1997) Nitric oxide inhibits apoptosis by preventing increases in caspase-3-like activity via two distinct mechanisms. J Biol Chem 272:31138–31148
99. Ceneviva GD et al (1998) Nitric oxide inhibits lipopolysaccharide-induced apoptosis in pulmonary artery endothelial cells. Am J Phys 275:L717–L728
100. Mannick JB, Asano K, Izumi K, Kieff E, Stamler JS (1994) Nitric oxide produced by human B lymphocytes inhibits apoptosis and epstein-barr virus reactivation. Cell 79:1137–1146
101. Hussain AR et al (2015) Xiap over-expression is a poor prognostic marker in breast cancer and can be targeted to induce efficient apoptosis. Cancer Res 75
102. Ji J et al (2015) XIAP maintains the characteristics of cancer stem cells and is a therapeutic target in nasopharyngeal carcinoma. Cancer Res 75
103. Gu L et al (2016) Discovery of dual inhibitors of MDM2 and XIAP for cancer treatment. Cancer Cell 30:623–636
104. Yang J et al (1997) Prevention of apoptosis by Bcl-2: release of cytochrome c from mitochondria blocked. Science 275:1129–1132
105. Kim YM, Chung HT, Simmons RL, Billiar TR (2000) Cellular non-heme iron content is a determinant of nitric oxide-mediated apoptosis, necrosis, and caspase inhibition. J Biol Chem 275:10954–10961

106. Li H, Zhu H, Xu CJ, Yuan J (1998) Cleavage of BID by caspase 8 mediates the mitochondrial damage in the Fas pathway of apoptosis. Cell 94:491–501
107. Kim Y-M, Bergonia H, Lancaster JR (1995) Nitrogen oxide-induced autoprotection in isolated rat hepatocytes. FEBS Lett 374:228–232
108. Kim YM, de Vera ME, Watkins SC, Billiar TR (1997) Nitric oxide protects cultured rat hepatocytes from tumor necrosis factor-alpha-induced apoptosis by inducing heat shock protein 70 expression. J Biol Chem 272:1402–1411
109. Liu D et al (2000) Cytokines induce apoptosis in beta-cells isolated from mice lacking the inducible isoform of nitric oxide synthase (iNOS-/-). Diabetes 49:1116–1122
110. Rössig L et al (2000) Nitric oxide down-regulates MKP-3 mRNA levels: involvement in endothelial cell protection from apoptosis. J Biol Chem 275:25502–25507
111. Choudhari SK, Chaudhary M, Bagde S, Gadbail AR, Joshi V (2013) Nitric oxide and cancer: a review. World J Surg Oncol 11:118
112. Ziche M, Morbidelli L (2000) Nitric oxide and angiogenesis. J Neuro-Oncol 50:139–148
113. Jenkins DC et al (1995) Roles of nitric oxide in tumor growth. Proc Natl Acad Sci U S A 92:4392–4396
114. Morbidelli L, Donnini S, Ziche M (2004) Role of nitric oxide in tumor angiogenesis. Cancer Treat Res 117:155–167
115. Gallo O et al (1998) Role of nitric oxide in angiogenesis and tumor progression in head and neck cancer. J Natl Cancer Inst 90:587–596
116. Franchi A et al (2002) Inducible nitric oxide synthase expression in laryngeal neoplasia: correlation with angiogenesis. Head Neck 24:16–23
117. Hoeben A et al (2004) Vascular endothelial growth factor and angiogenesis. Pharmacol Rev 56.
118. Wiseman H, Halliwell B (1996) Damage to DNA by reactive oxygen and nitrogen species: role in inflammatory disease and progression to cancer. Biochem J 313:17–29
119. Sappayatosok K et al (2009) Expression of pro-inflammatory protein, iNOS, VEGF and COX-2 in oral squamous cell carcinoma (OSCC), relationship with angiogenesis and their clinico-pathological correlation. Med Oral Patol Oral Cir Bucal 14:E319–E324
120. Medeiros RM et al (2002) Outcome in prostate cancer: association with endothelial nitric oxide synthase Glu-Asp298 polymorphism at exon 7. Clin Cancer Res 8:3433–3437
121. Ghilardi G et al (2003) Vascular invasion in human breast cancer is correlated to T-->786C polymorphism of NOS3 gene. Nitric Oxide Biol Chem 9:118–122
122. Tatemichi M et al (2005) Increased risk of intestinal type of gastric adenocarcinoma in Japanese women associated with long forms of CCTTT pentanucleotide repeat in the inducible nitric oxide synthase promoter. Cancer Lett 217:197–202
123. Marangoni K, Araújo TG, Neves AF, Goulart LR (2008) The -786T>C promoter polymorphism of the NOS3 gene is associated with prostate cancer progression. BMC Cancer 8:273
124. Lee K-M et al (2009) Nitric oxide synthase gene polymorphisms and prostate cancer risk. Carcinogenesis 30:621–625
125. Gao X, Wang J, Wang W, Wang M, Zhang J (2015) eNOS genetic polymorphisms and cancer risk a meta-analysis and a case–control study of breast cancer. Medicine (Baltimore) 94:1–10
126. Jiao J, Wu J, Huang D, Liu L (2015) Lack of association of the iNOS gene polymorphism with risk of cancer: a systematic review and Meta-Analysis. Sci Rep 5:9889
127. Koppula S, Kumar H, Kim IS, Choi D-K (2012) Reactive oxygen species and inhibitors of inflammatory enzymes, NADPH oxidase, and iNOS in experimental models of Parkinson's disease. Mediat Inflamm 2012:823902
128. Godínez-Rubí M, Rojas-Mayorquín AE, Ortuño-Sahagún D (2013) Nitric oxide donors as neuroprotective agents after an ischemic stroke-related inflammatory reaction. Oxidative Med Cell Longev 2013:297357
129. Atochin DN et al (2016) A novel dual NO-donating oxime and c-Jun N-terminal kinase inhibitor protects against cerebral ischemia–reperfusion injury in mice. Neurosci Lett 618:45–49
130. Woodhouse L et al (2015) Effect of hyperacute administration (within 6 hours) of transdermal glyceryl trinitrate, a nitric oxide donor, on outcome after stroke. Stroke 46:3194–3201
131. Hickok JR, Thomas DD (2010) Nitric oxide and cancer therapy: the emperor has NO clothes. Curr Pharm Des 16:381–391
132. Kanayama N, Yamaguchi K, Nagasaki Y (2010) PEGylated polymer micelle-based nitric oxide (NO) photodonor with NO-mediated antitumor activity. Chem Lett 39:1008–1009
133. Kim J, Yung BC, Kim WJ, Chen X (2016) Combination of nitric oxide and drug delivery systems: tools for overcoming drug resistance in chemotherapy. J Control Release. doi:10.1016/j.jconrel.2016.12.026
134. Chakrapani H et al (2008) Synthesis, nitric oxide release, and anti-leukemic activity of glutathione-activated nitric oxide prodrugs: structural analogues of PABA/NO, an anti-cancer lead compound. Bioorg Med Chem 16:2657–2664
135. Kiziltepe T et al (2007) JS-K, a GST-activated nitric oxide generator, induces DNA double-strand breaks, activates DNA damage response pathways, and induces apoptosis in vitro and in vivo in human multiple myeloma cells. Blood 110:709–718
136. Dong R et al (2017) Effects of JS-K, a novel anti-cancer nitric oxide prodrug, on gene expression in human hepatoma Hep3B cells. Biomed Pharmacother 88:367–373. doi:10.1016/j.biopha.2017.01.080

137. Liu J et al (2009) Gene expression profiling for nitric oxide prodrug JS-K to kill HL-60 myeloid leukemia cells. Genomics 94:32–38
138. Hagos GK et al (2007) Colon cancer chemoprevention by a novel NO chimera that shows anti-inflammatory and antiproliferative activity in vitro and in vivo. Mol Cancer Ther 6:2230–2239
139. Gao J, Liu X, Rigas B (2005) Nitric oxide-donating aspirin induces apoptosis in human colon cancer cells through induction of oxidative stress. Proc Natl Acad Sci 102:17207–17212
140. Aliev G et al (2013) Link between cancer and Alzheimer disease via oxidative stress induced by nitric oxide-dependent mitochondrial DNA overproliferation and deletion. Oxidative Med Cell Longev 2013:962984
141. Stewart B, Wild CP (eds) (2014). International Agency for Research on Cancer, W World Cancer Rep 2014
142. International Agency for Research on Cancer and Cancer Research UK (2014) World cancer factsheet.
143. Fidler I, Timeline J (2003) The pathogenesis of cancer metastasis: the 'seed and soil' hypothesis revisited. Nat Rev Cancer 3:453–458
144. Nishida N, Yano H, Nishida T, Kamura T, Kojiro M (2006) Angiogenesis in cancer. Vasc Health Risk Manag 2:213–219

RNA Nuclear Export: From Neurological Disorders to Cancer

6

Guillaume M. Hautbergue

Abstract

The presence of a nuclear envelope, also known as nuclear membrane, defines the structural framework of all eukaryotic cells by separating the nucleus, which contains the genetic material, from the cytoplasm where the synthesis of proteins takes place. Translation of proteins in *Eukaryotes* is thus dependent on the active transport of DNA-encoded RNA molecules through pores embedded within the nuclear membrane. Several mechanisms are involved in this process generally referred to as RNA nuclear export or nucleocytoplasmic transport of RNA. The regulated expression of genes requires the nuclear export of protein-coding messenger RNA molecules (mRNAs) as well as non-coding RNAs (ncRNAs) together with proteins and pre-assembled ribosomal subunits. The nuclear export of mRNAs is intrinsically linked to the co-transcriptional processing of nascent transcripts synthesized by the RNA polymerase II. This functional coupling is essential for the survival of cells allowing for timely nuclear export of fully processed transcripts, which could otherwise cause the translation of abnormal proteins such as the polymeric repeat proteins produced in some neurodegenerative diseases. Alterations of the mRNA nuclear export pathways can also lead to genome instability and to various forms of cancer. This chapter will describe the molecular mechanisms driving the nuclear export of RNAs with a particular emphasis on mRNAs. It will also review their known alterations in neurological disorders and cancer, and the recent opportunities they offer for the potential development of novel therapeutic strategies.

G.M. Hautbergue (✉)
RNA Biology Laboratory, Sheffield Institute for Translational Neuroscience (SITraN), Department of Neuroscience, University of Sheffield,
385a Glossop Road, Sheffield S10 2HQ, UK
e-mail: g.hautbergue@sheffield.ac.uk

S. El-Khamisy (ed.), *Personalised Medicine*, Advances in Experimental Medicine and Biology 1007,
DOI 10.1007/978-3-319-60733-7_6

Keywords
RNA • Nuclear export • Nuclear Pore Complex (NPC) • TREX complex • NXF1 • Exportins • Neurodegenerative diseases • Cancer

6.1 Eukaryotic Expression of Genes

The tightly controlled expression of eukaryotic genes into RNA molecules and proteins is essential to cell survival and homeostasis. This is a complex process that integrates several mechanisms: activation, repression, cleavage, processing, directionality, surveillance and regulated degradation. The physiological expression of mammalian genes relies on a very large number of mRNAs (estimated between 100,000 and 1,000,000 molecules per cell), protein factors and ncRNAs implicated in the composition of ribosomes and the synthesis of proteins, as well as in the regulation of gene expression at the post transcriptional and translational levels.

6.1.1 Eukaryotic Expression of mRNAs and ncRNAs

Three nuclear RNA polymerases are implicated in the expression of genes embedded in chromosomes. In the nucleolus, RNA polymerase I transcribes the mammalian 45S pre-ribosomal RNA precursor that is subsequently processed into mature 28S, 18S and 5.8S ribosomal RNAs (rRNAs). Together with the 5S rRNA transcribed by RNA polymerase III in the nucleoplasm, they constitute the major catalytic and architectural components of the ribosome. RNA polymerase III is also involved in the transcription of other ncRNAs including U6/U6atac small nuclear RNAs (snRNAs) that form components of the splicing machinery and transfer RNAs (tRNAs) required for recognition of codons and attachment of the corresponding amino-acid moieties to the neo-synthesized polypeptide chain.

The nucleoplasmic RNA polymerase II (RNAPII) transcribes the largest portion of the genome synthesizing the precursors of mRNAs (pre-mRNAs) and multiple classes of ncRNAs. The later are subdivided into small and long ncRNA classes if larger than 200 nucleotides. Small ncRNAs include U1, U2, U4, U4atac, U5, U7, U11 and U12 snRNAs which participate in pre-mRNA splicing by the major (U2-dependent) or minor (U12-dependent) spliceosomes and small nucleolar RNAs (snoRNAs) involved in the processing and modification of rRNAs. RNAPII also transcribes the precursors of microRNAs (miRNAs), small-interfering RNAs (siRNAs) and piwi-interacting RNAs (piRNAs). These are implicated in the post transcriptional or translational silencing of mRNAs and proteins by respectively promoting the degradation of mRNAs or interfering with the translation process. Long ncRNAs (lncRNAs) comprise natural antisense transcripts (NATs) which are transcribed from the antisense DNA strand opposing 50–70% of protein coding genes. They regulate the expression of the sense gene at both transcriptional and translational levels. Other lncRNAs include very long intergenic non-coding RNAs (vlincRNAs). Their transcripts span approximately 10% of the human genome ranging from 50 kb to 1 Mb in size and are thought to also play a regulatory function. Long intergenic non-coding RNAs (lincRNAs) resemble mRNAs with capped and poly-adenylated transcripts that contain small open reading frames and co-purify with ribosomes. Eight thousand to 10,000 lincRNAs have been characterised so far. They have established regulatory functions at epigenetic and transcriptional control levels with roles reported in development, cell differentiation and diseases. The list of ncRNAs presented here is not exhaustive. It is important to note that the repertoire of ncRNAs is very diverse and expands quickly with the rise of Next Generation RNA sequencing technologies. Discovery of new RNA species keeps on challenging the complex classification of ncRNAs as some previously characterised species may become shared between several groups.

6.1.2 Eukaryotic Expression of mRNAs and Proteins: Mechanistic Overview

Remodeling of the tightly packed heterochromatin into relaxed euchromatin is often a prerequisite to transcriptional activation. It facilitates the recruitment of transcription factors along with an RNA polymerase onto the promoters of genes to form a closed-state complex named the pre-initiation complex (PIC). The RNA polymerase core enzymes are unable to recognize promoters or initiate transcription from a DNA template. They require general transcription factors for the local melting of the double helix of DNA near the transcription start site downstream of promoters. Recognition of the TATA box element by the TATA box binding protein (TBP) subunit of TFIID in the promoters of RNAPII-transcribed genes initiates the assembly of the pre-initiation complex. The TFIIA and TFIIB factors are recruited next to stabilize the DNA-TFIID complex allowing for recruitment of the hypo-phosphorylated form of the RNA polymerase II (RNAPIIA) in association with the other general transcription factors TFIIE, TFIIF, TFIIH and TFIIS. TFIIB interacts with both the promoter and RNAPII. It triggers bending of the DNA molecule near the transcription start site while the Ssl2/ERCC3 DNA helicase subunit of TFIIH unwinds the double helix to generate a flexible single strand of DNA that can reach the active cleft center for the polymerization of ribonucleotides and promoter escape [58]. Stable initiation of transcription by RNAPII requires the polymerization of approximately 25 nucleotides.

Transcription elongation and co-transcriptional processing of pre-mRNAs is orchestrated by the recruitment of several RNA-processing machineries via differential phosphorylation of the heptapeptide (YSPTSPS) repeats composing the carboxyl-terminal domain (CTD) of the RNAPII [33, 74]. TFIIH-dependent phosphorylation of serine 5 in the heptapeptide repeats of the CTD triggers the start of transcription and phosphorylation of serine 5 remains high for the first few hundred polymerized nucleotides. A 7-methylguanosine CAP (m7G) is added to the 5′-end of nascent transcripts shortly after transcription initiation (<100 nucleotides) by recruitment of the capping enzyme to the highly phosphorylated serine 5 residues in the CTD. The CAP structure protects against RNA degradation and plays additional roles by interacting with the CAP-binding complex, which provides 5–3′ directionality during the mRNA nuclear export process [7], and by recruiting the eukaryotic initiation factor 4E (eIF4E) for translation initiation [69]. The CDK9 kinase subunit of the elongation factor P-TEFb phosphorylates CTD-serine 2 residues and the elongation factor SPT4/SPT5 to maintain the processivity of transcription elongation for complete synthesis of the nascent pre-mRNAs (hyper-phosphorylated RNAPII under form IIO). Removal of introns by splicing and exon skipping by alternative splicing are linked to phosphorylation of the CTD predominantly on serine 2 but also on serine 5 residues. Pre-mRNA splicing occurs co-transcriptionally in the vicinity of nuclear speckles, small organelles enriched in pre-mRNAs and splicing factors, for approximately 80% of human transcripts [24]. The final stage of transcription is achieved by endonucleolytic cleavage of the transcript and addition of approximately 200 adenosines at poly-adenylation sites composed of the consensus sequence AAUAAA [63]. Nuclear export of the bulk mammalian mRNAs is coupled to co-transcriptional splicing [54] and release from nuclear speckles [24] via recruitment of the evolutionary conserved transcription-export (TREX) complex and the nucleoporin-interacting export receptor NXF1 [30, 87].

It remains unclear whether completion of the nuclear mRNA export is linked to the initiation of translation in the cytoplasm or whether translation is truly compartmentalized and independent of the nuclear biogenesis and processing of mRNAs. In specialized cells, such as neurons, mRNAs that encode factors involved in guiding the growth and repair of axons or dentrites require transport prior to localized translation [38]. Eukaryotic translation involves several coupled steps [12, 69]. The eukaryotic translation initiation factor eIF3 bridges the interactions between the 40S ribosome small subunit and the eIF4F factor, which is composed of the CAP-binding protein eIF4E, the DEAD box RNA helicase eIF4A and a scaffold protein eIF4G. This forms the 43S pre-initiation complex which allows scanning of the 5′-untranslated region (5′-UTR) of the mRNA until the initiating AUG codon is reached. In the 43S complex, the poly(A)-binding protein (PABP) also interacts with eIF4F to circularize the mRNA. Recruitment of the methionine-charged tRNA initiator in the large 60S ribosomal subunit by eIF5B leads to interactions with the 43S pre-initiation complex to form an 80S initiating complex. Linking of amino-acid moieties to the growing polypeptide chain occurs through eEF2 (eukaryotic translation elongation factor 2) dependent translocation of ribosomes onto the translating mRNA. Up to five to ten elongating ribosomes are associated to each mRNA molecule composing actively translating polysomes. Eukaryotic release factor 1 (ERF1) is involved in the disassembly of the ribosome subunits by recognition of all three terminator (or stop) codons. Release of the neo-synthesized protein anchored in the 60S subunit is assisted by factor ERF3. A simplified stepwise overview of the eukaryotic expression of mRNAs and protein-coding genes is represented in Fig. 6.1.

The physiological expression of genes also involves regulatory and proof-reading mechanisms such as binding of transcriptional activators or repressors on specific elements in promoters [6], specific degradation of proteins by the ubiquitin/proteasome pathway [66], RNA-interference mechanisms [91] and RNA surveillance for the maturation/degradation of damaged/unprocessed RNAs by the nuclear exosome [42] or the degradation of RNAs by nonsense mediated decay in the cytoplasm [79].

6.2 Nuclear Export of RNAs: Mechanisms and Regulation

The nuclear export of eukaryotic RNAs involves functionally linked mechanistic steps ensuring that only mature transcripts are delivered to the cytoplasm. The process starts with the biogenesis of RNA molecules and the formation of ribonucleoprotein complexes. It follows on with the co-transcriptional processing of transcripts and the recruitment of adaptor proteins for selective and active transport. It ends with docking and transport through the nuclear pore prior to the release of transported RNA cargoes into the cytoplasm.

6.2.1 Formation of Ribonucleoprotein Complexes (mRNPs)

Within a cell, RNA molecules are never left naked but they dynamically associate with various sets of proteins to form ribonucleoprotein particles (RNPs) [56]. Most eukaryotic cells contain hundreds of RNA-binding proteins with diverse biological activities. Approximately 1500 RNA-binding proteins are encoded from the human genome [23]. The changing composition of RNPs dictates the functionalities and fate of the RNA molecules. Formation of RNPs also protects against premature RNA degradation and is essential for driving forward the gene expression process in functionally linked steps. The biogenesis of messenger RNP complexes (mRNPs) has indeed been found to be orchestrated in separate but extensively coupled nuclear steps – transcription, processing (capping, splicing, cleavage/poly-adenylation) and nuclear export – to allow correct expression of the chromatin into mature mRNA molecules which are translated into proteins in the cytoplasm [51].

6.2.2 Molecular Mechanisms Driving the Human Nuclear Export of RNAs

6.2.2.1 The NXF1-Dependent Pathways Mediate the Nuclear Export of Bulk mRNAs

Evolutionary conserved Nuclear Export Factor 1 (NXF1) proteins form an essential family of nuclear export receptors with a modular structure which comprises an unstructured RNA-binding

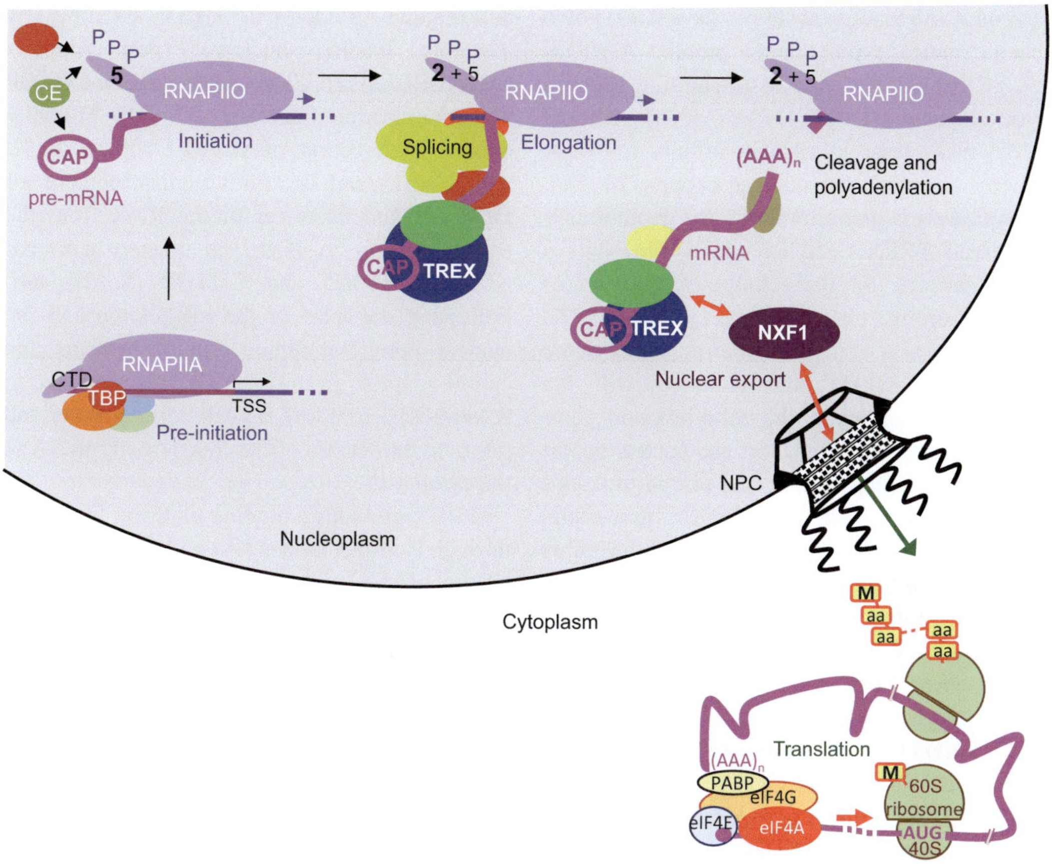

Fig. 6.1 Simplified eukaryotic expression of mRNAs and proteins. The diagram represents stepwise expression of protein-coding genes. Nuclear steps are in fact functionally linked to each other in order to ensure directionality of the biogenesis and processing of mRNAs. Remodeling of chromatin stimulates the recruitment of transcription factors including the TATA box binding protein (TBP) and the hypo-phosphorylated RNA polymerase under form IIA upstream of the transcription start site (TSS). The capping enzyme (CE) is recruited through phosphorylation of the CTD on serine 5 residues shortly after the initiation of transcription. Addition of the CAP onto the 5′-end of the mRNA is required to stabilize the nascent mRNA and provide 5–3′ directionality to the nuclear export process. It is also essential to the recruitment of translation initiation factors. Processivity of transcription elongation is dependent upon phosphorylation of the CTD on serine 2 residues and is maintained through recruitment of the spliceosome for splicing and of the cleavage and polyadenylation machinery to end transcription. Nuclear export of bulk mRNAs is linked to splicing in humans via the TREX complex which controls for the timely recruitment and activation of the nuclear export receptor NXF1 for the transport of fully processed transcripts through the nuclear pore complex (NPC). Transported mRNAs are circularized and subject to translation in the cytoplasm

domain linked to a pseudo RNA Recognition Motif not required for RNA-binding [28], a region containing Leucine Rich Repeats (LRRs), a stabilizing nuclear transport factor 2 (NTF2)-like domain that heterodimerizes with NTF2-related export protein 1 (NXT1 also known as p15) and a carboxyl terminal ubiquitin-associated (UBA) domain [31]. Both the NTF2-like and UBA domains are implicated in the direct association of NXF1 with the phenylalanine-glycine (FG) repeat regions of nucleoporins embedded in the nuclear pore complex (NPC).

NXF1 proteins exhibit poor RNA-binding activity. They mediate the nuclear export of mRNA through direct interactions with nuclear export adaptors, which avidly bind RNA, and were initially thought to bridge the interactions between RNA molecules and NXF1. However, structural and functional studies have later shown that the nuclear export adaptor proteins Aly/REF (ALYREF) [72] and some of the shuttling SR-rich splicing factors (SRSF1, 3, 7) [34] remodel NXF1 to increase in vitro its affinity for RNA thereby licensing the nuclear export [28, 86]. This process is orchestrated by the evolutionary conserved TREX complex which represents a major pathway for the eukaryotic transport of mRNA from the nucleus to the cytoplasm [71]. TREX interacts with the hyper-phosphorylated CTD of the RNAPII and associates with the CAP-binding complex, the exon-junction complex, 3′-end processing factors and nuclear export factors, thus harboring a pivotal role in functionally coupling co-transcriptional processing events to the nuclear export of mature transcripts [30, 87]. In human, TREX is co-transcriptionally deposited at the 5′-end of the mRNA during splicing [54]. It forms a multimeric complex [15] composed of THO, a stoichiometric and stable core comprising six subunits (THOC1, 2, 5–7 and TEX1/THOC3), the essential RNA/ATP-dependent DEAD-box RNA helicase 39B (DDX39B also known as UAP56 for U2AF65-associated protein 56), the nuclear export adaptor ALYREF (also known as THOC4) and a few other proteins including export adaptors UIF (UAP56-interacting factor) [29], LUZP4 (leucine zipper protein 4) [83] and co-adaptor CHTOP (chromatin target of PRMT1) [5].

Adaptors ALYREF, UIF and LUZP4 contain a conserved UBM (UAP56-binding motif) sequence which is required and sufficient for the direct binding of DDX39B. Direct interactions between ALYREF and DDX39B, which promotes the assembly of spliceosomes on nascent pre-mRNAs, trigger the recruitment of ALYREF onto spliced mRNAs prior to recruitment of the nucleopore-interacting receptor NXF1 [53]. DDX39B has also been implicated in the loading of ALYREF onto intronless vertebrate mRNAs in an ATP-dependent manner [76]. ALYREF-dependent activation of the ATPase and RNA helicase activities of RNA-bound DDX39B further lead to the handover of the RNA from the helicase to the nuclear export adaptor [5]. Successive cycles of ATP hydrolysis by DDX39B are thought to facilitate TREX assembly by therefore loading nuclear export adaptors (ALYREF, UIF, LUZP4) and co-adaptor CHTOP along processing transcripts [5, 30]. Mutually exclusive interactions of ALYREF with DDX39B and NXF1 lead to further displacement of DDX39B and handover of the RNA from the export adaptor to NXF1 in concert with co-adaptors THOC5 and CHTOP [5, 28, 84]. Following transport of the mRNP through the nuclear pore, the remodeling of proteins and export adaptors from the mRNPs is predicted to revert NXF1 to a low RNA-binding affinity and promote the release of the transported mRNA in the cytoplasm.

TREX provides a binding platform for NXF1 through its direct association with nuclear export adaptors (ALYREF, UIF, LUZP4) which interact with the RNA-binding domain of NXF1 and nuclear export co-adaptors (THOC5, CHTOP) that bind the NTF2-like domain [5, 28, 29, 41, 83]. In absence of interaction with ALYREF and THOC5, NXF1 adopts a closed conformation which silences its RNA-binding activity, whilst interactions with both ALYREF and THOC5 promote remodeling of NXF1 into an open conformation that exposes its RNA-binding domain [84] allowing efficient handover and binding to RNA. Coupling of the high RNA affinity remodeling of NXF1 with the co-transcriptional processing of transcripts offers in turn a retention mechanism to prevent the nuclear export of unprocessed transcripts in the cytoplasm [28, 86]. The nuclear export of human mRNAs is based upon successive RNA handover steps that link co-transcriptional splicing of pre-mRNAs and release from nuclear speckles to the nuclear export of mature mRNAs. A simplified diagram of the RNA handover process is presented in Fig. 6.2.

Assembly of TREX and activation of DDX39B is more complex than described above and the handover of RNA from the export adaptor to NXF1 is also facilitated by dynamic rearrangement of TREX and post-translational regulation events. The interaction of THOC5 with the NTF2-like domain of NXF1 is key to the remodeling of NXF1 however both co-adap-

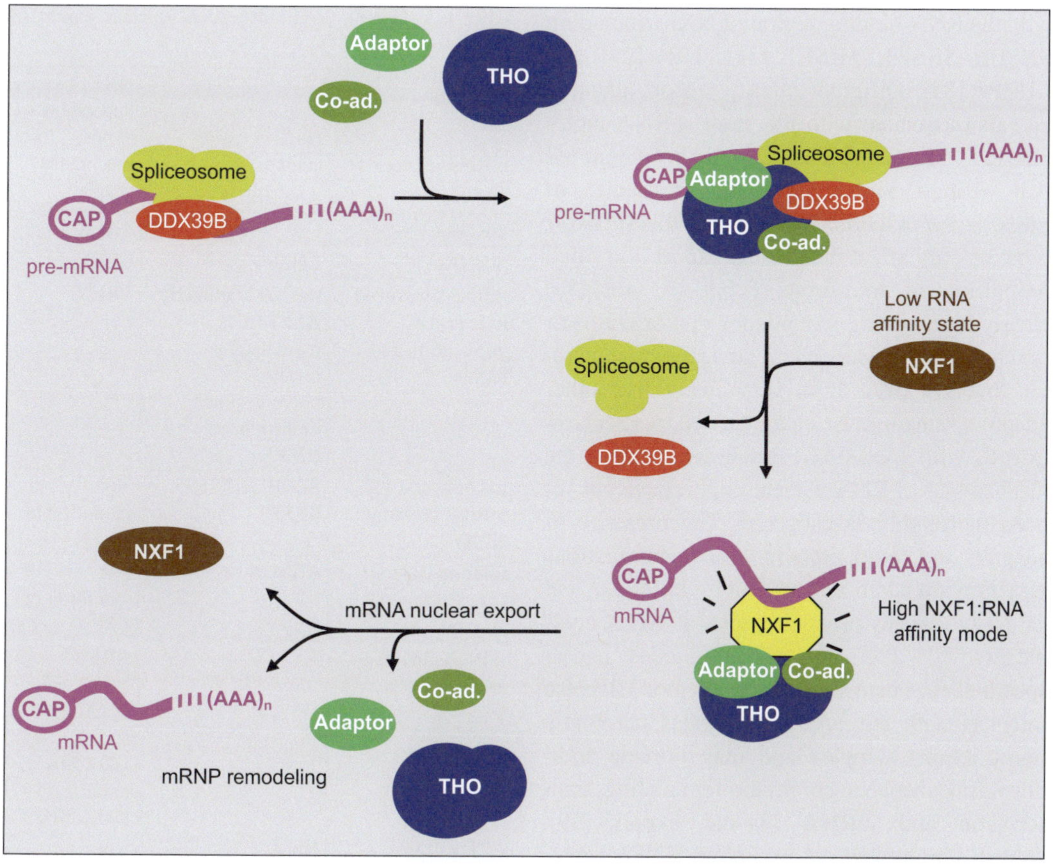

Fig. 6.2 Diagrammatic process of RNA handover during splicing and nuclear export. In the nucleoplasm, interaction of the DEAD box RNA helicase DDX39B with RNA promotes the assembly of spliceosomes on the nascent pre-mRNA synthesized by the RNA polymerase II. Direct interactions with nuclear export adaptors (ALYREF, UIF, LUZP4) and co-adaptor (Co-ad) CHTOP promote handover of the RNA from DDX39B and the loading of adaptor proteins onto pre-mRNAs. Successive cycles of ATP hydrolysis and recruitment of adaptors are thought to facilitate the assembly of TREX which is composed of the THO subcomplex, DDX39B, ALYREF and a few other proteins including the previously described adaptor proteins in various combinations. Direct interaction of NXF1 with the ternary RNA:ALYREF:DDX39B leads to the displacement of DDX39B and RNA handover onto NXF1. The high RNA affinity remodeling of NXF1 is achieved through direct interactions with both the adaptor (ALYREF and potentially UIF or LUZP4) and co-adaptors THOC5 or CHTOP within the TREX complex. On completion of transport through the nuclear pore, the mRNP is remodeled on the cytoplasmic side. Dissociation of adaptors are predicted to revert NXF1 to a low RNA binding activity that will promote the release of the transported mRNA in the cytoplasm

tors THOC5 and PRMT1 (protein arginine methyl transferase 1)-methylated CHTOP, which compete for the same binding domain of NXF1, are found in a single cellular protein complex [5, 84] indicating that TREX undergoes substantial remodeling during processing and export of mRNA. In addition, the methylation of ALYREF by PRMT1 has also been shown to decrease its RNA-binding affinity but not its interaction with NXF1 promoting in turn the handover of RNA from the nuclear export adaptor to the nuclear export receptor [35].

In contrast to yeast, multiple nuclear export adaptors have been characterised in higher *Eukaryote* organisms. The depletion of ALYREF in human cells does not significantly affect the global nuclear export of mRNA [41] and is dispensable to the development of *C. elegans* [49] and *D. melanogaster* [22]. Consistent with this, several other nuclear export adaptors interact with the RNA-binding region of NXF1 including SRSF1, SRSF3, SRSF7 [34], UIF [29] and LUZP4 [83]. Different nuclear export adaptors can also associate with the same mRNA molecule [29]. Moreover, it has recently been reported that despite interacting with thousands of mRNAs, the individual depletion of the SRSF1-7 proteins only affect the nuclear export of a small proportion of transcripts (<0.5–2% mRNAs) clearly highlighting redundancy and/or cooperation in the NXF1-dependent nuclear export adaptor function [60]. It is very likely that other adaptors remain to be characterised, particularly in cells with specialized functions in which the mechanisms of RNA nuclear export have not yet been thoroughly investigated. The presence of adaptors and co-adaptors in varied combinations may provide additional selectivity to the nuclear export process by producing several TREX complexes with alternative functionalities and/or specificities. For example, the adaptor UIF also interacts with the FACT (facilitates chromatin transcription) complex and may provide additional links between chromatin remodeling, transcription and mRNA nuclear export [29]. Table 6.1 highlights various known NXF1 dependent pathways and their associated mRNA cargoes and illustrates that not all NXF1 pathways involve TREX.

Table 6.1 Human NXF1-dependent nuclear export of mRNAs

mRNA cargoes	Nuclear export adaptor	NXF1-dependent export machinery
mRNAs	ALYREF	TREX
mRNAs	UIF	TREX
mRNAs	LUZP4	TREX
mRNAs involved in genome duplication and repair	mRNA binding by ALYREF is regulated by inositol polyphosphate multi-kinase (IMPK)	TREX
mRNAs and ITE mRNA (Histone H2A)	SRSF1, SRSF3, SRSF7	Not identified in TREX
RTE mRNAs (Transposons)	RBM15	Not identified in TREX
mRNAs involved in cytokinesis	?	AREX composed of CIP29 and DDX39A (a paralog of DDX39B)
CTE mRNAs (type D retrovirus)	None	Not identified in TREX
SSCR mRNAs (secretory proteins)	None	Not identified in TREX

NXF1 is either recruited by different nuclear export adaptors in the TREX/AREX (alternative mRNA export) complexes or directly by the constitutive transport element (CTE) in type D retroviral mRNAs or by the signal sequence-coding region (SSCR) found in secretory proteins. The RNA transport element (RTE) was identified in some mouse transposons and is similar to the CTE element. The Intronless Transport Element (ITE) is a 22-nucleotide element in the histone H2A mRNA which is recognized by SR-rich splicing factors SRSF3 and SRSF7

6.2.2.2 Exportin-Dependent Pathways Mediate the Nuclear Export of ncRNAs and Some mRNAs

The nuclear export of rRNAs, in association with ribosomal subunits, of snRNAs and of a few subsets of mRNAs depends on the karyopherin CRM1 (chromosome region maintenance 1, also known as exportin1 or XPO1). This shuttling transport receptor associates to the GTP-bound form of the small GTPase Ran and plays a major role in the nuclear export of proteins containing nuclear export signals (NES). CRM1 does not interact with RNA but with nucleoporins and NES-containing adaptor proteins that bind RNA [36, 44]. The nuclear-enriched form of GTP-bound Ran directly interacts with exportins to promote high affinity binding with protein/RNA cargoes and transport through the nuclear pore prior to release by GTP hydrolysis in the cytoplasm. The exportin is recycled back to the nucleus for additional rounds of Ran-GTP interactions and nucleocytoplasmic shuttling. Conversely, the GDP-bound form of Ran, which is predominant in the cytoplasm, directly binds importins to

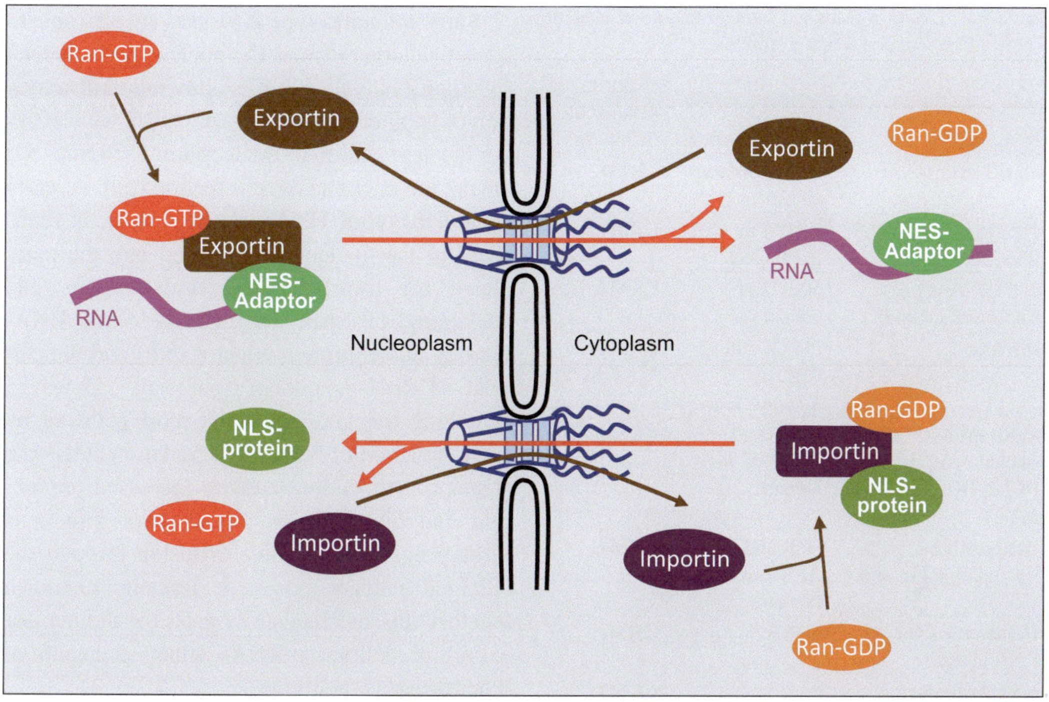

Fig. 6.3 Schematic representation of the nucleocytoplasmic transport mediated by exportins and importins. This active transport is dependent on the small Ran GTPase. The GTP bound state of Ran is enriched in the nucleus while the Ran-GDP form is cytoplasmic. The nuclear Ran-GDP exchange factor (Ran-GEF) and the cytoplasmic Ran-GTPase-activating protein (Ran-GAP) maintain the Ran-GTP/Ran-GDP gradient across the nuclear membrane generating the driving force for the nucleocytoplasmic transport process. Binding of Ran-GTP to the exportin (CRM1, Exp-t or Exp-5 for respective nuclear export of some mRNAs/proteins, tRNAs or miRNAs) trigger conformational changes that induce high affinity of the exportin for NES-containing adaptor proteins that can either be transported across the nuclear pore or bind specific subsets of RNAs. The exportins are also able to directly bind nucleoporins and license the nuclear process. GTP hydrolysis by the cytoplasmic Ran-GAP protein will remodel the exportins to a low affinity for their NES-adaptor proteins releasing the transported proteins or adaptor:RNA complexes into the cytoplasm. The free exportins are recycled back to the nucleus using the importin-dependent pathway. Conversely, interactions of the Ran-GDP with importins induce high affinity for NLS-containing proteins. The Ran-GEF factor will promote exchange of GDP for GTP in the nucleus triggering the release of the transported proteins

mediate the nuclear import of proteins with nuclear localization signal (NLS) and the release of transported proteins occur upon GTP exchange in the nucleus (Fig. 6.3). On the other hand, the nuclear export of tRNA and miRNA, which involves different exportins, is achieved through direct binding to exportin-t (Exp-t) and exportin-5 (Exp-5) respectively. Table 6.2 summarizes known RNA export pathways mediated by exportins and their adaptor proteins.

6.2.2.3 Alternative RNA Nuclear Export Pathways

It has recently been shown that mRNPs containing synaptic transcripts, too large to be transported through the channel of the nuclear pore, can exit the nucleus by budding through the nuclear membrane during the *Wnt* signaling development of synapses in *Drosophila* [70]. The budding process involves phosphorylation of lamin A by an atypical protein kinase C which

Table 6.2 Exportin-mediated nuclear export of specific RNAs and associated adaptor proteins

RNA cargoes	Adaptor proteins	Exportin-dependent pathways
5S rRNA	L5 in *Xenopus laevis*	CRM1
18S rRNA in pre-40S ribosomal subunit	RPS15 in metazoans?	CRM1
28S rRNA in pre-60S ribosomal subunit	NMD3 in human	CRM1
snRNAs	PHAX and CBC in *Xenopus laevis*	CRM1
4ESE mRNAs (including cyclin D1, BCL2, BCL6 and MYC)	eIF4E and LRPPRC in human	CRM1
ARE mRNAs (including c-Fos and CD83)	HuR and APRIL in human	CRM1
Unidentified polyA+ RNA in testis	NXF3	CRM1
mRNAs (human interferon alpha1, cyclooxygenase 2)	?	CRM1
tRNAs	None	Exp-t
miRNAs	None	Exp-5

Eukaryotic initiation translation factor 4E (eIF4E), the CAP-binding protein required for CAP-dependent translation of proteins, is also localized to the nucleus where it plays a role in the nuclear export of a subset of capped mRNAs that contain a 50-nucleotide 4E-sensitivity element (4ESE) in the 3′-untranslated region (3′-UTR). The 4ESE RNA element is bound by the leucine-rich pentatricopeptide repeat containing (LRPPRC) protein which also interacts with eIF4E and CRM1. Human antigen R (HuR) plays various roles in the processing and stability of RNA molecules through interactions with the AU-rich element (ARE) commonly found in the 3′-UTR of various transcripts. The NES-containing APRIL factor directly interacts with HuR and bridges the interactions between the HuR:RNA complex and CRM1. NXF3 belongs to the NXF1 family of proteins but has tissue specific expression with strong expression in testis. It lacks the carboxyl terminal nucleoporin-binding region and use CRM1 for translocation through the nuclear pore

induces the invagination of the inner nuclear membrane prior to the fusion of a vesicle with the outer membrane. This allows cytoplasmic release in a similar mechanism used for the nuclear exit of *Herpes* viruses.

Some influenza type A viruses are also able to induce enlargement of the nuclear pore channel (by approximately a third) following viral activation of apoptotic cellular caspases 3/7 which trigger the degradation of nucleoporin 153 (Nup153) during the later stages of infection [59]. At early stages, the viral RNA genome, which is replicated in the nucleus, is exported into the cytoplasm for translation of viral proteins and packaging of virus through the viral RNA-binding nucleoprotein adaptor (NP) and the cellular CRM1-dependent pathway. However, switching the viral nuclear export pathway by viral induction of Nup153 degradation at the late stages of replication leads to increased production and high efficiency release of infectious virus progeny by passive diffusion through the enlarged nuclear pores. It remains unknown whether this mechanism is used for the nuclear export of cellular mRNAs either in health or other disease conditions.

6.2.3 The Nucleocytoplasmic Transport of RNPs

6.2.3.1 The Nuclear Pore Complex

Vertebrate nuclear pore complexes form large 125-MDa protein assemblies stably embedded in circular holes created by fusion of the inner and outer nuclear membranes. They constitute aqueous transport channels which mediate and regulate the bidirectional exchange of macromolecules between the nucleus and cytoplasm [43]. Small molecules under 40 kDa (or approximately 5 nm in size) freely shuttle between the nucleus and cytoplasm by passive diffusion, while larger molecules and mRNPs require active transport mechanisms which depend on either NXF1 or exportins and importins.

The NPC has a symmetrical octagonal structure that contains a nuclear basket made of eight rod-shaped filaments associated to a distal ring on the nucleoplasmic side and eight extended flexible fibrils at the cytoplasmic side. Nucleoporin fibers from the central core of the NPC protrude inside the pore opening to form a

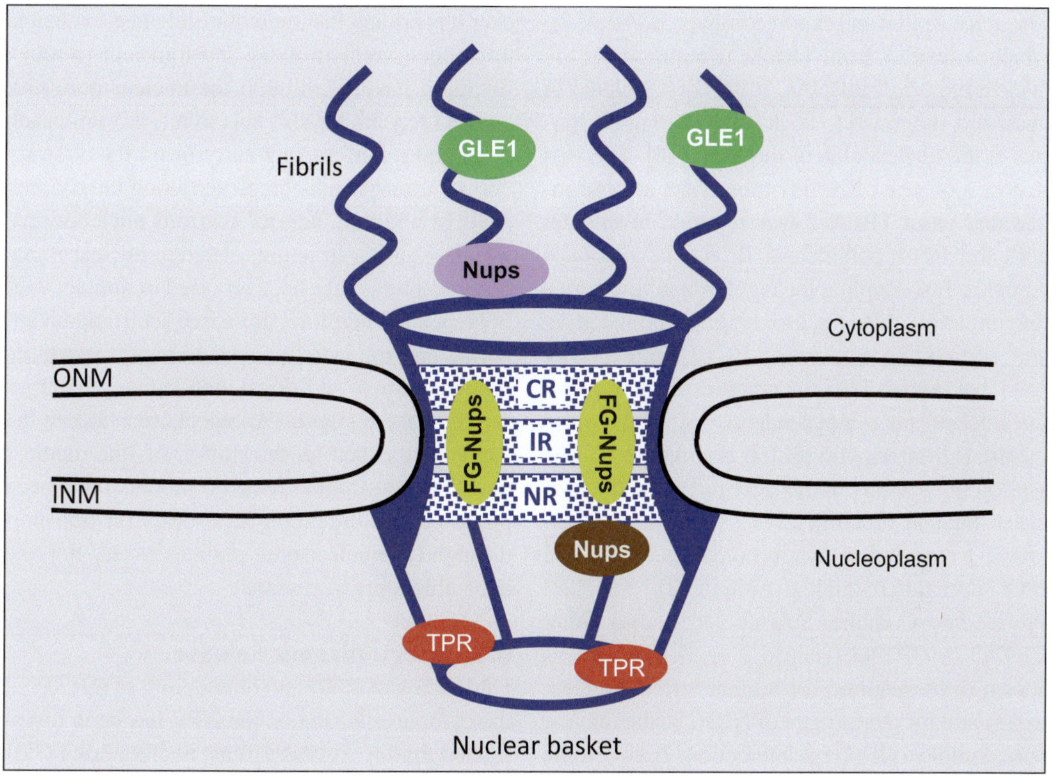

Fig. 6.4 Schematic representation of the nuclear pore complex (NPC). The NPC forms a stable symmetrical structure composed of a central core, a nuclear basket and eight flexible fibrils on the cytoplasmic side built through interactions of approximately 30 different nucleoporins. The central core appears to contain three porous rings by electron microscopy: *NR* nucleoplasmic ring, *IR* inner ring, *CR* cytoplasmic ring. The interspersed unstructured FG-repeat regions of some nucleoporins protrude within the channel of the pore to form a semi-permeable hydrogel-like environment that allows for selective transport. The NPC is anchored in pores created through fusion of the inner nuclear membrane (INM) and outer nuclear membrane (ONM)

selective semi-permeable barrier. The structure is well conserved among all metazoans. Approximately 30 different nucleoporins in multiple copies compose the NPC that contains between 500 and 1000 protein molecules in the fully assembled state. An essential Y-shaped sub-complex composed of six to ten nucleoporins constitute the basic scaffolding unit of the nuclear and cytoplasmic rings composing the central NPC core. Additional nucleoporins together with Y-shaped sub-complexes might be involved in the formation of the inner ring structure. Some of the scaffold nucleoproteins are the most long-lived proteins in cells with half-life of months and years, accounting for the very high structural stability of the NPC core. Other trans-membrane nucleoporins anchor the NPC to the fused nuclear membrane. The nuclear basket is made of specific nucleoporins and TPR (Translocated Promoter Region) while the cytoplasmic fibrils are composed of additional nucleoporins including GLE1 (RNA export mediator). Protruding channel fibres that make the semi-permeable barrier correspond to unstructured regions that extend from about ten nucleoporins. They are composed of approximately 50 interspersed phenylalanine-glycine (FG) repeats which form a size-selective hydrogel-like environment within the nuclear pore (Fig. 6.4).

6.2.3.2 Docking of mRNPs to the Nuclear Pore Complex

The nuclear export of mRNPs appears to involve a specific mechanism for docking at the NPC.

The transcription and export complex 2 (TREX-2), which is distinct from TREX, is required for the nuclear export of mRNAs. It was first isolated in yeast and suggested to dock mRNPs to nucleoporins at the nuclear side of the NPC [16]. The vast majority of yeast RNAPII transcripts are intronless and yeast TREX-2 was reported to interact with the RNA polymerase II via the mediator complex thus coupling the regulation of transcription initiation to the nuclear export of both coding and non-coding transcripts [67]. On the other hand, the human TREX-2 complex is recruited at the nuclear pore independently of RNA polymerase II transcription [81]. It is composed of the scaffolding subunit GANP (germinal centre-associated nuclear protein), ENY2 (enhancer of yellow 2 transcription factor homologue), PCID2 (PCI domain-containing protein 2), the 26S Proteasome Complex Subunit DSS1 and either CETN2 or CETN3 (centrin 2 or 3). GANP was shown to be required for human mRNA nuclear export and for recruitment of NXF1 to the nuclear pore complex via direct interactions between the carboxyl terminal region of NXF1 and the amino terminal domain of GANP which contains a cluster of 6 nucleoporin-like FG repeats [88]. The ENYP subunit and carboxyl terminal region of GANP have been shown to associate with TPR and Nup153 at the nuclear basket of the NPC [81] allowing for docking of NXF1-containing mRNP complexes at the nuclear pore, potentially by association of GANP with NXF1-containing mRNP complexes downstream of TREX. TREX-2 might also play additional roles in coupling transcription or RNA processing to the nuclear export of specific subsets of transcripts. It is however unclear whether mRNAs can directly be transferred from TREX-2 to NXF1. Whether TREX and TREX-2 act on same or different transcripts is a long-standing question that remains yet to be answered.

6.2.3.3 Transport of RNPs Through the Nuclear Pore

The nuclear transport receptors (exportins, importins and NXF1) have intrinsic affinity for the FG-repeat regions of the nucleoporins that protrude in the central channel of the NPC, however it is critical that these multiple fast-exchange interactions remain weak and transient to allow for rapid passage through the nuclear pore [32, 55]. FG repeats are also able to interact with each other and might prevent entry or on the contrary "brush" transported complexes along the channel [48]. In addition, several scaffold nucleoporins, which exhibit a structure related to nuclear transport receptors, have been reported to interact with FG repeats. Therefore, these free scaffold nucleoporins and unloaded nuclear transport receptors might confer an additional mobile layer that transiently interacts with FG-repeats to regulate the connectivity and permeability of the nuclear pore. Several thermodynamic models have been proposed and the biophysical basis for transport through the nuclear pore remains a very hot and debatable topic of research.

6.2.3.4 Cytoplasmic Release

Unwinding of RNA and remodeling of mRNPs at the cytoplasmic side on the NPC has been investigated mainly in yeast. Yeast nucleoporins Gle1 and Nup159 (Nup214 in human) have been implicated in this process together with the yeast DEAD-box protein RNA helicase Dbp5 (DDX19 in human) in association with inositol hexakisphosphate (IP6), which spatially regulates the activity of Dbp5 at the cytoplasmic side of the NPC [18]. IP6-bound Gle1 stabilizes the interaction with Dbp5 and stimulates ATP binding, leading therefore to the recruitment of Dbp5 onto mRNAs. Multiple rounds of ATP binding appear to be sufficient to promote unwinding of secondary RNA structures and remodeling of mRNPs by displacement of bound protein factors, while ATP hydrolysis is required for RNA release and recycling of Dbp5. Yeast Mex67p, the ortholog of NXF1, has been shown to be remodeled by Dbp5 [52]. Remodeling of nuclear export adaptors and Mex67p/NXF1 by Dbp5/DDX19 is predicted to revert NXF1 to a low affinity RNA-binding affinity mode that will promote mRNA release into the cytoplasm.

A summary diagram representing the molecular mechanisms involved in the co-transcriptional processing and NXF1-dependent nuclear export of bulk mRNAs is presented in Fig. 6.5.

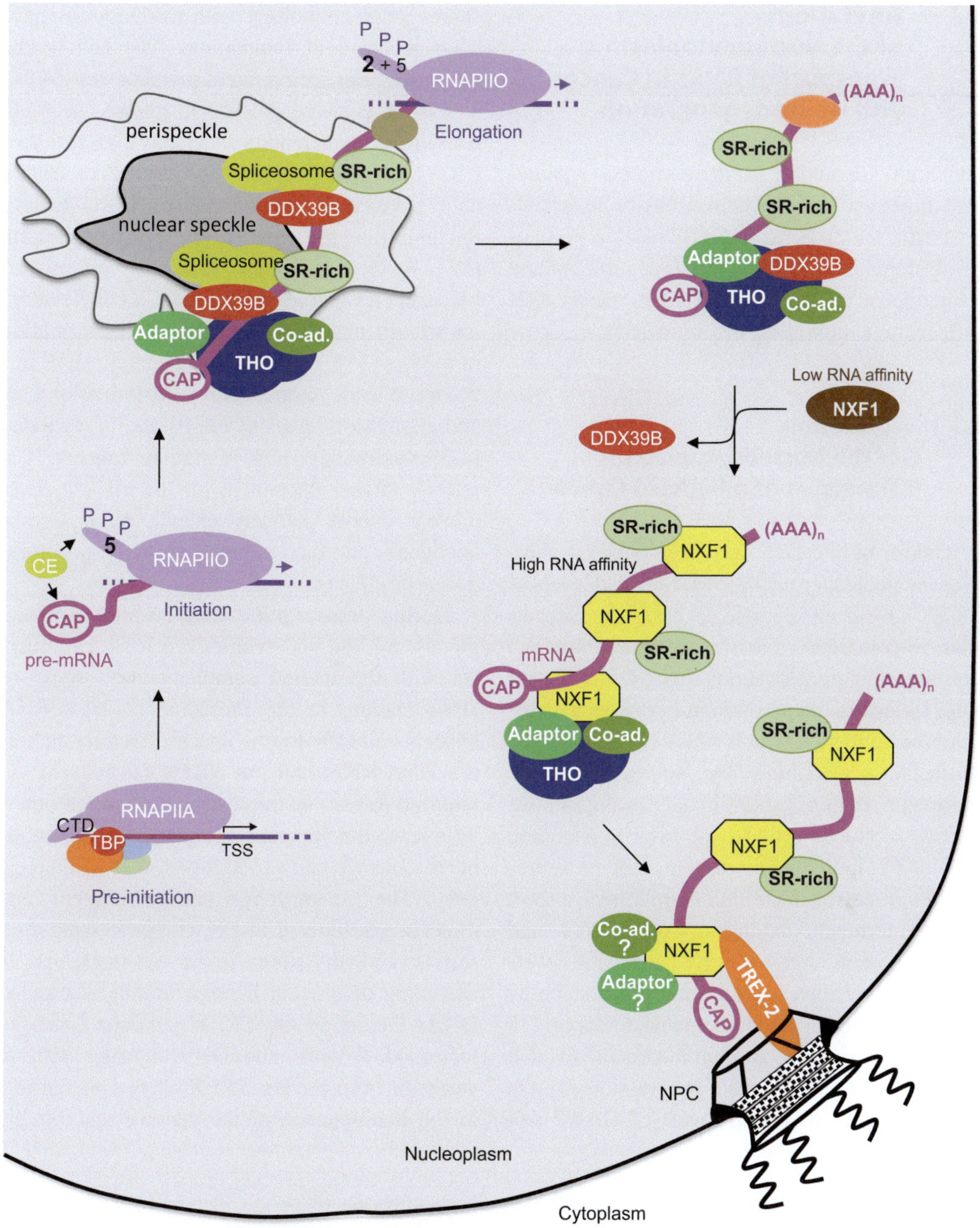

Fig. 6.5 Model for the biogenesis, processing and nuclear export of bulk mRNAs in humans. The remodeling of compact heterochromatin into relaxed euchromatin is usually required for transcriptional activation by facilitating recruitment of transcription factors and the hypophosphorylated form of the RNA polymerase IIA upstream of the transcription start site (TSS). Phosphorylation on serine 5 residues of the CTD is associated with initiation of transcription and recruitment of the capping enzyme which lead to the addition of a cap onto the 5′end of the nascent transcript. Loading of the RNA helicase DDX39B onto the pre-mRNA promotes the assembly of the spliceosome complex and splicing/processing occurs in the vicinity of nuclear speckles in the perispeckle space. The direct interaction of nuclear export adaptors (ALYREF, UIF, LUZP4) and co-adaptor CHTOP with DDX39B leads to RNA handover and deposition of adaptor proteins onto the spliced exon junction to promote the assembly of the TREX complex. TREX is composed of the stable hexameric core THO, DDX39B, ALYREF

6.3 Alteration of the Nucleocytoplasmic Transport of RNAs in Cancer and Neurodegeneration

Mutations disrupting RNP particles, whether they directly affect a protein, RNA or an assembly factor, are prone to cause disease. In particular, dysregulation of RNA-binding proteins and formation of mRNPs is affected in cancer [92] and several neurological disorders [64].

6.3.1 Alteration of the Nucleocytoplasmic Transport of mRNAs in Cancer

Several forms of cancer have been linked to alterations of nucleoporins [45, 93]. Elevated levels of Nup88 have been reported in breast, hepatocellular, colorectal and ovarian tumors. Chromosomal translocations in TPR, Nup98 and Nup214 lead to the production of oncogenic chimeric nucleoporins which cause carcinogenesis, particularly leukemias, by up-regulating the expression levels of proto-oncogenes. Alternative splicing of Nup98 produce a transcript encoding a Nup98-Nup96 fusion protein that is subsequently processed into either Nup98, with a short carboxyl-terminal extension, or Nup98 and Nup96 proteins. Interestingly, expression levels of Nup96 contribute to cell cycle progression by regulating the differential nuclear export of mRNAs encoding key protein factors involved in the control of the cell cycle progression [4]. On the other hand, increased levels of GANP that shares some homology with nucleoporins have been reported in lymphomas [20] and in the malignant transformation of melanocytes [39].

CRM1 is overexpressed in glioma, cervical, ovarian and pancreatic cancers, as high levels of CRM1 are required for the survival of cancer cells. Conversely, the depletion of CRM1 leads to the inhibition of cervical cancer cell proliferation [82]. A clear link has also been established between elevated levels of eIF4E, a CRM1 adaptor protein, and the in vitro and in vivo formation of tumors [25]. The overexpression of eIF4E furthermore leads to oncogenic transformation [10] and expression levels of eIF4E are up regulated in approximately 30% of human cancers. The mRNA targets dependent on the eIF4E:CRM1 nuclear export pathway encode many known oncogenes and factors involved in cell proliferation [9].

During transcription and co-transcriptional processing, the neo-synthesized RNA can interact with the melted complementary strand of DNA leading to the formation of DNA/RNA hybrids called R-loops. Specific factors such as the DNA/RNA helicase SETX (senataxin) are required to resolve these structures which otherwise leave the opposing strand of DNA susceptible to cleavage and varied forms of DNA damage [90]. The co-transcriptional recruitment and direct interactions of TREX with processing transcripts is ideally suited to prevent inappropriate annealing of nascent RNA with single-stranded DNA. Depletion of TREX subunits leads to increased R-loops and DNA damage both in yeast and human cells. TREX plays a pivotal role in the maintenance of the genome stability by

Fig. 6.5 (continued) and a few other proteins that may produce different TREX complexes with various selectivity for various subsets of mRNAs. SR-rich splicing factors SRSF1, 3 and 7 proteins (SR-rich) also act as NXF1-dependent nuclear export adaptors however they have not been isolated in TREX. They are co-transcriptionally recruited and deposited along the processing transcript at the spliced exon junctions during alternative splicing. Export adaptors bound onto spliced transcripts further allow recruitment of NXF1, displacing in turn DDX39B upon mutually exclusive interactions with NXF1. Within TREX, simultaneous interactions of a nuclear export adaptor and co-adaptor THOC5 further remodel NXF1 into an open structural conformation exposing its RNA-binding domain which was silenced by intra-molecular interactions. The high RNA-binding affinity state of NXF1 triggers the handover of the RNA from the nuclear export adaptor. The methylated CHTOP co-adaptor is also involved in this process by interacting with NXF1 in an exclusive manner with THOC5 promoting further events of remodeling within TREX. The SR-rich adaptors SRSF1, 3, 7 are also able to remodel NXF1 to directly induce its RNA-binding affinity in absence of TREX. The TREX-2 complex interacts with NXF1 and will allow docking of the mRNP at the nuclear pore complex (NPC) and interaction of NXF1 with the FG-repeats of the nucleoporins that protrude in the channel of the nuclear pore

regulating the selective nuclear export of mRNAs encoding proteins involved in genome duplication and DNA repair (including RAD51, CHK1, FANCD2). This selective nuclear export pathway involves differential regulation of the RNA-binding activity of ALYREF by the inositol polyphosphate multikinase (IPMK) [89]. Formation of R-loops, genome instability and alteration of TREX components have consistently been implicated in many types of cancer [90]. The THOC1 subunit of TREX is up regulated in ovarian, colon and lung cancers but down regulated in testis and skin cancers [14]. Phosphorylation of THOC5 by the leukemogenic protein tyrosine kinase (PTK) has been involved in chronic myeloid leukemia [26]. On the other hand, the interaction of the nuclear export co-adaptor CHTOP with the methylosome complex promotes PRMT1-dependent di-methylation of histone H4 on arginine 3 in gene promoters and intragenic regions, leading to the transcriptional activation of cancer-related genes involved in glioblastoma [75]. Expression levels of nuclear export adaptor ALYREF are dysregulated in colon, stomach, pancreatic and testis tumors with down regulation observed in high-grade cancers [14]. Expression of the adaptor LUZP4, which is normally restricted to testis, is up regulated in tumors from various tissues, and its expression is essential to the proliferation of melanoma cells [83]. Depletion of ALYREF [65], THOC1 [47] and LUZP4 [83] inhibit the proliferation of cancer cells and may therefore provide novel therapeutic strategies to treat some forms of cancer [11].

6.3.2 Alteration of the Nucleocytoplasmic Transport of mRNAs in Neurodegeneration

6.3.2.1 Neurological Disorders Caused by Genetic Mutations in TREX Subunits

Mutations in the core THO subunits of the TREX complex affect neuronal development and cause rare diseases. A chromosomal translocation that produces a chimeric inactive PTK2-THOC2 protein fusion leads to cognitive impairment, cerebellar hypoplasia and congenital ataxia in childhood [13]. The protein tyrosine kinase 2 (PTK2) is involved in axonal and neurite growth however depletion alone does not cause this phenotype, indicating that the disease is due to the loss-of-function of THOC2. In addition, THOC2 missense mutations that affect protein stability have been implicated in X-linked intellectual disability [46]. In addition, the expression levels of THOC1, THOC3, THOC5 and THOC7 proteins, but not of ALYREF, DDX39B and CHTOP, were also decreased, supporting a loss-of-function mechanism by global alteration of the THO subcomplex. A homozygous missense mutation in THOC6 has also been reported in patients from two related Hutterite families, an isolated population of 40,000 individuals living in the North American prairies, which present with intellectual disability [2]. The mutation causes the THOC6 protein to mislocalize to the cytoplasm from the nucleus where it physiologically associates with THO in the TREX complex.

6.3.2.2 Mutations in Gle1 Cause Motor Neuron Diseases

Loss-of-function mutations in the mRNA export mediator Gle1 were shown to cause severe neurodegeneration that results in amyotrophic lateral sclerosis (ALS) [40] and fetal motor neuron disease (LCCS1, Lethal congenital contracture syndrome 1) [61]. ALS is an invariably fatal adult onset disease with an annual incidence rate of approximately 2 cases per 100,000 individuals. It leads to progressive loss of upper and lower motor neurons invariably resulting in progressive paralysis and death usually within 2–3 years from symptom onset. The autosomal recessive disease LCCS1 is caused by a *Fin major* mutation inherited in Finnish families with an incidence rate of 1 in 25,000 births. It leads to severe atrophy of spinal motor neurons and skeletal muscles and total immobility of the fetus, which lead to multiple joint contractures and pre-natal death. The *Fin major* mutation specifically impairs the nuclear export of bulk mRNAs in human cells, but not the Gle1 functions associated with translation, triggering loss of localization to the nuclear pore and nuclear accumulation of polyadenylated RNA [17]. The mRNA targets and the pathophysiological mechanisms by which Gle1 loss-of-function leads to neurodegeneration remains uncharacterised due to the severity of the disease phenotype and the lack of experimental animal and cell models.

6.3.2.3 Altered Nucleocytoplasmic Transport of mRNAs in Microsatellite Repeat Expansion Disorders

The nucleocytoplasmic transport of RNA and proteins is affected in several neurodegenerative diseases caused by repetition of microsatellite expansions. These have been subdivided into poly-glutamine (poly-Q) and non-poly-glutamine disorders. Poly-Q sequences encoded by CAG trinucleotide-repeat expansions have been reported in Huntington disease (HD) and several subtypes of spinocerebellar ataxia (SCA1-3, 6, 7, 17). SCA8 and myotonic dystrophy type 1 (DM1) further involve bi-directional transcription of CUG-sense and CAG-antisense trinucleotide-repeat transcripts. Non-poly-Q disorders are caused by expansions ranging from trinucleotide to hexanucleotide repeats including: (i) CGG repeats in Fragile X-associated mental retardations; (ii) pentanucleotide (ATTCT, TGGAA) and hexanucleotide (GGCCTG) expansions in SCA10, 31 and 36 respectively; (iii) bi-directionally transcribed GGGGCC-sense and GGCCCC-antisense hexanucleotide-repeat expansions in chromosome 9 open reading frame 72 (C9ORF72) related amyotrophic lateral sclerosis (ALS) [50, 62, 85].

Repeat expansions are found both in non-coding (5′-UTR, intronic, 3′UTR) and coding regions of mRNAs. They cause neurodegeneration through a complex pathogenesis involving protein loss-of-function and protein/RNA toxic gain-of-function mechanisms through sequestration of proteins by RNA repeat sequences and production of toxic polymeric repeat proteins by repeat-associated non-ATG (RAN) translation [50, 85]. This unconventional form of translation does not require canonical AUG start codons and can be initiated in all frames at various positions within the length of the repeat expansion. The molecular mechanism(s) of RAN translation remain poorly characterised but are dependent on the formation of secondary RNA structures that may recruit ribosomes similarly to internal ribosome entry site elements used by virus. The RAN translation of CAG-repeat transcripts lacking start codons into homo-polymeric proteins in all frames (poly-glutamine, poly-serine and poly-alanine) was discovered in cell models and SCA8/DM1 human brain tissue [94]. RAN translation of non-coding transcript regions was subsequently highlighted to occur from CGG repeats in the 5′-UTR of the *FMR1* (fragile X mental retardation 1) gene in fragile X–associated tremor and ataxia syndrome (FXTAS) [77] and from GGGGCC sense/antisense intronic repeats in C9ORF72-ALS [57, 95]. Moreover, RAN translation through coding CAG-repeat expansions in the Huntingtin (*HTT*) gene was reported in HD [1].

Exonic CAG-repeat expansions found in polymorphic glutamine regions in autosomal-dominant cerebellar ataxias and HD lead to the translation of abnormal proteins with extended poly-Q domains that promote misfolding/aggregation, abnormal binding to other protein factors and reduced interactions with protein partners. Strikingly, mechanisms of pathogenicity in microsatellite repeat expansion disorders are shared between the nuclear retention of repeat transcripts that form characteristic RNA foci which sequester RNA-processing proteins and the cytoplasmic production of aggregating repeat proteins by RAN translation. However the pathophysiological contribution of each of these alterations remains debatable and is to be precisely determined for each neurodegenerative disease. The mechanisms driving and regulating the nuclear export of repeat transcripts are therefore expected to play a key role in delineating pathological outcomes induced by nuclear retention of repeat transcripts and RAN translation in the cytoplasm.

Indeed, manipulating the expression levels of mRNA nuclear export factors either exacerbates or suppresses neurodegeneration in cellular and animal models of DM1 [21], C9ORF72-ALS [19] and poly-Q diseases [73, 80]. Manipulating the expression of nuclear pore complex components is also a modifier of neurodegeneration in C9ORF72-ALS. On the other hand, nucleocytoplasmic alterations of protein trafficking have been extensively reported in HD, DM1, C9ORF72-ALS and upon expression of expanded poly-Q proteins [3], but will not be reviewed in this chapter which focuses on RNA nuclear export.

The accumulation of intranuclear RNA foci in Poly-Q diseases, SCAs, DM1, HD and C9ORF72-ALS suggest resistance to the nuclear export of repeat transcripts however the occurrence of RAN translation in the cytoplasm implies that a fraction is at least transported through the nuclear pore. CAG-repeat transcripts were shown to directly bind U2AF65 which serves as a nuclear export adaptor by interacting with NXF1 [80]. Consistent with this, the nuclear export of CAG-repeat transcripts is enhanced by overexpression of U2AF65 in HD models, while it is inhibited by overexpression of MBLN1 (muscleblind-like protein 1) which is sequestered on RNA repeats [73]. Reduced levels of Ref1, the *Drosophila* orthologue of ALYREF in mammals, exacerbate neurodegeneration in a DM1 model of *Drosophila* [21] suggesting that ALYREF is involved in the nuclear export of CUG-repeat transcripts.

In ALS, GGGGCC-repeat expansions are found in intron 1 of the *C9ORF72* gene. Nuclear retention of pre-mRNA repeat transcripts would therefore be expected however RAN translation of dipeptide-repeat proteins indicates transport through the nuclear pore. The nuclear export adaptors ALYREF and SRSF1 were shown to directly interact with GGGGCC-repeat RNA and sequestration of adaptors was suggested to play a role in the abnormal nuclear export of *C9ORF72* repeat transcripts by triggering abnormal interactions with NXF1 [8]. Interestingly, depleting the non-essential ALYREF factor in a C9ORF72-ALS *Drosophila* model ameliorates the rough eye phenotype [19]. Reduced levels of NXF1 and CHTOP intriguingly enhanced neurodegeneration in this model [19] however this might be caused by indirect effects due to global alterations of the nuclear export of mRNAs. CHTOP has also been implicated in multiple other cellular functions which would be altered upon depletion.

Widespread dysregulation of gene expression associated with these alterations of the nucleocytoplasmic transport in neurodegeneration present challenges but also opportunities for therapeutic intervention [27]. Evaluating the pathogenic contributions between repeat protein production and RNA-mediated toxicity by nuclear retention of transcripts will be fundamental to the successful development of neuroprotective strategies. If expression of repeat proteins can kill cells in vitro, it is difficult to evaluate which levels are translated in patients and whether these are sufficient to trigger toxicity depending on the repeat expansion, disease and cell type. There are however growing evidences for a pathogenic role of RAN-translation. For example, FXTAS was initially thought to be caused by intranuclear retention of transcripts and sequestration of splicing factors [37, 68] however the discovery of RAN translation in the same model challenged this view [77]. Similarly in C9ORF72-ALS, increasing tenfold the number of intranuclear RNA foci does not significantly alter cell survival or global RNA processing while expression of dipeptide repeat proteins causes neurodegeneration [78].

The nuclear export of repeat transcripts appears to involve the NXF1 pathway and various export adaptors such as ALYREF or U2AF65 in DM1 [21], poly-Q-related diseases [73, 80] and C9ORF72-ALS [19]. In FXTAS, PUR-alpha might play a role in the nuclear export of CGG-repeat transcripts [37] however the nuclear export receptor remains yet to be characterised. The partial depletion of individual RNA nuclear export adaptors does not appear to be essential to the functioning of higher eukaryote cells due to high level of redundancy. Therefore, they might constitute new therapeutic targets for inhibiting the nuclear export of repeat transcripts and the production of toxic repeat proteins, particularly in disease where RAN translation appears to have a prominent role over the nuclear retention of transcripts.

Acknowledgments G.M.H. acknowledges support from the Motor Neurone Disease Association (grant Apr16/846-791), the Medical Research Council (MRC grant MR/M010864/1) and the Thierry Latran Foundation (grant FTLAAP2016/Astrocyte secretome).

References

1. Bañez-Coronel M, Ayhan F, Tarabochia AD, Zu T, Perez BA, Tusi SK et al (2015) RAN translation in Huntington disease. Neuron 88(4):667–677
2. Beaulieu CL, Huang L, Innes AM, Akimenko M-A, Puffenberger EG, Schwartz C et al (2013) Intellectual disability associated with a homozygous missense mutation in THOC6. Orphanet J Rare Dis 8:62
3. Boeynaems S, Bogaert E, Van Damme P, Van Den Bosch L (2016) Inside out: the role of nucleocytoplasmic transport in ALS and FTLD. Acta Neuropathol 132(2):159–173
4. Chakraborty P, Wang Y, Wei J-H, van Deursen J, Yu H, Malureanu L et al (2008) Nucleoporin levels regulate cell cycle progression and phase-specific gene expression. Dev Cell 15(5):657–667
5. Chang C-T, Hautbergue GM, Walsh MJ, Viphakone N, van Dijk TB, Philipsen S et al (2013) Chtop is a component of the dynamic TREX mRNA export complex. EMBO J 32(3):473–486
6. Charoensawan V, Janga SC, Bulyk ML, Babu MM, Teichmann SA (2012) DNA sequence preferences of transcriptional activators correlate more strongly than repressors with nucleosomes. Mol Cell 47(2):183–192
7. Cheng H, Dufu K, Lee C-S, Hsu JL, Dias A, Reed R (2006) Human mRNA export machinery recruited to the 5′ end of mRNA. Cell 127(7):1389–1400
8. Cooper-Knock J, Walsh MJ, Higginbottom A, Robin Highley J, Dickman MJ, Edbauer D et al (2014) Sequestration of multiple RNA recognition motif-containing proteins by C9orf72 repeat expansions. Brain 137(Pt 7):2040–2051
9. Culjkovic B, Topisirovic I, Skrabanek L, Ruiz-Gutierrez M, Borden KLB (2006) eIF4E is a central node of an RNA regulon that governs cellular proliferation. J Cell Biol 175(3):415–426
10. Culjkovic-Kraljacic B, Baguet A, Volpon L, Amri A, Borden KLB (2012) The oncogene eIF4E reprograms the nuclear pore complex to promote mRNA export and oncogenic transformation. Cell Rep 2(2):207–215
11. Culjkovic-Kraljacic B, Borden KLB (2013) Aiding and abetting cancer: mRNA export and the nuclear pore. Trends Cell Biol 23(7):328–335
12. Dever TE, Green R (2012) The elongation, termination, and recycling phases of translation in eukaryotes. Cold Spring Harb Perspect Biol 4(7):a013706
13. Di Gregorio E, Bianchi FT, Schiavi A, Chiotto AMA, Rolando M, Verdun di Cantogno L et al (2013) A de novo X;8 translocation creates a PTK2-THOC2 gene fusion with THOC2 expression knockdown in a patient with psychomotor retardation and congenital cerebellar hypoplasia. J Med Genet 50(8):543–551
14. Domínguez-Sánchez MS, Sáez C, Japón MA, Aguilera A, Luna R (2011) Differential expression of THOC1 and ALY mRNP biogenesis/export factors in human cancers. BMC Cancer 11:77
15. Dufu K, Livingstone MJ, Seebacher J, Gygi SP, Wilson SA, Reed R (2010) ATP is required for interactions between UAP56 and two conserved mRNA export proteins, Aly and CIP29, to assemble the TREX complex. Genes Dev 24(18):2043–2053
16. Fischer T, Strässer K, Rácz A, Rodríguez-Navarro S, Oppizzi M, Ihrig P et al (2002) The mRNA export machinery requires the novel Sac3p-Thp1p complex to dock at the nucleoplasmic entrance of the nuclear pores. EMBO J 21(21):5843–5852
17. Folkmann AW, Collier SE, Zhan X, Aditi O, Wente SR (2013) Gle1 functions during mRNA export in an oligomeric complex that is altered in human disease. Cell 155(3):582–593
18. Folkmann AW, Noble KN, Cole CN, Wente SR (2011) Dbp5, Gle1-IP6 and Nup159: a working model for mRNP export. Nucleus 2(6):540–548
19. Freibaum BD, Lu Y, Lopez-Gonzalez R, Kim NC, Almeida S, Lee K-H et al (2015) GGGGCC repeat expansion in C9orf72 compromises nucleocytoplasmic transport. Nature 525(7567):129–133
20. Fujimura S, Xing Y, Takeya M, Yamashita Y, Ohshima K, Kuwahara K et al (2005) Increased expression of germinal center-associated nuclear protein RNA-primase is associated with lymphomagenesis. Cancer Res 65(13):5925–5934
21. Garcia-Lopez A, Monferrer L, Garcia-Alcover I, Vicente-Crespo M, Alvarez-Abril MC, Artero RD (2008) Genetic and chemical modifiers of a CUG toxicity model in Drosophila. PLoS One 3(2):e1595
22. Gatfield D, Izaurralde E (2002) REF1/Aly and the additional exon junction complex proteins are dispensable for nuclear mRNA export. J Cell Biol 159(4):579–588
23. Gerstberger S, Hafner M, Tuschl T (2014) A census of human RNA-binding proteins. Nat Rev Genet 15(12):829–845
24. Girard C, Will CL, Peng J, Makarov EM, Kastner B, Lemm I et al (2012) Post-transcriptional spliceosomes are retained in nuclear speckles until splicing completion. Nat Commun 3:994
25. Graff JR, Konicek BW, Carter JH, Marcusson EG (2008) Targeting the eukaryotic translation initiation factor 4E for cancer therapy. Cancer Res 68(3):631–634
26. Griaud F, Pierce A, Gonzalez Sanchez MB, Scott M, Abraham SA, Holyoake TL et al (2013) A pathway from leukemogenic oncogenes and stem cell chemokines to RNA processing via THOC5. Leukemia 27(4):932–940
27. Hautbergue GM (2016) Widespread RNA dysregulation in neurodegeneration: challenges and opportunities. Austin Neurol 1(1):1002
28. Hautbergue GM, Hung M-L, Golovanov AP, Lian L-Y, Wilson SA (2008) Mutually exclusive interactions drive handover of mRNA from export adaptors to TAP. Proc Natl Acad Sci U S A 105(13):5154–5159

29. Hautbergue GM, Hung M-L, Walsh MJ, Snijders APL, Chang C-T, Jones R et al (2009) UIF, a new mRNA export adaptor that works together with REF/ALY, requires FACT for recruitment to mRNA. Curr Biol 19(22):1918–1924
30. Heath CG, Viphakone N, Wilson SA (2016) The role of TREX in gene expression and disease. Biochem J 473(19):2911–2935
31. Herold A, Suyama M, Rodrigues JP, Braun IC, Kutay U, Carmo-Fonseca M et al (2000) TAP (NXF1) belongs to a multigene family of putative RNA export factors with a conserved modular architecture. Mol Cell Biol 20(23):8996–9008
32. Hough LE, Dutta K, Sparks S, Temel DB, Kamal A, Tetenbaum-Novatt J et al (2015) The molecular mechanism of nuclear transport revealed by atomic-scale measurements. elife 15:4
33. Hsin J-P, Manley JL (2012) The RNA polymerase II CTD coordinates transcription and RNA processing. Genes Dev 26(19):2119–2137
34. Huang Y, Gattoni R, Stevenin J, Steitz JA (2003) SR splicing factors serve as adapter proteins for TAP-dependent mRNA export. Mol Cell 11(3):837–843
35. Hung M-L, Hautbergue GM, Snijders APL, Dickman MJ, Wilson SA (2010) Arginine methylation of REF/ALY promotes efficient handover of mRNA to TAP/NXF1. Nucleic Acids Res 38(10):3351–3361
36. Hutten S, Kehlenbach RH (2007) CRM1-mediated nuclear export: to the pore and beyond. Trends Cell Biol 17(4):193–201
37. Jin P, Duan R, Qurashi A, Qin Y, Tian D, Rosser TC et al (2007) Pur alpha binds to rCGG repeats and modulates repeat-mediated neurodegeneration in a Drosophila model of fragile X tremor/ataxia syndrome. Neuron 55(4):556–564
38. Jung H, Yoon BC, Holt CE (2012) Axonal mRNA localization and local protein synthesis in nervous system assembly, maintenance and repair. Nat Publ Group 13(5):308–324
39. Kageshita T, Kuwahara K, Oka M, Ma D, Ono T, Sakaguchi N (2006) Increased expression of germinal center-associated nuclear protein (GANP) is associated with malignant transformation of melanocytes. J Dermatol Sci 42(1):55–63
40. Kaneb HM, Folkmann AW, Belzil VV, Jao L-E, Leblond CS, Girard SL et al (2015) Deleterious mutations in the essential mRNA metabolism factor, hGle1, in amyotrophic lateral sclerosis. Hum Mol Genet 24(5):1363–1373
41. Katahira J, Inoue H, Hurt E, Yoneda Y (2009) Adaptor Aly and co-adaptor Thoc5 function in the Tap-p15-mediated nuclear export of HSP70 mRNA. EMBO J 28(5):556–567
42. Kilchert C, Wittmann S, Vasiljeva L (2016) The regulation and functions of the nuclear RNA exosome complex. Nat Rev Mol Cell Biol 17(4):227–239
43. Knockenhauer KE, Schwartz TU (2016) The nuclear pore complex as a flexible and dynamic gate. Cell 164(6):1162–1171
44. Köhler A, Hurt E (2007) Exporting RNA from the nucleus to the cytoplasm. Nat Rev Mol Cell Biol 8(10):761–773
45. Köhler A, Hurt E (2010) Gene regulation by nucleoporins and links to cancer. Mol Cell 38(1):6–15
46. Kumar R, Corbett MA, van Bon BWM, Woenig JA, Weir L, Douglas E et al (2015) THOC2 mutations implicate mRNA-export pathway in X-linked intellectual disability. Am J Hum Genet 97(2):302–310
47. Li Y, Lin AW, Zhang X, Wang Y, Wang X, Goodrich DW (2007) Cancer cells and normal cells differ in their requirements for Thoc1. Cancer Res 67(14):6657–6664
48. Lim RYH, Fahrenkrog B, Köser J, Schwarz-Herion K, Deng J, Aebi U (2007) Nanomechanical basis of selective gating by the nuclear pore complex. Science 318(5850):640–643
49. Longman D, Johnstone IL, Cáceres JF (2003) The Ref/Aly proteins are dispensable for mRNA export and development in *Caenorhabditis elegans*. RNA 9(7):881–891
50. Loureiro JR, Oliveira CL, Silveira I (2016) Unstable repeat expansions in neurodegenerative diseases: nucleocytoplasmic transport emerges on the scene. Neurobiol Aging 39:174–183
51. Luna R, Gaillard H, González-Aguilera C, Aguilera A (2008) Biogenesis of mRNPs: integrating different processes in the eukaryotic nucleus. Chromosoma 117(4):319–331
52. Lund MK, Guthrie C (2005) The DEAD-box protein Dbp5p is required to dissociate Mex67p from exported mRNPs at the nuclear rim. Mol Cell 20(4):645–651
53. Luo ML, Zhou Z, Magni K, Christoforides C, Rappsilber J, Mann M et al (2001) Pre-mRNA splicing and mRNA export linked by direct interactions between UAP56 and Aly. Nature 413(6856):644–647
54. Masuda S, Das R, Cheng H, Hurt E, Dorman N, Reed R (2005) Recruitment of the human TREX complex to mRNA during splicing. Genes Dev 19(13):1512–1517
55. Milles S, Mercadante D, Aramburu IV, Jensen MR, Banterle N, Koehler C et al (2015) Plasticity of an ultrafast interaction between nucleoporins and nuclear transport receptors. Cell 163(3):734–745
56. Mitchell SF, Parker R (2014) Principles and properties of eukaryotic mRNPs. Mol Cell 54(4):547–558
57. Mori K, Arzberger T, Grässer FA, Gijselinck I, May S, Rentzsch K et al (2013) Bidirectional transcripts of the expanded C9orf72 hexanucleotide repeat are translated into aggregating dipeptide repeat proteins. Acta Neuropathol 126(6):881–893
58. Murakami K, Tsai K-L, Kalisman N, Bushnell DA, Asturias FJ, Kornberg RD (2015) Structure of an RNA polymerase II preinitiation complex. Proc Natl Acad Sci U S A 112(44):13543–13548
59. Mühlbauer D, Dzieciolowski J, Hardt M, Hocke A, Schierhorn KL, Mostafa A et al (2015) Influenza virus-induced caspase-dependent enlargement of nuclear pores promotes nuclear export of viral ribonucleoprotein complexes. J Virol 89(11):6009–6021

60. Müller-McNicoll M, Botti V, de Jesus Domingues AM, Brandl H, Schwich OD, Steiner MC et al (2016) SR proteins are NXF1 adaptors that link alternative RNA processing to mRNA export. Genes Dev 30(5):553–566
61. Nousiainen HO, Kestilä M, Pakkasjärvi N, Honkala H, Kuure S, Tallila J et al (2008) Mutations in mRNA export mediator GLE1 result in a fetal motoneuron disease. Nat Genet 40(2):155–157
62. Orr HT, Zoghbi HY (2007) Trinucleotide repeat disorders. Annu Rev Neurosci 30:575–621
63. Proudfoot NJ (2011) Ending the message: poly(A) signals then and now. Genes Dev 25(17):1770–1782
64. Ramaswami M, Taylor JP, Parker R (2013) Altered ribostasis: RNA-protein granules in degenerative disorders. Cell 154(4):727–736
65. Saito Y, Kasamatsu A, Yamamoto A, Shimizu T, Yokoe H, Sakamoto Y et al (2013) ALY as a potential contributor to metastasis in human oral squamous cell carcinoma. J Cancer Res Clin Oncol 139(4):585–594
66. Schmidt M, Finley D (2014) Regulation of proteasome activity in health and disease. Biochim Biophys Acta 1843(1):13–25
67. Schneider M, Hellerschmied D, Schubert T, Amlacher S, Vinayachandran V, Reja R et al (2015) The nuclear pore-associated TREX-2 complex employs mediator to regulate gene expression. Cell 162(5):1016–1028
68. Sofola OA, Jin P, Qin Y, Duan R, Liu H, de Haro M et al (2007) RNA-binding proteins hnRNP A2/B1 and CUGBP1 suppress fragile X CGG premutation repeat-induced neurodegeneration in a Drosophila model of FXTAS. Neuron 55(4):565–571
69. Sonenberg N, Hinnebusch AG (2009) Regulation of translation initiation in eukaryotes: mechanisms and biological targets. Cell 136(4):731–745
70. Speese SD, Ashley J, Jokhi V, Nunnari J, Barria R, Li Y et al (2012) Nuclear envelope budding enables large ribonucleoprotein particle export during synaptic Wnt signaling. Cell 149(4):832–846
71. Strässer K, Masuda S, Mason P, Pfannstiel J, Oppizzi M, Rodríguez-Navarro S et al (2002) TREX is a conserved complex coupling transcription with messenger RNA export. Nature 417(6886):304–308
72. Stutz F, Bachi A, Doerks T, Braun IC, Séraphin B, Wilm M et al (2000) REF, an evolutionarily conserved family of hnRNP-like proteins, interacts with TAP/Mex67p and participates in mRNA nuclear export. RNA 6(4):638–650
73. Sun X, Li PP, Zhu S, Cohen R, Marque LO, Ross CA et al (2015) Nuclear retention of full-length HTT RNA is mediated by splicing factors MBNL1 and U2AF65. Sci Rep 5:12521
74. Svejstrup JQ (2013) RNA polymerase II transcript elongation. Biochim Biophys Acta 1829(1):1
75. Takai H, Masuda K, Sato T, Sakaguchi Y, Suzuki T, Suzuki T et al (2014) 5-Hydroxymethylcytosine plays a critical role in glioblastomagenesis by recruiting the CHTOP-methylosome complex. Cell Rep 9(1):48–60
76. Taniguchi I, Ohno M (2008) ATP-dependent recruitment of export factor Aly/REF onto intronless mRNAs by RNA helicase UAP56. Mol Cell Biol 28(2):601–608
77. Todd PK, Oh SY, Krans A, He F, Sellier C, Frazer M et al (2013) CGG repeat-associated translation mediates neurodegeneration in fragile X tremor ataxia syndrome. Neuron 78(3):440–455
78. Tran H, Almeida S, Moore J, Gendron TF, Chalasani U, Lu Y et al (2015) Differential toxicity of nuclear RNA foci versus dipeptide repeat proteins in a drosophila model of C9ORF72 FTD/ALS. Neuron 87(6):1207–1214
79. Trcek T, Sato H, Singer RH, Maquat LE (2013) Temporal and spatial characterization of nonsense-mediated mRNA decay. Genes Dev 27(5):541–551
80. Tsoi H, Lau CK, Lau KF, Chan HYE (2011) Perturbation of U2AF65/NXF1-mediated RNA nuclear export enhances RNA toxicity in polyQ diseases. Hum Mol Genet 20(19):3787–3797
81. Umlauf D, Bonnet J, Waharte F, Fournier M, Stierle M, Fischer B et al (2013) The human TREX-2 complex is stably associated with the nuclear pore basket. J Cell Sci 126(Pt 12):2656–2667
82. van der Watt PJ, Maske CP, Hendricks DT, Parker MI, Denny L, Govender D et al (2009) The Karyopherin proteins, Crm1 and Karyopherin beta1, are overexpressed in cervical cancer and are critical for cancer cell survival and proliferation. Int J Cancer 124(8):1829–1840
83. Viphakone N, Cumberbatch MG, Livingstone MJ, Heath PR, Dickman MJ, Catto JW et al (2015) Luzp4 defines a new mRNA export pathway in cancer cells. Nucleic Acids Res 43(4):2353–2366
84. Viphakone N, Hautbergue GM, Walsh M, Chang C-T, Holland A, Folco EG et al (2012) TREX exposes the RNA-binding domain of Nxf1 to enable mRNA export. Nat Commun 3:1006
85. Walsh MJ, Cooper-Knock J, Dodd JE, Stopford MJ, Mihaylov SR, Kirby J et al (2015) Invited review: decoding the pathophysiological mechanisms that underlie RNA dysregulation in neurodegenerative disorders: a review of the current state of the art. Neuropathol Appl Neurobiol 41(2):109–134
86. Walsh MJ, Hautbergue GM, Wilson SA (2010) Structure and function of mRNA export adaptors. Biochem Soc Trans 38(Pt 1):232–236
87. Wickramasinghe VO, Laskey RA (2015) Control of mammalian gene expression by selective mRNA export. Nat Rev Mol Cell Biol 16(7):431–442
88. Wickramasinghe VO, McMurtrie PIA, Mills AD, Takei Y, Penrhyn-Lowe S, Amagase Y et al (2010) mRNA export from mammalian cell nuclei is dependent on GANP. Curr Biol 20(1):25–31
89. Wickramasinghe VO, Savill JM, Chavali S, Jonsdottir AB, Rajendra E, Grüner T et al (2013) Human inositol polyphosphate multikinase regulates transcript-selective nuclear mRNA export to preserve genome integrity. Mol Cell 51(6):737–750

90. Wickramasinghe VO, Venkitaraman AR (2016) RNA processing and genome stability: cause and consequence. Mol Cell 61(4):496–505
91. Wilson RC, Doudna JA (2013) Molecular mechanisms of RNA interference. Annu Rev Biophys 42:217–239
92. Wurth L (2012) Versatility of RNA-binding proteins in cancer. Comp Funct Genomics 2012:178525
93. Xu S, Powers MA (2009) Nuclear pore proteins and cancer. Semin Cell Dev Biol 20(5):620–630
94. Zu T, Gibbens B, Doty NS, Gomes-Pereira M, Huguet A, Stone MD et al (2011) Non-ATG-initiated translation directed by microsatellite expansions. Proc Natl Acad Sci U S A 108(1):260–265
95. Zu T, Liu Y, Bañez-Coronel M, Reid T, Pletnikova O, Lewis J et al (2013) RAN proteins and RNA foci from antisense transcripts in C9ORF72 ALS and frontotemporal dementia. Proc Natl Acad Sci U S A 110(51):E4968–E4977

Can Astrocytes Be a Target for Precision Medicine?

7

Chloe F. Allen, Pamela J. Shaw,
and Laura Ferraiuolo

Abstract

Astrocytes are the most abundant non-neural cell type residing within the central nervous system (CNS) displaying tremendous heterogeneity depending on their location. Once believed to be 'passive support cells for electrically active neurons', astrocytes are now recognised to play an active role in brain homeostasis by forming connections with the surrounding neurons, microglia and endothelial cells. Most importantly, they provide an optimum microenvironment for functional neurons through regulation of the blood brain barrier, energy supply and removal of debris and toxic waste.

Their dysfunction has been identified as a potential contributing factor for several neurodegenerative disorders, from Alzheimer's Disease to Amyotrophic Lateral Sclerosis.

In this chapter, we will explore the implications of astrocyte dysfunction in neurodegenerative diseases and how these cells can be used as therapeutic targets in precision medicine.

Keywords

Astrocytes • Neurodegeneration • Inflammation • Non-cell autonomous mechanism • Biomarkers • Transcriptomic analysis • High-throughput screening • Precision medicine

7.1 Astrocyte Function and Dysfunction in the Central Nervous System

Current research is discovering that many neurological diseases have shared pathological mechanisms; for example, neuroinflammation and

C.F. Allen • P.J. Shaw • L. Ferraiuolo (✉)
Department of Neuroscience, Sheffield Institute for Translational Neuroscience, University of Sheffield, Sheffield S10 2HQ, UK
e-mail: l.ferraiuolo@Sheffield.ac.uk

S. El-Khamisy (ed.), *Personalised Medicine*, Advances in Experimental Medicine and Biology 1007,
DOI 10.1007/978-3-319-60733-7_7

neuronal death in concomitance with accumulation of misfolded and oxidised protein aggregates are common features of Alzheimer's disease (AD), Parkinson's disease (PD) and Amyotrophic Lateral Sclerosis (ALS) [1–3]. Most of these phenomena have been associated not only with motor neuron degeneration, but also with astrocyte dysfunction. In the next few sections, some of the studies providing evidence for astrocytes role in maintaining CNS function will be summarised along with studies highlighting how failure in those same functions is involved in neurological diseases.

7.1.1 Brain Homeostasis

Astrocytes maintain brain homeostasis through strict regulation of ion distribution, osmotic balance and recycling of glutamate, the main excitatory neurotransmitter in the CNS [4]. Glutamate uptake by astrocytes is an essential process as a high extracellular concentration of glutamate causes over-activation of neurons which could lead to excitotoxicity or cell death. Glutamate is taken into the astrocytes by sodium-dependent glutamate transporter proteins which are present on the cell membrane. Within the astrocyte, glutamate is converted to glutamine by the enzyme glutamine synthase and is then converted back to glutamate at the synaptic terminal [5]. This uptake of glutamate stimulates glycolysis within astrocytes, resulting in the secretion of lactate to the surrounding neurons [6], which is an important source of energy.

The function of glutamate transporters can be impaired either by altered function, reduced expression or disrupted RNA synthesis of the protein; this leads to increased synaptic glutamate levels which cause excitotoxicity and neuronal death [7] (Fig. 7.1). Studies performed by Rothstein [8] and Bruijn [9] documented that astrocytes from the motor cortex and spinal cord of patients with sporadic or familial ALS, as well as mutant SOD1 (mSOD1) mouse models, had a reduced expression of the glutamate transporter EAAT2 (GLT-1 in mouse). Rothstein [10] discovered that complete knockdown of the glutamate transporter caused paralysis and motor neuron degeneration. In agreement with the finding that glutamate handling is impaired in ALS, the only treatment currently available for this disease is the antiglutamatergic drug Riluzole, the main function of which is to reduce the presynaptic release of glutamate to protect neurons from excitotoxicity [7].

7.1.2 Neuronal Development and Support

Astrocytes regulate neurite outgrowth through the production of growth promoting molecules, such as laminin, fibronectin, N-cadherin and neural cell adhesion molecule (NCAM), which guide the direction of growth during development or after injury [11]. They secrete growth factors essential for normal brain function, including neuronal growth factor (NGF), glial cell line-derived neurotrophic factor (GDNF), brain-derived growth factor (BDNF), glial maturation factor (GMF) and vascular endothelial growth factor (VEGF) [12]. Astrocytes have an important role in the protection of neuronal cells from oxidative damage and neurotoxins. Healthy astrocytes will increase their metabolic activity after brain injury or during disease to promote regenerative processes [12].

Studies using chimeric mice for mSOD1 discovered that there was a higher loss of motor neurons when they were surrounded by mSOD1 astrocytes than wild type astrocytes [13]. Multiple in vitro studies using post-mortem astrocytes from patients [14] or reprogrammed astrocytes from fibroblasts [15] have shown that astrocytes from ALS patients induce death of healthy motor neurons. Several pathways have been associated to this toxicity, but many aspects are still unknown. The study by Ferraiuolo [16] demonstrated that astrocytes derived from mSOD1 mouse models have altered lactate and nerve growth factor (NGF) processing which increases neuronal death signalling and vulnerability (Fig. 7.1).

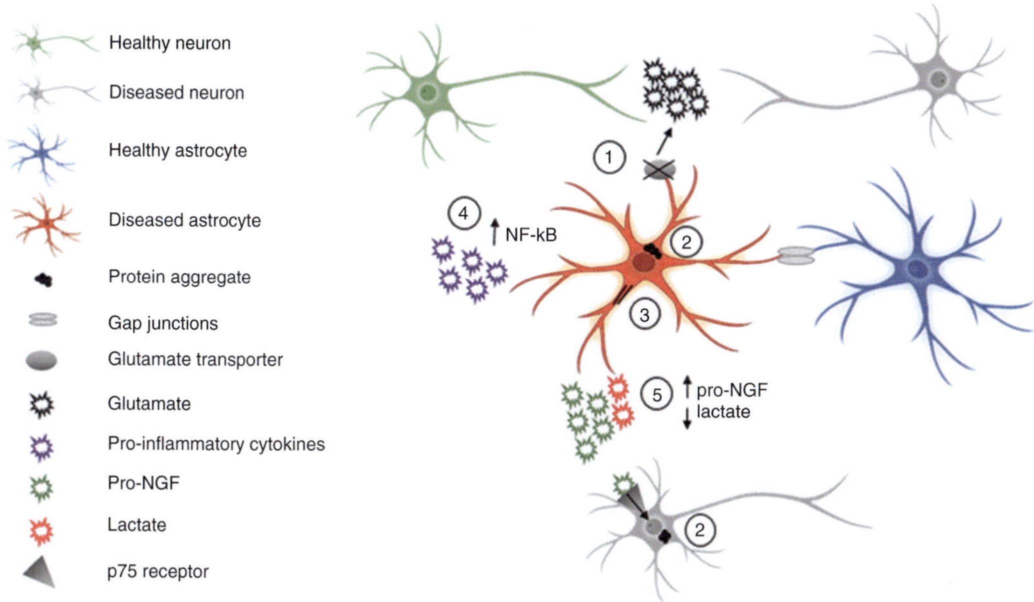

Fig. 7.1 Potential mechanisms of disease in astrocytes. (*1*) Dysregulation of glutamate transporters in astrocytes results in the accumulation of glutamate within the synaptic cleft and excitotoxicity. (*2*) The accumulation of protein aggregates, such as amyloid-β or misfolded SOD1, in neurons and astrocytes. (*3*) Upregulation of GFAP is a common feature of reactive astrocytes. (*4*) Increased NF-kB signalling promotes expression of pro-inflammatory cytokines leading to neuroinflammation. (*5*) Suggested increase in pro-NGF which binds to p75 receptor on neurons, increasing death signalling. Reduced lactate processing in astrocytes contributes to astrocyte toxicity to neurons

On the other hand, human and mouse studies appear to support the theory that astrocytes have a neuroprotective role in Parkinson's disease (PD). Depletion of nitric oxide and glutathione are common pathological hallmarks of PD. Exposure of astrocytes to nitric oxide seems to stimulate glutathione production in the astrocytes and it is thought that glutathione availability makes neurons less susceptible to reactive nitrogen species [7]. Data from patients with PD support this theory as the dopaminergic neurons were preserved when surrounded by glutathione-containing cells [17]. However, the role of astroglia in PD is still controversial and unexplained.

7.1.3 Blood Brain Barrier

The blood brain barrier (BBB) is a physical barrier of cells that prevents the exchange of molecules of a specific size and charge between the brain and the blood. The astrocytes form this barrier with the endothelial cells and pericytes of the brain microvessels [18]. They also regulate cerebral blood flow in response to neuronal activity by releasing potassium ions through their end feet onto the blood vessels [4]. Permeability of the BBB is regulated by tight junctions which are activated by NF-kB upregulation in astrocytes; astrocytes also regulate blood vessel dilation through the release of prostaglandins which stimulate calcium influx [18].

High-density lipoproteins move through the BBB to transport lipids into the brain tissue [19]. Astrocytes are responsible for the synthesis of the most abundant apolipoproteins in the CNS; ApoE and ApoJ [20]. Halliday [21] demonstrated that AD patients that were carriers for the APOE4 gene displayed accelerated pericyte degeneration at the BBB. APOE4 also contributed to the activation of the LRP1-dependent CypA–MMP-9 BBB-degrading pathway in the endothelial cells and pericytes, causing extensive damage to the BBB [21].

7.1.4 Inflammation and Immune Response

Since the brain has a limited capacity for regeneration, astrocytes must control inflammation and immune responses to prevent neuronal damage. They release neuroprotective factors towards endothelial cells to increase permeability of the BBB, including cytokine IL-1 and IL-6, macrophage inflammatory protein, endothelin-1 and tumour necrosis factor (TNF) [12]. Astrocytes regulate inflammation through the release of pro-inflammatory cytokines (IL-1, IL-6, and TNF) or anti-inflammatory molecules (prostaglandin E2 and transforming growth factor) [12]. They suppress the activity and induce apoptosis of T lymphocytes which are a source of neuroinflammation toxic to the CNS [22].

When astrocytes detect lesions in the brain, they undergo 'reactive astrogliosis'; the astrocytes become hypertrophic and rapidly proliferate, increasing glial fibrillary acidic protein (GFAP) expression which is the main marker for the astrogliotic response (Fig. 7.1). Reactive astrogliosis is often seen in the later stages of disease and can be triggered by either the deposition of toxic amyloid-β protein aggregates or dysfunctional neuronal signalling [4]. Transgenic AD animal models have demonstrated altered calcium signalling in astrocytes associated with these plaques [23]. These activated astrocytes undergo apoptosis, forming more amyloid plaques positive for common astrocyte markers GFAP and S100β [4].

Neuroinflammation is also a classic hallmark of ALS seen across both mouse models and human patients with familial and sporadic cases. Astrocytes and microglia positive for mSOD1 have been shown to express a multitude of pro-inflammatory genes [24]. Haidet-Phillips [14] found that the NF-kB pathway was the master regulator of inflammation in ALS astrocytes derived from post-mortem tissue using microarray analysis. Frakes [25] demonstrated that NF-kB signalling is activated in glia during disease progression in a mSOD1 mouse model, suggesting that NF-kB signalling regulates microglial activation in ALS.

7.2 Current Application of Personalised Medicine in Neurological Disorders

Since many neurological disorders share common pathological hallmarks, identifying the shared etiopathological mechanisms between diseases will allow the development of stratified therapeutics for more than one neurological disorder [26]. For example, cytoplasmic accumulation of TAR DNA-binding protein 43 (TDP-43) is seen in multiple neurodegenerative disorders; from ALS to frontotemporal dementia (FTD), thus creating a new spectrum of diseases called TDP-43 proteinopathies [27]. The study by Tan et al. [28], where the authors assessed the severity of TDP-43 pathology in selected brain regions of patients with ALS, FTD and AD, also proposed that the regional concentration of TDP-43 could potentially characterise these distinct clinical disorders. Advances in genetics have allowed medical professionals to make a start at personalising treatment for neurological disorders; however, these are still early days. To date the main efforts towards precision medicine have focused on a better classification of the patient population through the identification of disease-specific biomarkers, as highlighted in the following sections.

7.2.1 Alzheimer's Disease

AD is caused by a complex interplay of genetic, epigenetic and environmental factors that result in neuronal shrinkage and cell death, leading to progressive loss of cognition and memory. The main diagnostic hallmark is the accumulation of extracellular amyloid plaques which consist of amyloid-β and aggregated tau protein [29]. Due to the aging population, disease prevalence of AD is predicted to triple by 2050 [30].

Neurons that are surrounded by reactive astrocytes develop intracellular protein aggregates and axonal pathology which makes them more susceptible to cell death. In AD, it has been proposed that amyloid-β aggregates interfere with the gap junctions between astrocytes which could alter calcium signalling and glial communication [29]. Studies suggest that astrocytes are responsible for the clearance of the Aβ peptide to prevent the accumulation of these plaques [31].

Positron emission tomography (PET) technology is being used by clinicians to visualise these amyloid plaques in AD patients to assist in diagnosis and treatment [32]. Radioactive PET ligand 1 ([^{18}F]florbetapir) is used in the brain imaging of patients with cognitive defects to confirm a diagnosis of AD or other forms of dementia [33], while PET ligands 2 ([^{18}F]flutemetamol) and 3 ([18F]florbetaben) detect the presence of amyloid plaques [34, 35]. These ligands have a great potential to improve patient treatment through the monitoring of patients undergoing therapy, patient-risk analysis and patient selection for Aβ-targeting therapy. However, recent studies suggest that the abnormal aggregation of the tau protein has a greater contribution to neurodegeneration in AD, therefore detecting the severity of tau pathology may be a more effective biomarker than amyloid plaques [36]. One PET tau imaging agent has been clinically validated [37] and three more have reached clinical trials [38–40].

7.2.2 Parkinson's Disease

The cognitive impairment and dysfunctional control of movement in PD arises as the result of progressive dopaminergic neuron degeneration in the substantial nigra pars compacta and striatum [26]. On average, by the time of diagnosis patients will have already lost 60–70% of dopaminergic neurons [41], hence the need for biological indicators of disease progression early on.

In PD, microRNAs (miRNAs) are essential for neuron survival and previous studies have witnessed miRNA downregulation in the substantial nigra, frontal cortex and cerebellum of PD patients [42]. The study by Khoo and colleagues [41] identified 9 pairs of miRNAs that are predictive of PD and 13 differentially expressed miRNAs which could be potential biomarkers. After qPCR, replication and validation steps, this number was cut down to three candidate markers that showed the highest predictive biomarker performance: k-TSP1(miR-1826/miR-450b-3p), miR-626, and miR-505. Although the role of these miRNAs in PD pathogenesis is still unknown, previous studies have witnessed an upregulation of miR-1826 in the blood plasma of MS patients [43], miR-626 is overexpressed in the blood of glioblastoma patients [44] and miR-505 has been called a potential 'informative' biomarker present in the CSF of AD patients [45]. These diagnostic biomarkers are desperately required seeing as current diagnosis of PD relies on the clinical assessment of symptoms which occur once the neurons are heavily damaged [41]. Biofluids such as blood plasma and CSF are great resources for biomarkers however they have yet to be fully validated for use in clinical assessment [26].

7.2.3 Amyotrophic Lateral Sclerosis

ALS is associated with the progressive loss of motor neurons from the motor cortex, brain stem and spinal cord. It is estimated that 5–10% of patients have the hereditary form, known as familial ALS (fALS), while most patients are sporadic (90–95%). Devastatingly, 60% of patients die within 3 years of diagnosis normally due to respiratory failure and there is still only one treatment available, Riluzole, which provides only a modest benefit. Current research has discovered 23 genes associated with ALS; these account for approximately two-third of fALS and 10% of sporadic cases [46].

Mutant genes associated with ALS pathology, including TDP-43 and FUS, are directly involved in messenger RNA (mRNA) processing, indicating that miRNAs may play a role in the disease. The study by Butovsky [47] demonstrated that the inhibition of pro-inflammatory miR-155 in mSOD1 mice rescued mice from the disease phenotype through restoration of abnormal microglia, hinting the therapeutic potential of miRNAs in ALS.

Interestingly, miR-125b is expressed by microglia and has been shown to activate NF-kB signalling in the CNS through targeting the tumour necrosis factor alpha-induced protein 3 (TNFAIP3) A20. This microRNA has also been shown to regulate NF-κB-dependent inflammatory and oxidative stress pathways in both models of AD [48] and ALS [49], thus indicating that miR-125b may be a potential biomarker and therapeutic target in both diseases.

7.3 Astrocytes Driving the Future of Precision Medicine

As summarised in the previous section, astrocytes contribute to a series of toxic mechanisms affecting neuronal function and survival. Therefore, these cells are vital in the development of precision medicine either for cell replacement, genomics, biomarker identification and drug discovery.

7.3.1 Sources of Astrocytes

Studies show that transplanted astrocyte progenitor cells can survive and differentiate within the host brain, and have even been shown to slow down disease progression in ALS and Alzheimer animal models [50, 51]. However, these protocols require the isolation of astrocyte progenitor cells from the neonatal brain from which there is only a small supply. These cells also have a different immunoprofile to the host, causing rejection and immune response to transplantation, meaning that they have limited use in cell therapies [52].

In 2006, history was made when Takahashi and Yamanaka [53] demonstrated how to reprogram adult somatic cells into induced pluripotent stem cells (iPSCs) using four transcription factors; Klf4, Oct3/4, Sox2 and cMyc. This opened up a world of opportunities in the derivation of a huge supply of stem cells directly from diseased patients [4]. For example, the study by Chestkov [54] derived iPSC lines from ALS patient fibroblasts carrying the SOD1 mutation using either Sendai or lentivirus and further differentiated these lines into motor neurons.

Many studies have been able to reprogram astrocytes from human derived IPSCs [55, 56]. However, the problem is that these protocols are time-consuming, complex and are highly variable in the maturation time of the astrocytes (Table 7.1). Therefore, a promising alterative to iPSC resources is the direct reprogramming of fibroblasts into astrocytes from an immunomatched host [57].

Instead of generating IPSCs, direct reprogramming involves the use of cell-lineage transcription factors to convert adult somatic cells into another cell type [15]. This technology has been used to generate sub-specific neural lineages such as cholinergic, dopaminergic and motor neurons [62–64]. Meyer [15] decided to use direct reprogramming technology to derive astrocytes from ALS patient fibroblasts. Using the protocol from Kim [65], they generated tripotent induced neural progenitor cells (iNPCs) from ALS patients and controls within 1 month. When these cells were differentiated into astrocytes, they displayed similar toxicity towards motor neurons in co-cultures as autopsy-derived astrocytes [14], making them useful tools in the development of drug screens.

7.3.2 Astrocytes in Cellular Transplantation Therapy

Further effort is being invested in the development of cellular replacement therapy for neurodegenerative disease as it can provide therapeutic benefit through not only cell replenishment but also by reducing inflammation and protein aggregates [57].

Both microglia and astrocytes are capable of phagocytosing and degrading amyloid-β deposits in the brain [31, 66]. In the study by Pihlaja et al. [51], the authors transplanted both mature and neonatal mouse astrocytes into the brains of AD

Table 7.1 Protocols for astroglial differentiation from stem cells

Cell source	Method of differentiation	Key transcription/growth factors	Astrocyte outcome	References
hESCs	Neurospheres	Heparin: 2 μg/ml FGF2: 20 ng/ml BDNF/GDNF: 10 ng/ml cAMP: 1 μM Ascorbic acid: 200 μM	Astrocytes appeared after 9 weeks	[58]
hESCs and iPSC	Embryoid bodies	Retinoic acid: 0.5 μm FGF8: 50 ng/ml SHH: 500 ng/ml EGF/FGF2: 10 ng/ml CNTF/LIF: 10 ng/ml	Populations of immature astrocytes	[59, 60]
hESCs and hIPSC	Embryoid bodies	SB43152: 10 μM Noggin: 500 ng/ml	55–70% GFAP+ cells after 5 weeks	[61]
hIPSC	Neurospheres/EZ spheres	EGF/FGF2: 20 ng/ml CNTF: 10 μl/ml	90% GFAP+ cells after 9 weeks	[56]
mESC, hESC and hIPSC	Monolayer	LDN193189: 0.2 μM SB43152: 10 μM Ascorbic acid: 0.4 μg/ml Retinoic acid: 1 μM BDNF/GDNF: 10 ng/ml	100% S100β+ and 70% GFAP+ cells after 80 days	[55]
mEF, hfibroblast	Direct reprogramming	Lentiviral vectors: NFIA, NFIB, SOX9 TFs	Astrocytes derived from fibroblasts after 2–3 weeks	[52]
hfibroblast	Direct reprogramming	Retroviral vectors: Klf4, Oct3/4, Sox2 and c-Myc FGF2/EGF: 20 ng/ml Heparin: 5 μl/ml DMEM: 10% FBS and 0.3% N2	iAstrocytes generated from patients in less than 4 weeks	[15]

mouse models and ex vivo human AD brain sections. In these brain sections, only adult astrocytes were able to internalise the amyloid-β deposits, however both adult and neonatal astrocytes were able to remove aggregates in vivo within 1–7 days of transplantation. This study suggests that therapeutic strategies looking into the transplantation of amyloid-β-clearing astrocytes or promoting endogenous astrocytes to degrade these toxic aggregates [51] might lead to positive results.

Experimental therapies for PD are focused on preventing dopaminergic neuron loss using pharmacological compounds or transplantation of new dopaminergic neurons [67]. The transplantation of astrocytes derived from glial-restricted precursor cells exposed to bone morphogenetic protein (GDA^{BMP}) into injured spinal cord have promoted the survival of multiple neuron populations [68]. Proschel [67] demonstrated that the delayed transplantation of rat or human GDA^{BMP} cells into an experimental model of PD rescued parvalbumin-positive GABAergic interneurons, a population that has not been rescued by any other experimental treatment, and restored synaptophysin expression which is essential for synaptic function. Unlike previous cell transplantation methods in PD, GDA^{BMP} do not require genetic modification prior to transplantation since they intrinsically produce multiple therapeutic molecules against PD symptoms, including BDNF, GDNF [68], neurotrophic factors, synaptogenic modulators and the antioxidant glutathione. The ability of these cells to target multiple problems within the PD model indicate the potential of using astrocytes as a vehicle for restoration of the CNS [67].

Human derived neural stem/progenitor cells (NSC/NPC) are a promising tool for cell replacement due to their plasticity and the ability to differentiate into neurons, astrocytes and oligodendrocytes. The study by Das [69] injected young and aged rats with human NPCs derived from the foetal brain to investigate if cell replacement therapy could rescue motor neuron function in aging. There was a short-term motor neuron rescue seen in young rats receiving NPC injections, although there was a much more robust NPC survival and migration towards the aged motor neurons. Unfortunately, the implantation of NPCs had no positive effect on motor neuron function as they were unable to provide protection to neuromuscular junction (NMJ) innervation, preventing motor neurons from innervating and stimulating the muscle [69].

Human IPSCs represent an alternative source to human derived-NSCs. Transplantation of human IPSC-derived neural progenitor cells into mSOD1 mice have been shown to differentiate into healthy astrocytes, upregulate expression of neurotrophic factors and increase survival of mice [70]. A second study by Nizzardo [71] also found that the transplantation of neural stem cells enhanced neuronal survival and maintained NMJ integrity in mSOD1 mice. The authors suggest that the implanted NSCs secrete growth factors that inhibit the GSK3β pathway, preventing motor neuron death. Cellular transplantation of NSC might directly protect motor neurons from degeneration and indirectly by antagonising the toxic effects of astrocytes [71].

One question that arises is why did the IPSC-derived NPCs in Nizzardo's study improved motor function and the human-derived NSCs in Das's study did not? Das [69] suggests that the dysfunctional microenvironment in ALS is more susceptible to NSC survival than the wildtype environment due to the higher availability of space, more permissible factors or the weakened immune system of the model, indicating the NSCs are more likely to survival and exert beneficial effects within the ALS model.

The promising results from these studies in rodents have led to attempts to translate this into clinical trials for patients (https://clinicaltrials.gov/ct2/home). Clinical trials using transplantation of glia progenitors for ALS and other diseases are listed in Table 7.2.

7.3.3 Astrocytes in Genomics and Transcriptomics

As highlighted in the previous sections, astrocytes have been identified as key players in disease development in several neurodegenerative disorders. Gene expression profiling has greatly contributed to uncover the molecular mechanisms underlying the progression of neurodegenerative diseases, helping us identify specific biochemical pathways and cellular processes that are altered by disease. Gene expression profiles of the CNS are difficult to comprehend due to the complex interplay of microglia and astrocytes interspersed between different neuronal subtypes. This means that cell specific gene expression changes cannot be detected when analysing the whole brain tissue [72].

To overcome this problem, several studies have used laser capture microdissection (LCM) in order to isolate single cells from brain or spinal cord and obtain a highly enriched cell population for transcriptomic analysis [16, 73–75]. These studies led to the identification of pathways specifically activated/altered in astrocytes during disease.

In a longitudinal study analysing astrocytes isolated from the spinal cord of mSOD1 mice throughout disease, the lactate shuttle between astrocytes and neurons was identified as altered at the pre-symptomatic stage of ALS for the first time [16]. As disease progresses, inflammatory pathways and cytokine production increase, along with astrocytic lysosomal and phagocytic activity [73].

Simpson et al. [76], by analysing different post-mortem brain areas from AD patients, identified dysregulation of genes associated with cell proliferation, apoptosis, and ubiquitin-mediated proteolysis at low Braak stages, while they found

Table 7.2 Current clinical trials using transplantation of glia progenitors for ALS and other neurological diseases (https://clinicaltrials.gov/ct2/home)

Study name	Condition	Intervention
Safety of the injection of human glial restricted progenitor cells into subjects with ALS	ALS	Transplantation of human glia progenitor cells
Dose escalation and safety study of human spinal cord derived neural stem cell transplantation in ALS patients	ALS	Transplantation of human spinal cord stem cells
Transplantation of human neural progenitor cells secreting GDNF for the treatment of ALS	ALS	Transplantation of human glia progenitor cells
Safety and tolerability of fetal mesencephalic dopamine neuronal precursor cells for Parkinson's disease	PD	Transplantation of mesencephalic neuronal precursor cells
Embryonic dopamine cell implants for Parkinson's disease	PD	Transplantation of embryonic dopamine cell implants
Infusion of recombinant-Methionyl human GDNF for the treatment of idiopathic PD	PD	Administration of recombinant-methionyl human GDNF
Infusion of recombinant-Methionyl human GDNF to treat progressive Supranuclear palsy (PSP)	PSP	Administration of recombinant-methionyl human GDNF

that altered regulation of intracellular signaling pathways, including insulin, phosphatidylinositol 3-kinase (PI3K)/Akt, and mitogen-activated protein kinase (MAPK) pathways were primarily associated with high levels of Alzheimer-type pathology, and occurred at lower Braak stages in individuals with the APOEε4 allele. These studies identified valuable therapeutic targets, either based upon timing of disease [16, 73] or brain regions associated with specific genetic mutations [76].

One of the limitations of LCM is the length of the process as well as the potential contamination with surrounding cells. Srinivasan and coleagues [72] generated a method of isolating neuronal and non-neuronal cell types simultaneously from brain tissue without these limitations. All enzymatic incubations were performed at 4 °C or on ice and specific cell types were immunolabelled, for example, anti-GFAP label for astrocytes, anti-CD11b for microglia and anti-NeuN for neurons. The authors generated sequencing data from specific cell type populations derived from the brain tissue of mouse models and human patients with FTD, ALS and AD [72]. From this data, they determined that the different patterns of gene expression in disease is due to the altered cellular composition of the brain tissue rather than changes in transcriptional regulation patterns. In ALS and FTD, there was a recurring trend of lower neuronal RNA expression and higher levels of astrocytic and microglia RNA which reflected the altered neuron to glia ratio due to neuronal loss. However, the authors were unsure as to how representative the population of purified cells are to the tissue as transcripts were only derived from the cell body; dendrites and axons were lost during dissociation [72].

Gene expression analysis is often used to identify therapeutic targets, however, an interesting approach has been undertaken by Aronica et al. [77] The authors performed whole-genome expression analysis of post-mortem cortex tissue from sporadic ALS (sALS) patients and normal controls to explore the entire spectrum of genetic and molecular pathways in ALS pathology. Using these data, they were able to distinguish between patient and control samples, and then further subdivide the patients into two groups which had similar expression profile changes. However, the authors argue that a much larger sample size is required in order to categorise patients by clinical characteristics [77]. Molecular taxonomy of patients through gene expression analysis has been used in cancer to diagnose and develop personalised therapies [78]. This taxonomy could also be used in sALS patients to uncover hidden pathogenic mechanisms and develop personalised treatment [77].

A similar approach was also taken by Wang and colleagues [79]. The authors analysed the transcription profile of 19 cortical regions from 125 individuals with a severity spectrum of dementia and neuropathology of AD. Comparing their data with single-cell RNA-sequencing data, the authors determined that the cells mainly contributing to the transcriptional alterations were neurons, astrocytes and oligodendrocytes. Their contribution was different in different brain regions, thus suggesting that pathology is driven by selective regional vulnerability. By analysing the data in terms of degree of severity, the authors observed that most of the transcriptional changes occur early in the disease and astrocytes and oligodendrocyte play a crucial role in neuronal death.

7.3.4 Astrocytes in Diagnostic and Prognostic Biomarkers

Biomarkers are proteins, lipids or mutant transcripts associated with disease that can be used to tract normal or abnormal biological processes [80]. They can be divided into three subcategories; prognostic (determine stage of disease), therapeutic (determine the right drug at the right dose) and predictive (the effectiveness of treatment) [81]. A good biomarker is tested on the sensitivity, specificity and positive predictive value; new technology such as genomics, proteomics and bioinformatics can be used to help develop more accurate biomarkers [82]. This is important for the advancement of medicine as novel biomarkers increase treatment efficiency and safety and reduce the cost of diagnostic methods and treatments [81].

An effective way of monitoring neurological disease would be using serum biomarkers. This minimally invasive technique is able to detect brain-specific pathology and is reflective of the health status of the glial cells [83]. Previous studies have detected GFAP in the blood serum both before and after traumatic brain injury [84]. Using GFAP as a clinical biomarker could be a cost-effective replacement to expensive imaging scans while retaining diagnostic sensitivity [83]. Another astrocyte marker S100β has also been detected in the blood of patients with neurological disorders [85]. This gene is mainly expressed by mature astrocytes and is responsible for regulation of calcium signalling and apoptosis in the surrounding glial cells [83]. A comparison study between S100β and GFAP found that S100β rose and peaked within the serum at 2 h post-injury while GFAP rose more steadily over the first 4 h after injury [84]. Shepheard et al. [86] validated the use of the extracellular domain of the neurotrophin receptor p75 (p75NTR^{ECD}) as a candidate marker for ALS; there were increased levels of p75NTR^{ECD} detected in the urine of human ALS patients and mSOD1 mice. This links back to the study by Ferriauolo [16] which demonstrated that the increased activation of pro-nerve growth factor and p75 signalling were important components of astrocyte toxicity in ALS.

During reactive astrogliosis, there is a wide variety of gene expression changes which could be used as medical biomarkers to tract disease progress. PET tracers can detect neuroinflammation and microglial activation through the expression of the translocator protein (TSPO) on the outer mitochondrial membrane [87]. Studies show that TSPO expression is globally nonexistent in a healthy brain, but the expression rapidly increases during astrocytic/microglial activation and neuroinflammation [88], making TSPO an attractive biomarker for targeting reactive gliosis in cerebral inflammation and imaging microglial activation [87].

Another potential biomarker is the type 2 cannabinoid receptor (CB2R) which is virtually undetectable in healthy tissue but greatly expressed in activated astrocyte and microglial cells [89]. This receptor is also found in macrophages and peripheral T lymphocytes as it is involved in central and peripheral inflammatory

Table 7.3 Patient response to L-dopa mediation variation based on individual genetic mutations

Gene	Polymorphism	Drug response to L-dopa	References
BDNF	rs6265 (Val66Met)	Significantly higher risk of developing dyskinesias early on in course	[99]
ACE	rs4646994	Risk of L-dopa-induced psychosis	[100]
APOE	rs429358 rs7412 (e2, e3, e4)	No association with L-dopa-induced dyskinesias	[101]
OPRMI	rs1799971 (118A>G, Asn40Asp)	Increased risk of earlier onset of dyskinesia	[102]
MAOB	rs1799836 intron 13	No association with L-dopa dosage.	[96]
GBA	Various mutations	Higher risk of L-dopa induced dyskinesias	[103, 104]

responses [90]. Previous studies have discovered PET ligands of CB2 receptors that could be potential biomarkers for multiple sclerosis (MS) [91, 92].

Monoamine oxidase type B, located the outer mitochondrial membrane, is also greatly expressed in reactive astrocytes in neurological disease [93]. It is responsible for the modulation of neurotransmitter concentrations, making it a major drug target for movement disorders [94]. Gulyas et al. [95] reported increased monoamine oxidase type B expression in reactive astrocytes of AD patients and it is currently beginning investigated in MS [94].

7.3.5 Astrocytes in Drug Screening

Over the previous decades, research has been focusing on how genetic differences between individuals can lead to variations in patient drug response, giving rise to pharmacogenetics which aims to tailor drug choice and dosage based on the individual patient's genome for optimal therapeutic benefit. Neurodegenerative diseases demonstrate widespread genetic variability, hence there is a broad range of patient responses to prescribed medications, in both terms of efficiency and adverse reactions [96]. The acetylcholinesterase inhibitor Donepezil is the main prescribed drug treatment for AD, providing a modest benefit on cognitive function, behaviour and disease progression in both moderate and severe AD patients [97]. Approximately 15–20% of patients demonstrate abnormal metabolism of the drug, depending on the function of CYP-related enzymes CYP2D6, CYP3A4, and CYP1A2. The CYP2D6 locus has more than 100 different polymorphisms which define whether a patient is a poor, normal or ultra-rapid metaboliser of the drug [97]. In PD, 80% of patients treated with levodopa demonstrate positive benefits to initial therapy, but 45% of these patients develop levodopa-induced dyskinesias within 5 years of treatment [98]. Genetic research has identified multiple genetic polymorphisms as strong candidates for determination of safety and efficiency of levodopa treatment, see table, however many of these are still controversial [96] (Table 7.3).

CNS drug development has slowed down since the 1990s as the candidate drugs often fail at the later stages of clinical trials. Almost all experimental drugs for ALS have failed clinical trials, potentially due to the unreliability and species differences of current animal models [105] or the heterogeneity of the patient population included in the trial. To overcome this problem, Isobe [106] used hESC-derived motor neurons with identical genetic backgrounds but differing mutations in SOD1 to investigate whether different SOD1 mutations might lead to different drug response. Surprisingly, through this model, they discovered mutant-specific morphological alterations within the motor neurons and differential drug responses. This result indicates that most likely heterogeneous patient populations will not benefit from the same drug treatment, thus indicating that there is a great need for targeted precision medicine.

Consistently, the study by Shichinohe [107] found that the compound MCI-189 only provided neuroprotective effects to motor neurons expressing the G93A-SOD1 variant. This suggests that neuroprotective drugs may be effective at treating ALS phenotypes with specific SOD1 mutations. There are currently no reports that astrocytes also display these SOD1 mutation-dependent drug responses but this question should be addressed if we are to attempt to classify ALS into treatment-responsive categories.

Studies using transgenic AD mouse models have found that GFAP expression changes in astrocytes between different regions in the brain and at different stages of disease progression [108, 109], reinforcing that subpopulations of astrocytes play separate roles in disease. Barbeito and collaborators [110] isolated an astrocyte subpopulation from the spinal cord of transgenic mSOD1 rats, which he referred to as 'aberrant astrocytes' due to their fierce proliferation capacity. These aberrant cells were morphologically different to primary neonatal astrocytes, lacked detectable GLT-1 expression and their condition medium was specifically toxic to motor neurons [110]. These astrocytes are considered a distinct subpopulation of highly toxic astrocytes which could represent an additional cellular target for future treatment of ALS [111].

Drug screening in cellular cultures is a process traditionally mainly used by pharmaceutical companies to identify candidate compounds for further investigation but with the development of new automated systems and widespread availability of screening facilities, academic sites have also embarked in high-throughput drug screening [112].

Most drugs have a targeted approach; companies develop drugs that target only one gene or biological pathway which selectively helps to treat the disease while avoiding adverse effects. However, drugs with a selective target do not always deliver an effective treatment, as target engagement and phenotypic effect do not always match, due to the complexity of neurological diseases. For this reason, more effort has been invested in developing phenotypic screenings with a disease-relevant readout.

These cell culture models normally consist of 2D cultures containing neuronal-like cells such as neuroblastoma [113] or patient derived IPS cells [114]. However, 3D cultures of interacting cell types from different tissues are needed to be fully representative of the organ system, as the establishment of cell-cell and cell-extracellular matrix interactions in in vitro 3D models tries to mimic the tissue microenvironment [115]; reducing the gap between animal models and human trials [116].

Whilst high content imaging, combined with high-throughput drug screening, has been applied to primary neurons [117, 118], iPSC-derived neural progenitors [119] and motor neurons [120], very few studies so far have focused on astrocytes and neurons co-cultures [121, 122] and only one used cells from ALS patients [122].

Rinaldi and colleagues [122] described a robust 96-well assay to identify drugs that can dampen ALS astrocyte toxicity against motor neurons Z-score (0.679), thus supporting the idea that astrocytes and co-culture screenings can be used for precision medicine.

The identification of pharmacological agents for PD has proved slow going due to the limited availability of human cell-based neuronal models. The study by Efremova [123] combined immortalized mesencephalic neuronal precursors differentiated into post-mitotic dopaminergic neurons and immortalized murine astrocytes to create a potential new co-culture model to test experimental neuroprotective compounds against the toxic compound MPTP (1-methyl-4-phenyl-1,2,3,6-tetrahydropyridine). The most striking finding from this study was the different efficacy of the neuroprotective compounds between mono- and co-cultures. This lack of protection in the co-culture assays could be explained by compounds being metabolised or modified by the astrocytes or that neuronal metabolism and cell death mechanisms might be altered in the presence of astrocytes, potentially indicating that astrocytes respond differently to different drugs [123].

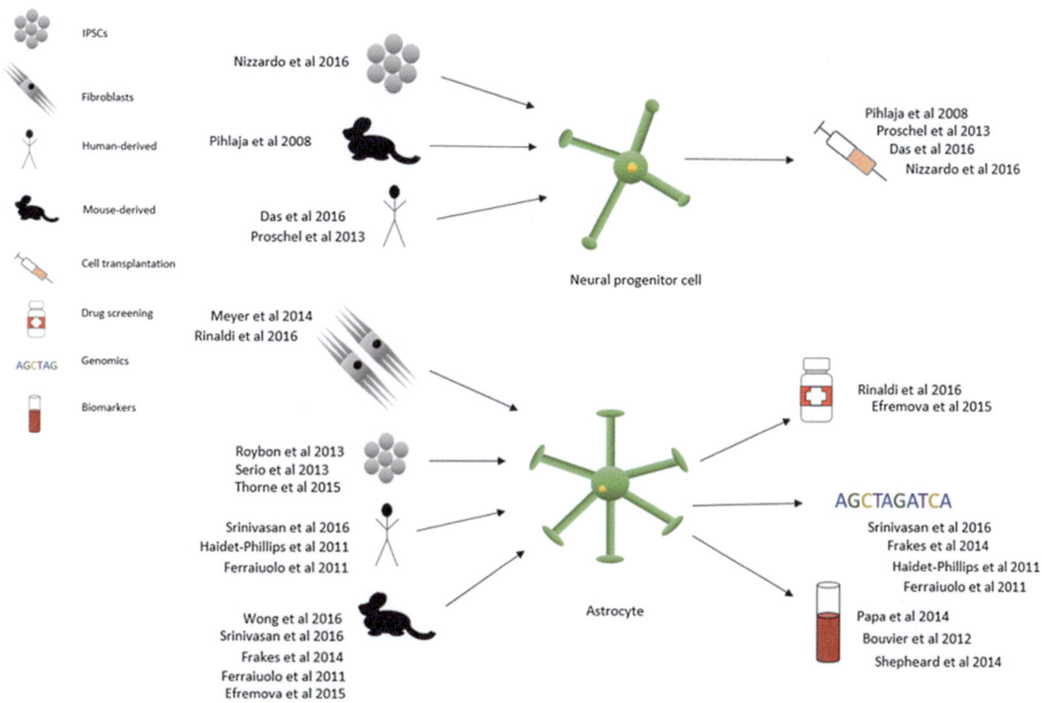

Fig. 7.2 Astrocytes as a target for personalised medicine. Astrocytes and NPCs can be harvested from mice or human brain or spinal cord or derived from fibroblasts or stem cells using differentiation and reprogramming technologies. They have a wide variety of uses in cellular transplantation theraphy, drug screening, screening, genomic expression and biomaker studies

7.4 Conclusion

More personalised approaches to medicine are being investigated in neurological disease because of the gap between patient disease variability and categorisation, possibly resulting in overall failure of clinical trials [26]. The desperate need for better patient classification and effective drugs converge in the concept of precision medicine, where patients with a certain "profile" can be identified as responders or non-responders to a treatment. An overwhelming amount of evidence has indicated that glial cells [79, 124, 125] contribute to the early phases of neurodegeneration.

Astrocytes are the cellular backbone of the CNS, providing support to the neurons through formation of the blood brain barrier, glutamate regulation, cellular communication, inflammation and the immune response. Therefore, it is not surprising that neurodegenerative diseases occur in concomitance with astrocytes dysfunction. In this book chapter we have tried to highlight the many pathways controlled by astrocytes and how their failure contributes to neurological disease in a wide variety of ways; dysfunction of glutamate transport, reactive astrogliosis and neuroinflammation, altered metabolism and growth factor secretion to mention a few.

In terms of precision medicine, astrocytes could be used to predict disease susceptibility, monitoring disease progression and developing the right drug at the right dose for treatment of patients (Fig. 7.2). The technology generated by Takahasi and Yamanaka [53] has opened up a world of opportunities in the derivation of a huge supply of stem cells directly from diseased patients which could help treat and understand disease. Cellular reprogramming could be used to derive patient fibroblasts into astrocytes and these astrocytes would behave uniquely to that patient phenotype. Patient astrocytes could be used in drug screening to identify new target compounds and understand the underlying mechanisms of drug treatment [122] (Fig. 7.2). These methods could be used to either individualise drug treatment or stratify it to a subgroup with similar mutations or genetic setup. To provide further evidence to back up the drug screening analysis, astrocytes could be used to study what genes the patient expresses, identify possible drug treatments and discover drug mechanisms through RNA sequencing post drug treatment (Fig. 7.2). Biomarkers allow us to tract the abnormal biological processes that arise during disease. Identification of these protein aggregates in fibroblast-derived patient astrocytes could be used as diagnostic biomarkers or prognosis in response to treatment.

Precision medicine is moving medicine away from the 'one size fits all' therapy, which is important for complex mainly sporadic disorders like ALS, AD and PD where the patient gene expression profile is as unique as a fingerprint. Further experimental investigation of patient-derived astrocytes is required to explore their potential as a tool for precision medicine, but their overpowering number and varied functions make them the ideal therapeutic target. Astrocyte manipulation can, in fact, lead to a complete modification of the environment surrounding injured neurons, thus potentially halting degeneration.

References

1. Lashley T, Rohrer JD, Mead S, Revesz T (2015) Review: an update on clinical, genetic and pathological aspects of frontotemporal lobar degenerations. Neuropathol Appl Neurobiol 41:858–881
2. Li W et al (2016) Neuropharmacologic approaches to restore the Brain's microenvironment. J NeuroImmune Pharmacol 11:484–494
3. Renton AE et al (2012) A hexanucleotide repeat expansion in C9ORF72 is the cause of chromosome 9p21-linked ALS-FTD. Neuron 72:257–268
4. Chandrasekaran A, Avci HX, Leist M, Kobolák J, Dinnyés A (2016) Astrocyte differentiation of human pluripotent stem cells: new tools for neurological disorder research. Front Cell Neurosci 10:215
5. Parpura V, Verkhratsky A (2012) Astrocytes revisited: concise historic outlook on glutamate homeostasis and signaling. Croat Med J 53:518–528
6. Pellerin L, Magistretti PJ (2012) Sweet sixteen for ANLS. J Cereb Blood Flow Metab 32:1152–1166
7. Maragakis NJ, Rothstein JD (2006) Mechanisms of disease: astrocytes in neurodegenerative disease. Nat Clin Pr Neurol 2:679–689
8. Rothstein JD, Martin LJ, Kungl RW (1992) Decreased glutamate transport by the brain and spinal cord in amyotrophic lateral sclerosis. N Engl J Med 326:1464–1468
9. Bruijn LI et al (1997) ALS-linked SOD1 mutant G85R mediates damage to astrocytes and promotes rapidly progressive disease with SOD1-containing inclusions. Neuron 18:327–338
10. Rothstein JD et al (1996) Knockout of glutamate transporters reveals a major role for astroglial transport in excitotoxicity and clearance of glutamate. Neuron 16:675–686
11. Wang DD, Bordey A (2008) The astrocyte odyssey. Prog Neurobiol 86:342–367
12. Jurič DM, Kržan M, Lipnik-Stangelj M (2016) Histamine and astrocyte function. Pharmacol Res 111:774–783
13. Clement AM et al (2003) Wild-type nonneuronal cells extend survival of SOD1 mutant motor neurons in ALS mice. Science (80-) 302:113–117
14. Haidet-Phillips AM et al (2012) Astrocytes from familial and sporadic ALS patients are toxic to motor neurons. Nat Biotechnol 29:824–828
15. Meyer K et al (2014) Direct conversion of patient fibroblasts demonstrates non-cell autonomous toxicity of astrocytes to motor neurons in familial and sporadic ALS. Proc Natl Acad Sci U S A 111:829–832
16. Ferraiuolo L et al (2011) Dysregulation of astrocyte-motoneuron cross-talk in mutant superoxide dismutase 1-related amyotrophic lateral sclerosis. Brain 134:2627–2641
17. Heales S, Lam A, Duncan A, Land J (2004) Neurodegeneration or neuroprotection: the pivotal role of astrocytes. Neurochem Res 29:513–519
18. Abbott NJ, Rönnbäck L, Hansson E (2006) Astrocyte–endothelial interactions at the blood–brain barrier. Nat Rev Neurosci 7:41–53
19. Erdő F, Denes L, de Lange E (2017) Age-associated physiological and pathological changes at the blood–brain barrier: a review. J Cereb Blood Flow Metab 37:4–24
20. Wang H, Eckel RH (2014) What are lipoproteins doing in the brain? Trends Endocrinol Metab 25:8–14
21. Halliday MR et al (2016) Accelerated pericyte degeneration and blood-brain barrier breakdown in apolipoprotein E4 carriers with Alzheimer's disease. J Cereb Blood Flow Metab 36:216–227
22. Gimsa U, Mitchison NA, Brunner-Weinzierl MC (2013) Immune privilege as an intrinsic CNS prop-

erty: astrocytes protect the CNS against T-cell-mediated neuroinflammation. Mediat Inflamm 2013
23. Kuchibhotla KV, Lattarulo CR, Hyman BT, Bacskai BJ (2009) Synchronous hyperactivity and intercellular calcium waves in astrocytes in Alzheimer mice. Science (80-) 323:1211–1215
24. Philips T, Rothstein J (2014) Glial cells in amyotrophic lateral sclerosis. Exp Neurol 262PB:111–120
25. Frakes AE et al (2014) Microglia induce motor neuron death via the classical NF-kB pathway in amyotrophic lateral sclerosis. Neuron 81:1009–1023
26. Gotovac K, Hajnšek S, Pašić MB, Pivac N, Borovečki F (2014) Personalized medicine in neurodegenerative diseases: how far away? Mol Diagn Ther 18:17–24
27. Geser F, Lee VMY, Trojanowski JQ (2010) Amyotrophic lateral sclerosis and frontotemporal lobar degeneration: a spectrum of TDP-43 proteinopathies. Neuropathology 30:103–112
28. Tan RH et al (2015) TDP-43 proteinopathies: pathological identification of brain regions differentiating clinical phenotypes. Brain 138:3110–3122
29. Cruz NF, Ball KK, Dienel GA (2010) Astrocytic gap junctional communication is reduced in amyloid-β-treated cultured astrocytes, but not in Alzheimer's disease transgenic mice. ASN Neuro 2:e00041
30. Hebert LE, Weuve J, Scherr PA, Evans DA (2013) Alzheimer disease in the United States (2010–2050) estimated using the 2010 census. Neurology 80:1778–1783
31. Wyss-Coray T et al (2003) Adult mouse astrocytes degrade amyloid-beta in vitro and in situ. Nat Med 9:453–457
32. Bolognesi ML, Gandini A, Prati F, Uliassi E (2016) From companion diagnostics to theranostics: a new avenue for Alzheimer's disease? J Med Chem. acs.jmedchem.6b00151. doi:10.1021/acs.jmedchem.6b00151
33. Yang L, Rieves D, Ganley C (2012) Brain amyloid imaging – FDA approval of florbetapir F18 injection. N Engl J Med 367:885–887
34. Mason NS, Mathis CA, Klunkc WE (2013) Positron emission tomography radioligands for in vivo imaging of Aβ plaques. J Label Compd Radiopharm 56:89–95
35. Abou-Gharbia M, Childers WE (2014) Discovery of innovative therapeutics: today's realities and tomorrow's vision. 2. Pharma's challenges and their commitment to innovation. J Med Chem 57:5525–5553
36. Villemagne VL, Fodero-Tavoletti MT, Masters CL, Rowe CC (2015) Tau imaging: early progress and future directions. Lancet Neurol 14:114–124
37. Maruyama M et al (2013) Imaging of tau pathology in a tauopathy mouse model and in Alzheimer patients compared to normal controls. Neuron 79:1094–1108
38. Xia CF et al (2013) [(18)F]T807, a novel tau positron emission tomography imaging agent for Alzheimer's disease. Alzheimers Dement 9:666–676
39. Villemagne VL et al (2014) In vivo evaluation of a novel tau imaging tracer for Alzheimer's disease. Eur J Nucl Med Mol Imaging 41:816–826
40. Harada R et al (2016) 18F-THK5351: a novel PET radiotracer for imaging neurofibrillary pathology in Alzheimer's disease. J Nucl Med 57:208–214
41. Khoo SK et al (2012) Plasma-based circulating microRNA biomarkers for Parkinson's disease. J Parkinsons Dis 2:321–331
42. Miñones-Moyano E et al (2011) MicroRNA profiling of Parkinson's disease brains identifies early downregulation of miR-34b/c which modulate mitochondrial function. Hum Mol Genet 20:3067–3078
43. Siege SR, MacKenzie J, Chaplin G, Jablonski NG, Griffiths L (2012) Circulating microRNAs involved in multiple sclerosis. Mol Biol Rep 39:6219–6225
44. Dong L et al (2014) miRNA microarray reveals specific expression in the peripheral blood of glioblastoma patients. Int J Oncol 45:746–756
45. Denk J et al (2015) MicroRNA profiling of CSF reveals potential biomarkers to detect Alzheimer's disease. PLoS One 10:1–18
46. Zou Z-Y, Liu C-Y, Che C-H, Huang H-P (2016) Toward precision medicine in amyotrophic lateral sclerosis. Ann Transl Med 4:27
47. Butovsky O et al (2016) Targeting miR-155 restores abnormal microglia and attenuates disease in SOD1 mice. Ann Neurol 77:75–99
48. Zhao Y et al (2014) Regulation of neurotropic signaling by the inducible, NF-kB-sensitive miRNA-125b in Alzheimer's disease (AD) and in primary human neuronal-glial (HNG) cells. Mol Neurobiol 50:97–106
49. Parisi C et al (2016) MicroRNA-125b regulates microglia activation and motor neuron death in ALS. Cell Death Differ 23:531–541
50. Lepore AC et al (2008) Focal transplantation-based astrocyte replacement is neuroprotective in a model of motor neuron disease. Nat Neurosci 11:1294–1301
51. Harrison JF et al (2007) Altering DNA base excision repair: use of nuclear and mitochondrial-targeted N-methylpurine DNA glycosylase to sensitize astroglia to chemotherapeutic agents. Glia 55:1416–1425
52. Caiazzo M et al (2015) Direct conversion of fibroblasts into functional astrocytes by defined transcription factors. Stem Cell Reports 4:25–36
53. Takahashi K, Yamanaka S (2006) Induction of pluripotent stem cells from mouse embryonic and adult fibroblast cultures by defined factors. Cell 126:663–676
54. Chestkov IV, Vasilieva EA, Illarioshkin SN, Lagarkova MA, Kiselev SL (2014) Patient-specific induced pluripotent stem cells for SOD1-associated amyotrophic lateral sclerosis pathogenesis studies. Acta Nat 6:54–60
55. Roybon L et al (2013) Human stem cell-derived spinal cord astrocytes with defined mature or reactive phenotypes. Cell Rep 4:1035–1048

56. Serio A et al (2013) Astrocyte pathology and the absence of non-cell autonomy in an induced pluripotent stem cell model of TDP-43 proteinopathy. Proc Natl Acad Sci U S A 110:4697–4702
57. Bucchia M et al (2015) Therapeutic development in amyotrophic lateral sclerosis. Clin Ther 37:668–680
58. Johnson MA, Weick JP, Pearce RA, Zhang S-C (2007) Functional neural development from human embryonic stem cells: accelerated synaptic activity via astrocyte coculture. J Neurosci 27:3069–3077
59. Krencika R, Zhang S-C (2011) Directed differentiation of functional astroglial subtypes from human pluripotent stem cells. Nat Protoc 6:1710–1717
60. Krencik R, Weick JP, Liu Y, Zhang Z, Zhang S-C (2011) Specification of transplantable astroglial subtypes from human pluripotent stem cells. Nat Biotechnol 29:528–534
61. Emdad L, D'Souza SL, Kothari HP, Qadeer ZA, Germano IM (2012) Efficient differentiation of human embryonic and induced pluripotent stem cells into functional astrocytes. Stem Cells Dev 21:404–410
62. Liu ML et al (2013) Small molecules enable neurogenin 2 to efficiently convert human fibroblasts to cholinergic neurons. Nat Commun 4:2183
63. Pfisterer U et al (2011) Direct conversion of human fibroblasts to dopaminergic neurons. Proc Natl Acad Sci U S A 108:10343–10348
64. Son E, Ichida J, Wainger B, Toma J (2011) Conversion of mouse and human fibroblasts into functional spinal motor neurons. Cell Stem Cell 9:205–218
65. Kim J et al (2011) Direct reprogramming of mouse fibroblasts to neural progenitors. PNAS 108:7838–7843
66. Koistinaho M et al (2004) Apolipoprotein E promotes astrocyte colocalization and degradation of deposited amyloid-beta peptides. Nat Med 10:719–726
67. Proschel C, Stripay JL, Shih CH, Munger JC, Noble MD (2014) Delayed transplantation of precursor cell-derived astrocytes provides multiple benefits in a rat model of Parkinsons. EMBO Mol Med 6:504–518
68. Davies SJA et al (2011) Transplantation of specific human astrocytes promotes functional recovery after spinal cord injury. PLoS One 6:e17328
69. Das MM et al (2016) Human neural progenitors differentiate into astrocytes and protect motor neurons in aging rats. Exp Neurol 280:41–49
70. Kondo T et al (2014) Focal transplantation of human iPSC-derived glial-rich neural progenitors improves lifespan of ALS mice. Stem Cell Reports 3:242–249
71. Nizzardo M et al (2016) iPSC-derived LewisX+CXCR4+β1-integrin+ neural stem cells improve the amyotrophic lateral sclerosis phenotype by preserving motor neurons and muscle innervation in human and rodent models. Hum Mol Genet 25:3152–3163
72. Srinivasan K et al (2016) Untangling the brain's neuroinflammatory and neurodegenerative transcriptional response. Nat Commun 7:11295
73. Baker DJ et al (2015) Lysosomal and phagocytic activity is increased in astrocytes during disease progression in the SOD1 (G93A) mouse model of amyotrophic lateral sclerosis. Front Cell Neurosci 9:410
74. Guillot F et al (2015) Transcript analysis of laser capture microdissected white matter astrocytes and higher phenol sulfotransferase 1A1 expression during autoimmune neuroinflammation. J Neuroinflammation 12:1–14
75. Waller R et al (2016) Gene expression profiling of the astrocyte transcriptome in multiple sclerosis normal appearing white matter reveals a neuroprotective role. J Neuroimmunol 299:139–146
76. Simpson JE et al (2011) Microarray analysis of the astrocyte transcriptome in the aging brain: relationship to Alzheimer's pathology and APOE genotype. Neurobiol Aging 32:1795–1807
77. Aronica E et al (2015) Molecular classification of amyotrophic lateral sclerosis by unsupervised clustering of gene expression in motor cortex. Neurobiol Dis 74:359–376
78. Biswas S, Holyoake D, Maughan TS (2016) Molecular taxonomy and tumourigenesis of colorectal cancer. Clin Oncol 28:73–82
79. Wang M et al (2016) Integrative network analysis of nineteen brain regions identifies molecular signatures and networks underlying selective regional vulnerability to Alzheimer's disease. Genome Med 8:104
80. Frangogiannis N, Biomarkers G (2012) Hopes and challenges in the path from discovery to clinical practice. Transl Res 159:197–204
81. Dosay-Akbulut M (2016) A review on determination and future of the predictive and personalized medicine. Int J Biol 8:32–41
82. Collins CD et al (2006) The application of genomic and proteomic technologies in predictive, preventive and personalized medicine. Vasc Pharmacol 45:258–267
83. Sajja VSSS, Hlavac N, VandeVord PJ (2016) Role of glia in memory deficits following traumatic brain injury: biomarkers of glia dysfunction. Front Integr Neurosci 10:1–9
84. Papa L et al (2014) GFAP out-performs S100β in detecting traumatic intracranial lesions on computed tomography in trauma patients with mild traumatic brain injury and those with extracranial lesions. J Neurotrauma 31:1815–1822
85. Bouvier D et al (2012) Serum S100B determination in the management of pediatric mild traumatic brain injury. Clin Chem 58:1116–1122
86. Shepheard SR, Chataway T, Schultz DW, Rush RA, Rogers ML (2014) The extracellular domain of neurotrophin receptor p75 as a candidate biomarker for amyotrophic lateral sclerosis. PLoS One 9:1–9

87. Ching ASC et al (2012) Current paradigm of the 18-kDa translocator protein (TSPO) as a molecular target for PET imaging in neuroinflammation and neurodegenerative diseases. Insights Imaging 3:111–119
88. Liu GJ et al (2014) The 18 kDa translocator protein, microglia and neuroinflammation. Brain Pathol 24:631–653
89. Cabral GA, Raborn ES, Griffin L, Dennis J, Marciano-Cabral F (2008) CB2 receptors in the brain: role in central immune function. Br J Pharmacol 153:240–251
90. Chiurchiù V et al (2014) Detailed characterization of the endocannabinoid system in human macrophages and foam cells, and anti-inflammatory role of type-2 cannabinoid receptor. Atherosclerosis 233:55–63
91. Turkman N et al (2011) Fluorinated cannabinoid CB2 receptor ligands: synthesis and in vitro binding characteristics of 2-oxoquinoline derivatives. Bioorg Med Chem 19:5698–5707
92. Vandeputte C et al (2011) A PET brain reporter gene system based on type 2 cannabinoid receptors. J Nucl Med 52:1102–1109
93. Veitinger M, Varga B, Guterres SB, Zellner M (2014) Platelets, a reliable source for peripheral Alzheimer's disease biomarkers? Acta Neuropathol Commun 2:65
94. Poutiainen P, Jaronen M, Quintana FJ, Brownell A-L (2016) Precision medicine in multiple sclerosis: future of PET imaging of inflammation and reactive astrocytes. Front Mol Neurosci 9:1–23
95. Gulyas B et al (2011) Activated MAO-B in the brain of alzheimer patients, demonstrated by [11C]-l-deprenyl using whole hemisphere autoradiography. Neurochem Int 58:60–68
96. Droździk M, Białecka M, Kurzawski M (2013) Pharmacogenetics of Parkinson's disease - through mechanisms of drug actions. Curr Genomics 14:568–577
97. Cacabelos R (2007) Donepezil in Alzheimer's disease: from conventional trials to pharmacogenetics. Neuropsychiatr Dis Treat 3:303–333
98. Rascol O et al (2000) A five-year study of the incidence of dyskinesia in patients with early Parkinson's disease who were treated with ropinirole or levodopa. N Engl J Med 342:1484–1491
99. Foltynie T et al (2009) BDNF val66met influences time to onset of levodopa induced dyskinesia in Parkinson's disease. J Neurol Neurosurg Psychiatry 80:141–144
100. Lin J-J, Yueh K-C, Lin S-Z, Harn H-J, Liu J-T (2007) Genetic polymorphism of the angiotensin converting enzyme and L-dopa-induced adverse effects in Parkinson's disease. J Neurol Sci 252:130–134
101. Molchadski I et al (2011) The role of apolipoprotein E polymorphisms in levodopa-induced dyskinesia. Acta Neurol Scand 123:117–121
102. Strong JA et al (2006) Genotype and smoking history affect risk of levodopa-induced dyskinesias in Parkinson's disease. Mov Disord 21:654–659
103. Clark L et al (2007) Mutations in the glucocerebrosidase gene are associated with early-onset Parkinson disease. Neurology 69:1270–1277
104. Lesage S et al (2011) Large-scale screening of the Gaucher's disease-related glucocerebrosidase gene in Europeans with Parkinson's disease. Hum Mol Genet 20:202–210
105. Limpert AS, Mattmann ME, Cosford NDP (2013) Recent progress in the discovery of small molecules for the treatment of amyotrophic lateral sclerosis (ALS). Beilstein J Org Chem 9:717–732
106. Isobe T, Tooi N, Nakatsuji N, Aiba K (2015) Amyotrophic lateral sclerosis models derived from human embryonic stem cells with different superoxide dismutase 1 mutations exhibit differential drug responses. Stem Cell Res 15:459–468
107. Shichinohe H et al (2004) Neuroprotective effects of the free radical scavenger Edaravone (MCI-186) in mice permanent focal brain ischemia. Brain Res 1029:200–206
108. Olabarria M, Noristani HN, Verkhratsky A, Rodríguez JJ (2010) Concomitant astroglial atrophy and astrogliosis in a triple transgenic animal model of Alzheimer's disease. Glia 58:831–838
109. Yeh C, Vadhwana B, Verkhratsky A, Rodríguez JJ (2011) Early astrocytic atrophy in the entorhinal cortex of a triple transgenic animal model of Alzheimer's disease. ASN Neuro 3:271–279
110. Diaz-Amarilla P et al (2011) From the cover: phenotypically aberrant astrocytes that promote motoneuron damage in a model of inherited amyotrophic lateral sclerosis. Proc Natl Acad Sci 108:18126–18131
111. Schitine C, Nogaroli L, Costa MR, Hedin-Pereira C (2015) Astrocyte heterogeneity in the brain: from development to disease. Front Cell Neurosci 9:76
112. McGivern JV, Ebert AD (2014) Exploiting pluripotent stem cell technology for drug discovery, screening, safety, and toxicology assessments. Adv Drug Deliv Rev 69–70:170–178
113. del Barrio L et al (2011) Neurotoxicity induced by okadaic acid in the human neuroblastoma SH-SY5Y line can be differentially prevented by a7 and b2* nicotinic stimulation. Toxicol Sci 123:193–205
114. Avior Y, Sagi I, Benvenisty N (2016) Pluripotent stem cells in disease modelling and drug discovery. Nat Rev Mol Cell Biol 17:170–182
115. Glajch KE et al (2016) MicroNeurotrophins improve survival in motor neuron-astrocyte co-cultures but do not improve disease phenotypes in a mutant SOD1 mouse model of amyotrophic lateral sclerosis. PLoS One 11:1–24
116. Terrasso AP et al (2016) Human neuron-astrocyte 3D co-culture-based assay for evaluation of neuroprotective compounds. J Pharmacol Toxicol Methods 83:72–79

117. Al-Ali H et al (2015) Rational polypharmacology: systematically identifying and engaging multiple drug targets to promote axon growth. ACS Chem Biol 10:1939–1951
118. Blackmore MG et al (2010) High content screening of cortical neurons identifies novel regulators of axon growth. Mol Cell Neurosci 44:43–54
119. Lorenz C et al (2017) Human iPSC-derived neural progenitors are an effective drug discovery model for neurological mtDNA disorders. Cell Stem Cell:1–16. doi:10.1016/j.stem.2016.12.013
120. Egawa N et al (2012) Drug screening for ALS using patient-specific induced pluripotent stem cells. Sci Transl Med 4:145ra104–145ra104
121. Anderl JL, Redpath S, Ball AJ (2009) A neuronal and astrocyte co-culture assay for high content analysis of neurotoxicity. J Vis Exp 27:1–6
122. Rinaldi F, Motti D, Ferraiuolo L, Kaspar BK (2016) High content analysis in amyotrophic lateral sclerosis. Mol Cell Neurosci. doi:10.1016/j.mcn.2016.12.001
123. Efremova L et al (2015) Prevention of the degeneration of human dopaminergic neurons in an astrocyte co-culture system allowing endogenous drug metabolism. Br J Pharmacol 172:4119–4132
124. Ferraiuolo L et al (2016) Oligodendrocytes contribute to motor neuron death in ALS via SOD1-dependent mechanism. Proc Natl Acad Sci U S A 113:E6496–E6505
125. Frakes AE, Braun L, Ferraiuolo L, Guttridge DC, Kaspar BK (2017) Additive amelioration of ALS by co-targeting independent pathogenic mechanisms. Ann Clin Transl Neurol 4:76–86

Mitochondrial Diseases as Model of Neurodegeneration

8

Laila A. Selim and Heba Hassaan

Abstract

"Mitochondria" partially autonomous sophisticated cellular organelle involved in a wide range of crucial cellular functions, well known as the power house of the cell where ATP (adenosine triphosphate) production takes place, that is the cellular source of energy.

Mitochondria has its own genome, however proper functioning of the mitochondria is dependent upon the coordinated expression of both nuclear and mitochondrial encoded gene products. Peculiar maternal inheritance of mitochondrial DNA has led the scientists to think about mitochondrial donation as a solution to maternally inherited mitochondriopathy "Three parent baby", raising many ethical and scientific issues, concerns about safety of the procedure, long term outcome and effect of genetic modification are still questionable.

Mitochondrial DNA has a higher mutation rate compared to nuclear DNA. Mitochondrial research has revealed a lot about methods of its DNA repair emphasizing the role of nuclear encoded products in this process.

Mitochondrial diseases are clinically and genetically diverse, fortunately next generation sequencing (NGS) technologies have made a breakthrough in mitochondrial disorders, the whole mitochondrial genome has been sequenced with more than 250 nuclear encoded genes associated with mitochondrial syndromes identified to date, It unraveled the role of mitochondrial disorders in neurodegenerative disorders. However many pathogenic candidate genes remain uncharacterized even with whole exome sequencing (WES).

L.A. Selim (✉) • H. Hassaan
Kasr Al Ainy School of Medicine, Cairo University
Children Hospital, Cairo, Egypt
e-mail: lselim83@mail.com

S. El-Khamisy (ed.), *Personalised Medicine*, Advances in Experimental Medicine and Biology 1007,
DOI 10.1007/978-3-319-60733-7_8

In this chapter here we handle cases with various neurodegenerative diseases that have been genetically diagnosed thanks to NGS, revealing the role of mitochondrial dysfunction in neurodegeneration, offering a therapeutic target for these handicapping disorders.

Keywords
Mitochondria • Mitohondrial genome (mtDNA) • Mitochondrial dysfunction • Gene • Mutation • Sequencing • Neurodegeneration

8.1 Introduction

Mitochondrion, from the Greek μίτος, mitos, i.e. "thread", and χονδρίον, chondrion, i.e. "granule" or "grain-like" [1], is a highly sophisticated cellular organelle, and unlike any other structure in mammalian cells is partially autonomous, highly dynamic, possessing its own genome [2] with peculiar characteristics defining mitochondrial inherited diseases. Nevertheless proper functioning of mitochondria is dependent upon the coordinated expression and interaction of both nuclear and mitochondrial-encoded gene products [3].

Altmann, the first to recognize ubiquitous occurrence of mitochondria in 1890, was a German pathologist who described them as "elementary organisms", and called them "bioblasts" carrying out vital functions [4]. In the 1990s, the structure of mitochondria could be visualized by electron tomography revealing the striking three-dimensional (3D) images of their internal membrane system lacking molecular details which are now revealed by the Cryo-EM showing the architecture of mitochondrial membranes and their macromolecular components at increasing levels of detail [5].

There are about ten million billion mitochondria in the human body with 1–2 k in each liver cell [6]. It is well known that mitochondria are the main organelles involved in ATP supply to the cells through oxidative phosphorylation (OXPHOs). They also play a crucial role in the synthesis of key molecules and response to oxidative stress resulting from naturally occurring inefficiencies of oxidative phosphorylation generating reactive oxygen species. They are in continuous dynamic movements required for correction of respiratory activity through fusion and or fission [7]. Mitochondrial dysfunction has been implicated in premature aging, age-related diseases, tumor initiation and progression as well as pathogenesis of Diabetes Mellitus, Alzheimer's and Parkinson's diseases [8].

This chapter handles mitochondrial structure describing OXPHOS system and energy production, mitochondrial genome, peculiar mitochondrial inheritance, how the recent advances in technology helped in mitochondrial medicine, role of mitochondria in some neurodegenerative diseases especially in infancy and childhood illustrated with clinical cases.

8.2 Structure of the Mitochondrion

The mitochondrion is a cellular organelle with outer and inner membranes separated by an intermembrane space; outer smooth and inner highly folded one forming structures called cristae which allow large surface area of the inner mitochondrial membrane to accommodate enzymes of the mitochondrial energy-generating apparatus OXPHOS [9]. The number of cristae is related to the energy requirement for the vital functions of certain cell type as well as the number of mitochondria per cell [10].

The outer membrane is porous, freely traversed by ions with no membrane potential across, but it needs special translocases for larger molecules especially proteins to pass through. On the other hand the inner membrane forms a tight diffusion barrier that for any ion or molecule to get across it needs the aid of specific membrane

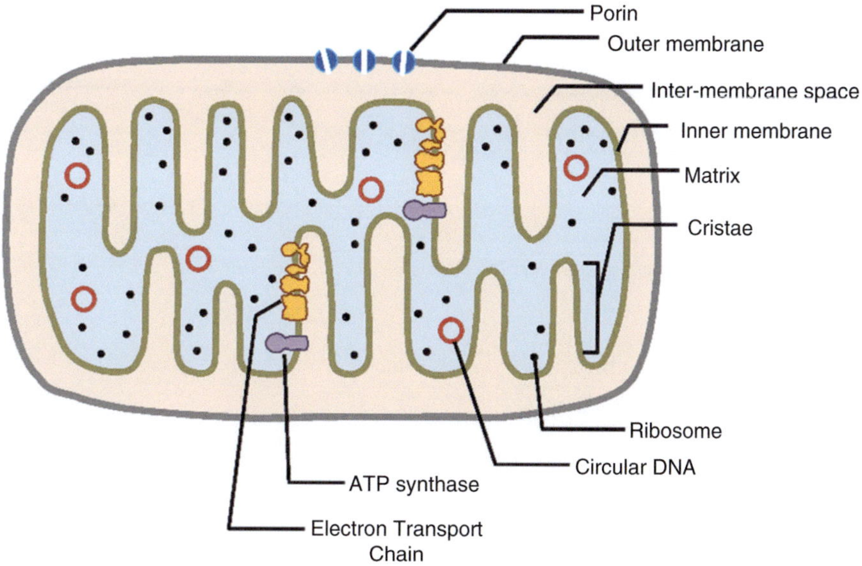

Fig. 8.1 Mitochondrion structure: inner and outer membranes with the inner one folded into cristae, carrying proteins of electon transport chain and enclosing the matrix [11]

transport protein, and as a result of ion selectivity, an electrochemical membrane potential is created across [5]. The inner mitochondrial membrane is enriched with the proteins involved in mitochondrial fusion, transport of nuclear-encoded proteins, oxidative phosphorylation (OXPHOS), iron-sulfur cluster biogenesis, protein synthesis and transport of mtDNA-encoded proteins [10]. Between the inner and outer mitochondrial membranes is the intermembrane space containing the chemical cytochrome C, its accidental or programmed leak can trigger cell death by apoptosis [6].

Mitochondrial DNA is present in the mitochondrial matrix; the site of organelle DNA replication, transcription, protein biosynthesis and numerous enzymatic reactions [5] (Fig. 8.1).

8.3 OXPHOS System and Energy Production

Mitochondria is well known as the power house of the cell where ATP is primarily synthesized in by oxidative phosphorylation (OXPHOS system) to be consumed throughout the cell [12], This OXPHOS system comprises five transmembrane complexes (I–V) consisting of ~90 protein subunits that are encoded by either the mitochondria's own genetic material (mtDNA) or the nuclear genome [8] (Fig. 8.2). Proper functioning of OXPHOS system further requires the assistance of nDNA-encoded assembly factors [13].

Electrons harvested from the catabolic processes of glycolysis, fatty acid oxidation and the tricarboxylic acid (TCA) cycle enter the electron transport chain (ETC) on the inner mitochondrial membrane where electron transfer is coupled to proton translocation out of the mitochondrial matrix creating electrochemical gradient that is used by complex five (ATP synthase) to form ATP (energy currency for the cell). In addition to the five multimeric complexes ubiquinone and soluble cytochrome c are mobile carriers embedded in inner mitochondrial membrane facilitating intra-protein electron transfer [12].

Complex I or NADH: ubiquinone oxidoreductase is the largest and most complicated one [15] which consists of 45 subunits, seven encoded by mitochondrial DNA and thirty eight by nuclear DNA [4] and over ten assembly factors [16] (Fig. 8.3). Complex I is the entry point for electrons from NADH, which are used to reduce ubiquinone (Q) to ubiquinol (QH2) that is

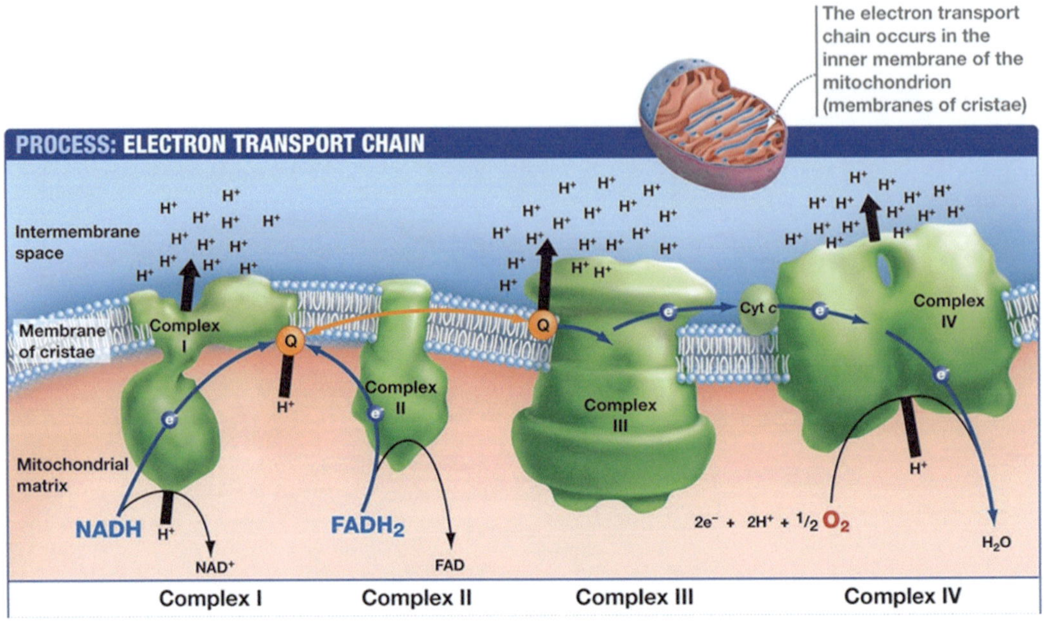

Fig. 8.2 OXYPHOS system showing four complexes of the mitochondrial respiratory chain embedded in the inner mitochondrial membrane where electron transfer is coupled to proton translocation out of the mitochondrial matrix [14]

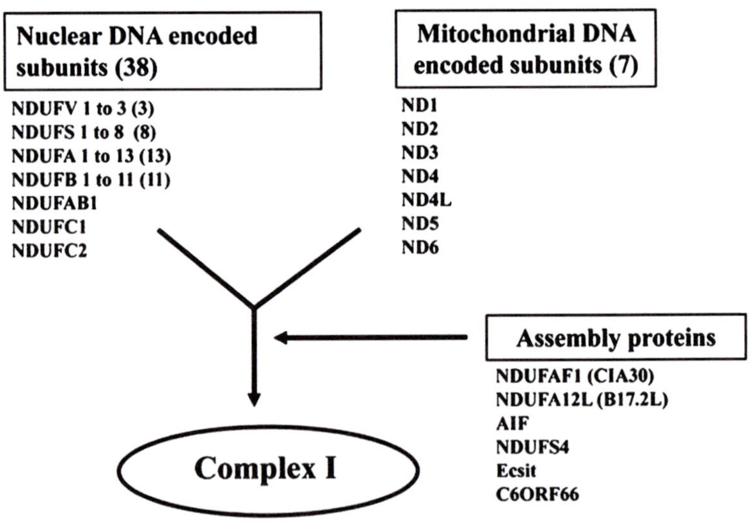

Fig. 8.3 Structure of Complex I; the largest of the electron transport chain with 45 subunits, 38 of which as well as the assembly proteins are encoded by nuclear DNA while seven only are encoded by mitochondrial DNA [21]

subsequently used by complex III to reduce cytochrome C in the intermembrane space (IMS), and complex IV uses cytochrome c to reduce molecular oxygen, which is the ultimate electron acceptor. Complex IV (also known as cytochrome c oxidase (COX)) is the terminal enzyme complex of the mitochondrial respiratory chain [17]. The human COX enzyme comprises 14 structural subunits, three of which are of mitochondrial origin and form the catalytic core [18, 19]. The remaining components are translated on cytosolic ribosomes and imported into mitochondria, over 20 different assembly factors are essential to form a mature complex IV [20].

For each NADH molecule oxidized, ten protons are translocated across the membrane from the matrix to the IMS. Complex five known as Adenosine triphosphate (ATP) synthases use the energy stored in a transmembrane proton-motive force to synthesize ATP from adenosine diphosphate (ADP) and inorganic phosphate [12].

Complex II consists entirely of nuclear-encoded proteins [22]. Complex II (succinate–quinone oxidoreductase) provides an additional entry point for electrons into the chain [12].

8.4 Mitochondrial Genome

Mitochondrion has its own genome with peculiar characteristics (Fig. 8.4). Pre and post fertilization events ensure uniparental inheritance of mitochondrial genome eliminating paternal one, and accordingly mitochondrial DNA is maternally inherited [23]. However Mitochondria need to import a lot of proteins encoded by nuclear genes to function properly, more than 1000 genes play a role in mitochondrial function [24]. This divided mitochondrial diseases genetically into two main categories, those due to defect in mitochondrial

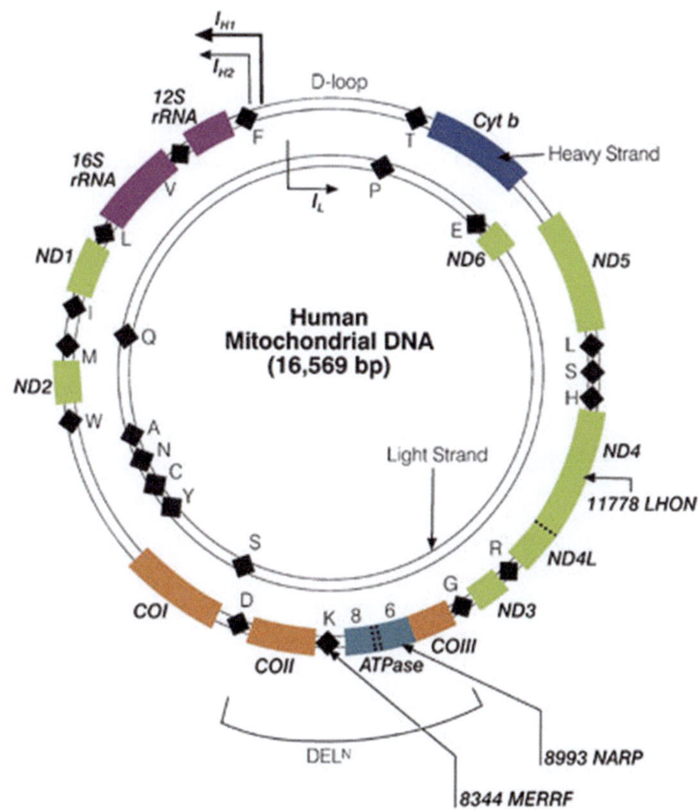

Fig. 8.4 The human mitochondrial genome. This small (16 569 bp) genome is almost completely transcribed from both strands, initiating from one of two promoters (IH1, IH2) on the Heavy (H-) strand or the single promoter (IL) on the Light (L-) strand. All of these promoters and elements involved in replication initiation are found in the displacement (D-) loop, the only major noncoding region. The genome encodes 22 mt-tRNA (black diamonds), 2 mt-rRNA genes (fuscia) and 13 protein-coding genes (olive, ND1-6 encoding members of NADH:ubiquinone oxido-reductase; blue, Cytb encoding apocytochrome b of ubiquinol:cytochrome c oxidoreductase; orange, COI-III encoding members of cytochrome c oxidase: aquamarine, ATPase 6, 8 encoding two members of Fo-F1 ATP synthase). Important mutations that are referred to in this article are indicated. Single letter code is given for each mt-tRNA-encoding gene [26]

DNA that are maternally inherited and others due to defect in nuclear genes controlling mitochondrial function which follow mendelian inheritance and a minor group resulting from disruption of the interplay between both mitochondrial and nuclear DNA as in mitochondrial neurogastrointestinal encephalopathy(MNGIE) as a prototype.

Table showing differences between mitochondrial and nuclear DNA

P.O.C	Mitochondrial DNA	Nuclear DNA
Number of base pairs	16,569	3.3 billion
Shape	Circular	Linear
Introns (non-coding segments)	3%	93%
Inheritance	Maternal	Mendelian
No. of DNA copies per cell	Thousands	One

The mitochondrial genome contains 37 genes that encode 13 proteins of the OXYPHOS system, 22 tRNA, 2 rRNA. Each mitochondrion has multiple copies of its DNA, and each cell contains hundreds to thousands of mitochondria. At the same time mitochondrial DNA has higher mutation rate, 100 folds compared to nuclear DNA, this results in a peculiar phenomenon of mitochondrial DNA, what is called heteroplasmy; the presence of heterogenous mitochondrial DNA population, normal and mutant copies. For a disease to be expressed mutant copies should exceed certain limit, Threshold, with the level of heteroplasmy at which disease symptoms typically appear can also vary based on the type of mitochondrial mutation [25].

Unlike nuclear DNA that is equally divided between cells, segregation of mitochondrial DNA is random, normal and mutant DNA are not equally distributed between daughter cells, which explains variable disease expression in offspring born to affected mother [9]. The transmission of heteroplasmic mtDNA is complicated by selective genome replication and genetic bottleneck [28], like the structure of many beverage bottles where the neck of the bottle regulates the amount of liquid that is poured at a time. While the overall quantity of mtDNA inherited might be small, some eggs may still end up with a significant amount [29] (Fig. 8.5). At the same time even if the presence of homoplasmic mutation guarantees its transmission to all offspring, it can't pre-

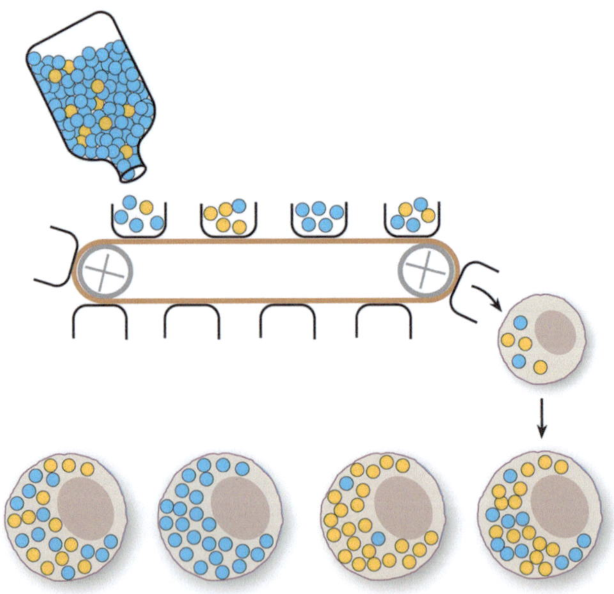

Fig. 8.5 Bottleneck theory of mitochondrial DNA and random segregation between wild and mutant DNA resulting in difficulty of disease prediction and variable severity [27]

dict disease expression and severity. This is attributed to complex interplay between mitochondrial and nuclear genome [9].

These facts about mitochondria inheritance explains limited role of preimplantation genetic diagnosis in mitochondrial diseases due to uncertainity in predicting disease [29].

Since mitochondria are the power house of the cell responsible for energy production the organs commonly affected in mitochondrial diseases are those with high energy demand; brain, skeletal and cardiac muscles and retina [30].

Mitochondrial dysfunction causes a range of diseases spanning from incurable neonatal neurodevelopmental diseases to adult-onset neurodegenerative diseases [31]. Pediatric-onset mitochondrial disease has an estimated incidence of 1 in 5000 [32]. Mitochondrial disorders are clinically and genetically diverse. Mutations in both structural and assembly genes and in genes involved in mtDNA maintenance, replication, transcription, and translation induce 'primary' OXPHOS disorders that are associated with neurodegenerative diseases [13].

Diseases due to defect in mitochondrial DNA are maternally inherited. Affected males do not transmit the disease to their offspring while the female carrying the mutant mitochondrial DNA whether asymptomatic or manifesting the disease will transmit the mutant DNA to all offspring with variable unpredictable disease expression. It occurs due to either point mutations or DNA damage manifesting in two molecularly distinct forms: mt DNA deletions typically manifesting in adulthood and mtDNA depletion syndromes, a quantitative loss of mtDNA copy number [33], occurring in childhood. Mitochondrial DNA depletion disorders are usually very severe, early onset diseases characterized by isolated organ or multisystem involvement [34].

Next-generation sequencing (NGS) technologies have made a breakthrough in identifying mutations in genes causing primary mitochondrial disorders, [35] The human mitochondrial genome has been completely sequenced and all the mitochondrial encoded genes have been identified and characterized [36] with more than 250 nuclear-encoded genes associated with mitochondrial syndromes identified to date [35]. Complex I deficiency is the most common biochemical phenotype observed in patients with mitochondrial disease [37] with all mutations of the seven mtDNA encoded structural subunits of complex I and 20 of nuclear encoded structural genes have been identified as well as defects in nine assembly factors. TMEM126B, a protein recently identified as a complex I assembly factor has been established as a candidate gene for complex one deficiency with a wide range of presentation from severe multisystem presentation in infancy to pure myopathy in later child- or adulthood [16]. However, given the size of the human mitochondrial proteome—comprising ~1300 gene products necessary to maintain mitochondrial function—many pathogenic candidate genes remain uncharacterized even with whole exome sequencing (WES) This is highlighted by the many patients with mitochondrial disease still requiring a diagnosis, where the defective gene has not yet been established [38]. Finding a genetic cause is important to families to find out what is wrong with their child. Genetic counseling is important to explain the genetic risks involved in spontaneous or assisted reproduction and the limits of prenatal and preimplantation testing [29].

8.4.1 Mitochondrial Donation

8.4.1.1 Three Parent Baby, Revolution for Mitochondrial Cure or Mysterious Future?

The peculiar maternal inheritance of mitochondrial DNA has led scientists to think about possibility of mitochondrial donation to replace the mutant one, what is now well known as "Three parent baby" with nuclear DNA formed by nucleus of a healthy father sperm together with that from an ovum of a mother carrying diseased mitochondria that is replaced with a healthy one from an ovum of a donating healthy mother, thus eliminating the risk of getting maternally inherited mitochondrial disease [39].

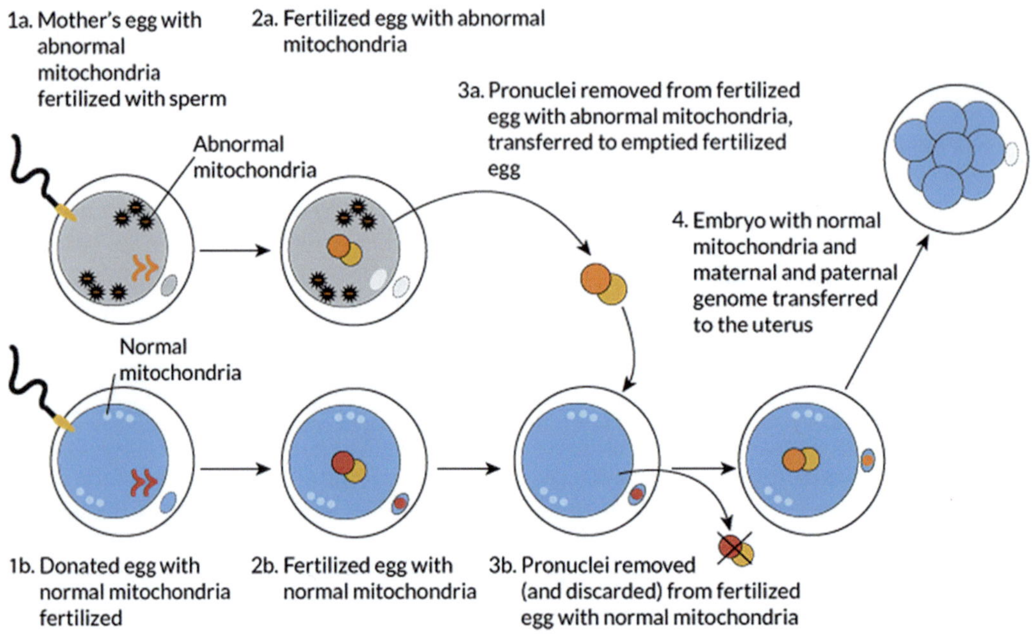

Fig. 8.6 Pronuclear transfer was the first technique that scientists tried in their attempts to keep diseases due to faulty mitochondria from being passed from a mother to her child [41]

Two approaches have been established: Pronuclear transfer and spindle nuclear transfer.

Pronuclear Transfer

The mother's egg and a donor egg are fertilized at the same time. The pronuclei removed from the donor's fertilized egg and discarded. Those from the mother's fertilized egg were sucked out and then injected into the empty donor egg. This procedure was claimed to be non ethical because of possibility to destroy two embryos, however it has been legally approved in UK [40].

Spindle Nuclear Transfer Approach

The nucleus from one of the mother's eggs (the spindle with maternally-derived chromosomes attached) is removed and inserted into a donor's egg that had its own nucleus removed, the resulting egg having nuclear DNA from the mother and mitochondria DNA from donor is then fertilized with the father's sperm [40].

John Zhang and his team at the New Hope Fertility Center in New York have led the successful experiment of the three parent baby for a couples with healthy mother who gave birth to two children with Leigh disease who died at 6 years and 8 month respectively could finally gave birth to healthy child by Spindle nuclear transfer procedure. Zhang's paper reveals that just 2% of the mitochondrial DNA of cells in the boy's urine came from the mother, but that figure rose as high as 9% in cells from the child's circumcised foreskin. Organs such as the heart or brain are impossible to test without invasive surgery. Still, there are ethical and safety concerns about this. The biggest concern whether the child's health will be affected by the traces of the mother's mitochondrial DNA that he carries. How far would this genetic modification affect subsequent generations. What is gonna be the outcome on the long run? [42].

After Zhang's successful event research has extended to use mitochondrial donation to treat infertility. A baby girl was born to infertile couple in Ukraine, conceived through mitochondrial donation as an experimental treatment for infer-

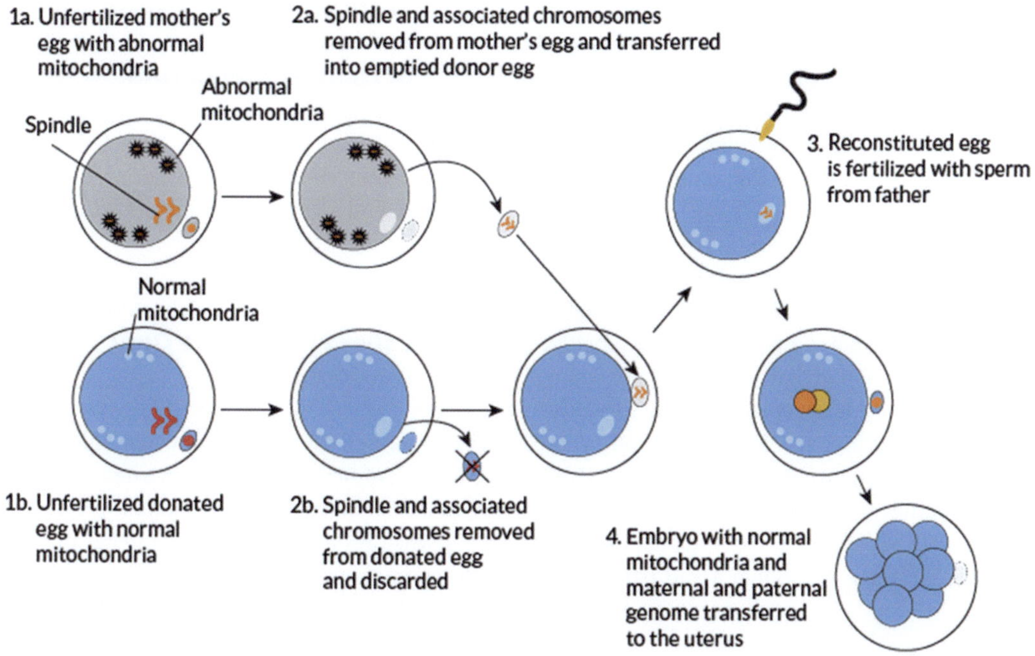

Fig. 8.7 The three-parent baby boy born last year was created using this technique, called spindle transfer [41]

tility using pronuclear transfer technique, the pronucleus is placed into cytoplasm of another woman's ovum. The success of the procedure suggests the presence of factors within a cell's cytoplasm that can hinder fertility causing embryo arrest, which happens when IVF embryos suddenly stop growing at around the two-cell stage [43].

This needs further follow up, being a girl means genetic modification is transmitted her generation. Though the United Kingdom approved pronuclear transfer, it's only legalized for women suffering mitochondrial disease [44].

8.4.2 Mitochondrial Genome Stability

The proximity of the mtDNA to the electron transport chain complexes increases its vulnerability to oxidative damage [45]. Mitochondrial DNA has higher mutation rate 100 folds compared to nuclear DNA [46]. Multiple mtDNA repair pathways have been identified including base excision repair, single-strand break repair, mismatch repair and possibly homologous recombination. They are mediated by enzymes similar in activity to those operating in the nucleus, encoded by nuclear genes [47]. A recent study has shown pivotal role for tyrosyl DNA phosphodiesterase (TDP1) a nuclear encoded enzyme in maintaining mitochondrial DNA transcription and bioenergetics, thereby controlling the level of free radical–induced DNA damage. This is completed through a functional interaction between TDP1 and both nuclear and mitochondrial topoisomerase ITOP1. Such research is putting increasing challenge to mitochondrial donation procedure which assume that there is very little interaction between the mitochondria and the nucleus [45].

Increased damage by reactive oxygen species (ROS) and defective DNA repair are the two causes proposed to explain the mitochondrial genome instability (mtGI) in cancer cells [48]. Mitochondria plays an important role in apoptosis, disturbance of which can result in cancer development and in the cellular response to anticancer agents [36]. Breast, colorectal, gastric and kidney cancers exhibit mitochondrial genome instability with a pattern of mitochondrial mutations specific for each tumor [46]. Identifying mitochondrial gene mutation in malignancy is offering a therapeutic target for cancer.

Mitochondrial dysfunction has been described in autosomal recessive neurodegenerative diseases inherited through Mendelian inheritance and this is the most common situation encountered in pediatric patients presenting with mitochondrial encephalomyopathies especially in Egypt and the MENA region where consanguineous marriage can reach up to 40%. Mitochondrial dysfunction has been also incriminated in pathogenesis of further diseases; Diabetes Mellitus, Alzheimer's and Parkinson's diseases.

8.5 Mitochondrial Diabetes

Beside mitochondrial diabetes that occurs due to mitochondrial DNA mutation mitochondrial dysfunction plays a role in both type 1 and 2 Diabetes Mellitus. For the former mitochondrial ATP production regulates acute insulin release from B cells of pancreatic islets which deteriorates with long term accumulation of mitochondrial reactive Oxygen species (ROS), while in type 2 Diabetes proper mitochondrial function is crucial for insulin sensitivity within muscle, liver and adipose tissue [49]. An inverse relationship was found between intramyocellular lipid (IMCL) content as measured by 1H MRS and insulin sensitivity, IMCL accumulation is linked to a reduction in mitochondrial oxidative-phosphorylation activity [50].

Mitochondrial diabetes is maternally inherited disease that typically present in middle age due to mutations in mitochondrial DNA, the most common is A3243G mutation of mitochondrial encoded tRNA (Leu, UUR) gene, often associated with hearing loss [49].

8.6 Mitochondrial Diseases as Model of Neurodegeneration

In the following part of the chapter, we will describe some of the mitochondrial disorders associated with neurodegeneration resulting from mitochondrial dysfunction.

8.6.1 Leber's Hereditary Optic Neuropathy

Leber's Hereditary optic neuropathy (LHON) is the most common maternally inherited blindness due to mutations in the mitochondrial genome. It is a disease prototype which highlights the link between energy production, oxidative stress and neurodegeneration. LHON is caused by mitochondrial degeneration of retinal ganglion cells (RGCs) and their axons that leads to an acute or subacute loss of central vision; usually sparing the pigmentary epithelium and photoreceptors and affecting predominantly young adult males. It is usually due to one of three pathogenic mitochondrial DNA (mtDNA) point mutations, at nucleotide positions 11778 G to A, 3460 G to A and 14484 T to C, respectively in the ND4, ND1 and ND6 subunit genes of complex I of the oxidative phosphorylation chain in mitochondria. Affected males cannot pass on the disease to their offspring [7].

Complex I mutation causing calcium dysregulation is implicated in the pathogenesis of LHON. Impaired axonal distribution of mitochondria in RCG is also presumed to result in local energy deprivation at most active sites where ATP is needed [51].

We present here in two cases with LHON who both presented with the main complaint of gradual progressive diminution of vision (Fig. 8.10). The first patient is a 21 year old male patient, whose condition started at 18 years of age by diminution of vision in the left eye, misdiagnosed as optic neuritis 2ry to disseminated sclerosis, for

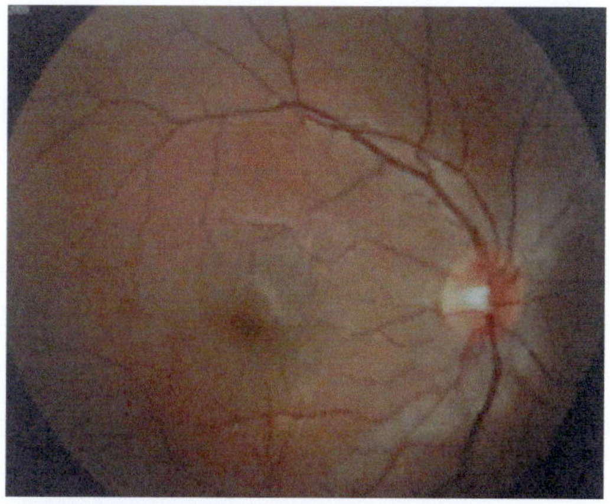

Fig. 8.8 Temporal pallor of optic disc from case 1 (Courtesy Dr. Dina Mehaney)

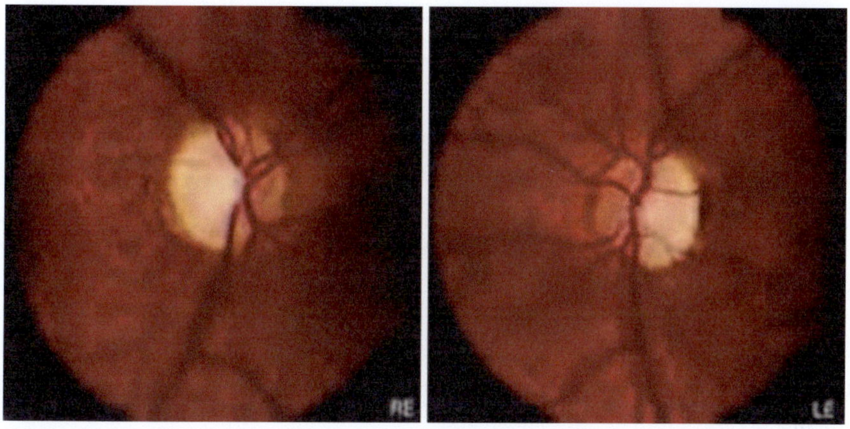

Fig. 8.9 Temporal pallor of optic disc from case 2 (Courtesy Dr. Dina Mehaney)

which he received steroid therapy. Five months following the onset, he developed defective vision in the right eye. Visual acuity was 6/12, 5/60 in the right and left eye respectively. Visual field examination revealed a central scotoma, more profound in the left eye. VEP showed a significant latency difference with relatively delayed response in the right eye compared to the left. No family history of similar condition (Fig. 8.8).

The second patient is a 44 years old male patient whose condition started at age 28 years by affection of the right eye followed 2 months later by the left eye. No family history of similar condition. Again, he was diagnosed as optic neuritis and received steroid therapy, visual acuity was 3/60 in both eyes. Fundus examination revealed bilateral temporal optic disc pallor. Visual field examination showed a deep central scotoma, VEP showed delay in P100 response at 120 msec. Brain MRI was normal (Fig. 8.9).

8.6.2 Autosomal Dominant Optic Atrophy(ADOA)

Autosomal dominant optic atrophy (ADOA) is one of the most common forms of hereditary optic neuropathy characterized by progressive bilateral visual loss, associated with optic disc pallor, visual field and color vision defects [52].

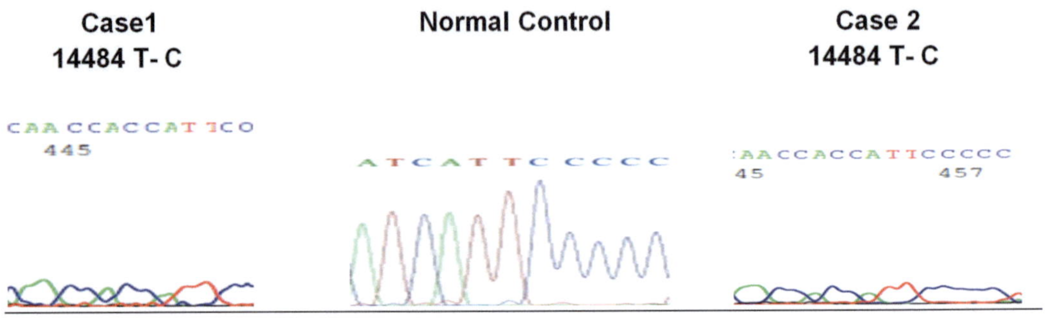

Fig. 8.10 Mitochondrial DNA point mutation detected in the 2 patients (Courtesy Dr. Dina Mehaney)

It is usually detected during the first decade of life during vision screening in school but may have a later onset visual impairment is usually moderate, and total blindness is rare. In about 20% of cases, extra-ocular signs are present, such as sensorineural hearing loss, myopathy, ataxia, peripheral neuropathy, chronic progressive external ophthalmoplegia (ADOA plus) [53, 54].

A majority of ADOA patients harbor mutations in the gene *OPA1* (3q29) which codes for an inner mitochondrial membrane protein, dynamin-related GTP protein, intricately involved in mitochondrial biogenesis, and plays a key role in the organization of the shape and structure of the mitochondria, in mitochondrial DNA replication and network stability and in regulation of apoptosis. The OPA1 protein is also involved in oxidative phosphorylation and plays a crucial role in the maintenance of mitochondrial DNA (mtDNA) [52].

Mutations in the *OPA1* gene lead to overall dysfunction of mitochondria altering the mitochondrial structure which become disorganized and cells become more susceptible to apoptosis. *OPA1* gene mutations lead to mitochondria with reduced energy-producing capabilities, impairing the maintenance of mtDNA, resulting in mtDNA mutations [55].

The diagnosis of ADOA is suspected in children with visual loss in the presence of family history. Fundus examination reveals bilateral and symmetrical pallor of the temporal side of the optic disk, atrophic optic nerve rim and presence of a temporal grey crescent, sometimes cupping of the disk (Fig. 8.11). Visual evoked potentials (VEP) are usually delayed and pattern electroretinogram shows an abnormal N95:P50 ratio, with reduction in the amplitude of the N95 waveform suggesting alterations of the ganglion cells layer. Optical Coherence Tomography (OCT) discloses a global reduction of the peripapillary retinal nerve fiber layer thickness, mainly in the infero-temporal quadrant. The diagnosis is confirmed by the genetic screening of *OPA1* [53, 54] (Fig. 8.12).

8.6.3 Charcot Marie- Tooth Disease

Charcot-Marie-Tooth hereditary neuropathy type 2A (CMT2A, OMIM#609260) is an early onset sensory motor peripheral neuropathy. Most affected individuals develop symptoms in the first or second decades of life, usually before 10 years [57]. It is characterized by early and more severe involvement of the lower than upper extremities, motor nerves are mainly affected than sensory ones and usually there is no delay in nerve conduction velocity [58]. CMT2A is inherited in an autosomal dominant manner caused by mutations in the MFN2 genes [58] [59], The MFN2 gene encode for an outer mitochondrial membrane protein called mitofusin 2 that have in cooperation with OPA1 gene and MFN1 gene an important role in regulating mitochondrial fusion [58]. MFN2 gene regulates the nuclear encoded respiratory chain subunits and hence can influence mitochondrial biogenesis [60]. It may also be involved in axonal transport of mitochondria

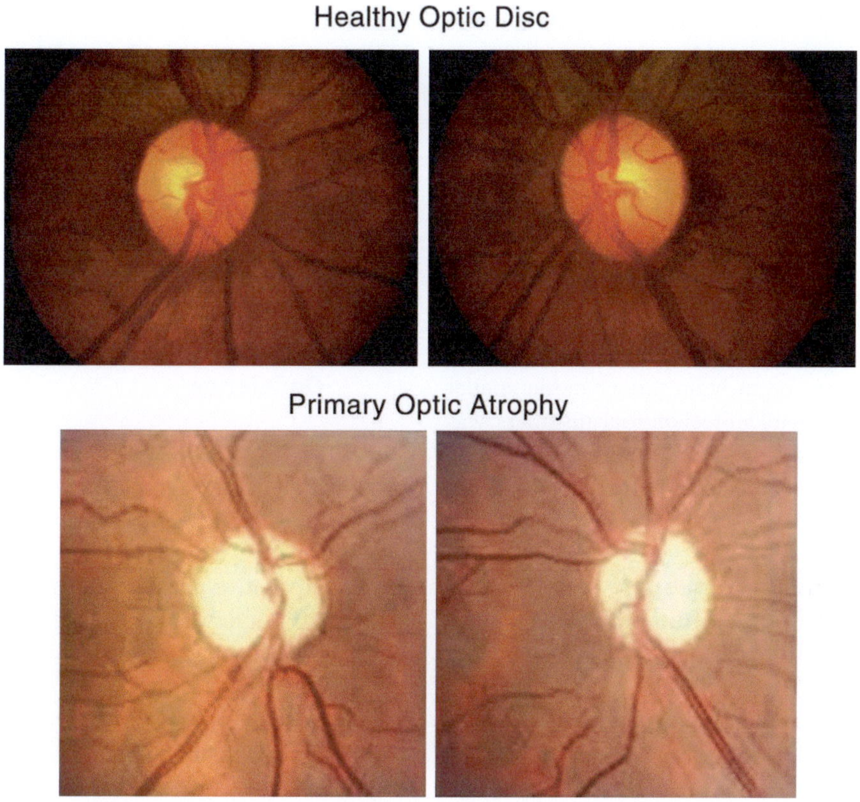

Fig. 8.11 Healthy optic disc and optic atrophy [56]

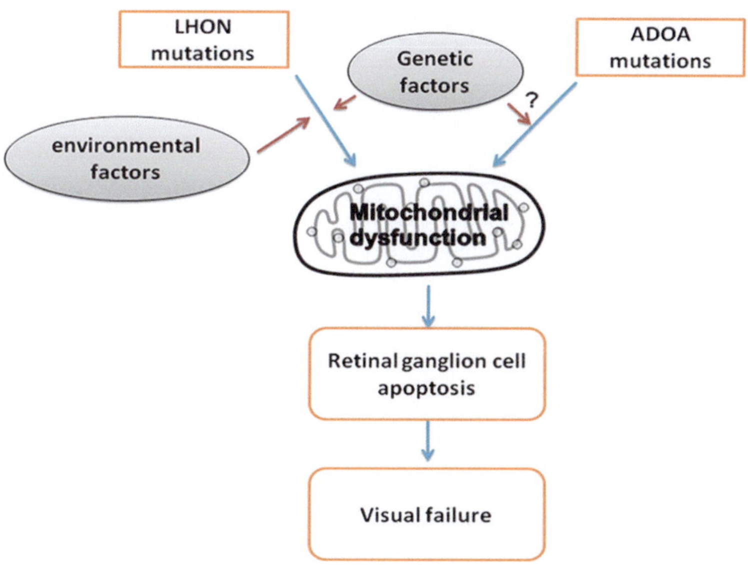

Fig. 8.12 Mitochondrial dysfunction in LHON and ADOA [57]

[58]. Neuropathological studies of patients with CMT2 disease revealed degeneration of long peripheral axons and small axonal mitochondria [61]. Abnormalities in mitochondrial fusion and fragmentation of mitochondria leading to respiratory chain and mitochondrial DNA repair defects were observed by Rousier et al. [62].

Loiseau et al. 2007 have demonstrated that fibroblasts from CMT2A patients show a mitochondrial coupling defect, with impaired membrane potential and reduced OXPHOS capacity [63]. Dysfunction of brain mitochondria similar to that of primary mitochondrial disorders was recently demonstrated in an Italian family with a new MFN2 gene mutation [53].

8.6.4 Myoclonic Epilepsy and Ragged-Red Fibres (MERRF)

MERRF (*m*yoclonic *e*pilepsy with *r*agged *r*ed *f*ibers) is a multisystem disorder characterized by myoclonus which is often the presenting symptom, followed by generalized epilepsy, ataxia, muscle weakness, and cognitive impairment. Onset is usually in childhood, patient experiences gradual progressive deterioration occurring after normal early development. Common findings are hearing loss, short stature, optic atrophy, and cardiomyopathy with Wolff-Parkinson-White (WPW) syndrome. Pigmentary retinopathy and lipomatosis are occasionally observed [64]. Cardiac involvement has been reported to be frequent in individuals with the m.8344A>G pathogenic variant in *MT-TK* [65]. The mitochondrial DNA gene MTTK is the most common pathogenic Variants and it is present in more than 80% of patients with MEERF with A to G Transition at nucleotide 8344. Patients harboring this mutation show degenerative changes in the olivocerebellar pathway with extensive neuronal loss involving the Purkinje fibers, the inferior olivary complex and dentate nucleus. Surviving neurons in the cerebellum often show bizarre and abnormal sized mitochondria containing inclusions [66].

Several studies demonstrated that the A > G 8834 mutation results in defective synthesis of mitochondrial protein resulting into malfunction of the respiratory chain. The impaired electron transport chain activity decreases mitochondrial membrane potential and decrease ATP production, modifies calcium homeostasis and ROS production evolving in increasing apoptosis [67].

8.6.5 Ataxia and Coenzyme Q Deficiency

Coenzyme Q10 (CoQ10) is an essential electron carrier in the mitochondrial respiratory chain and also acts as an antioxidant in various cell membranes [68]. CoQ deficiency syndrome is associated with oxidative phosphorylation dysfunction and in vitro studies demonstrated that CoQ deficiency has different biochemical consequences leading to cell apoptosis [69].

Human coenzyme Q_{10} (CoQ_{10}) deficiency (MIM 607426) is a clinically and genetically heterogeneous syndrome, about 100 patients has been so far published, and is associated with five major clinical phenotypes: encephalomyopathy [70, 71], severe infantile multisystemic disease [72–74], isolated nephropathy, especially steroid resistant nephrotic syndrome [75, 76], or associated with sensory hearing loss [77] cerebellar ataxia [78–80], and isolated myopathy [81, 82].

8.6.6 Neurodegeneration and POLG1 Deficiency

Polymerase gamma is the only DNA polymerase known to function in human mitochondria. It contains a large catalytic subunit, POLG1 (140 kDa), and two identical accessory subunits encoded by POLG2 (55 kDa) [83]. POLG1 consists of an exonuclease domain, a polymerase domain along with an intervening linker region [84]. Polymerase gamma contains DNA polymerase, 3′–5′ exonuclease and 5′-deoxyribose phosphate lyase activities and is involved in replication and repair of mtDNA [85].

Mutations in the POLG1 gene result in abnormal replication and impaired maintenance of mtDNA, resulting into significant decrease in mtDNA copy number, or multiple deletions in mtDNA which is expressed as mitochondrial dysfunction. These mutations have been associated with either dominant or recessive phenotypes. It has been observed that variants of the POLG1 CAG repeat encoding a polyglutamine tract is significantly associated with idiopathic sporadic Parkinson disease which is seen in the Finnish [86], in the North- American Caucasian [87] and in the Swedish population [88]. However, further genetic studies in cohorts from other geographical regions as well as functional studies of POLG1 poly-Q variants are needed.

Mancuso et al. [89] reported co-existence of parkinsonism and POLG1.

Mutations with mtDNA multiple deletions in several families, suggesting a possible role of POLG1 in inherited parkinsonism.

8.6.7 Mitochondrial Encephalopathy Lactic Acid Stroke (MELAS)

Mitochondrial encephalomyopathy, lactic acid and stroke (MELAS) is a devastating multisystem disease causing significant morbidity, disability and early death due to recurrent stroke like episodes evolving into progressive encephalopathy. Organ involvement is seen mainly in the CNS, Skeletal muscles, eye, cardiac muscles and rarely gastrointestinal tract and renal system are involved [90, 91]. The pathogenesis of stroke like episodes is not completely clear. They may be non vascular or due to oxidative phosphorylation dysfunction in the brain parenchyma [92]. Small vessel mitochondrial angiopathy is responsible for the mitochondrial abnormalities of the endothelial and smooth muscle cells of the blood vessels and is responsible for contrast enhancement on Brain MRI. Therefore the multisystem dysfunction in MELAS patients can be attributed to both parenchymal and vascular OXPHOS defect.

Alteration in nitric oxide homeostasis causing microvascular damage may explain the recurrent stroke like episodes and the higher morbidity observed in MELAS syndrome. By binding with cytochrome C oxidase- positive sites in the blood vessels present in the CNS, nitric oxide causes displacement of the Hem-bound oxygen resulting in decreased oxygen availability in the surrounding tissues and decreased free nitric oxide. The most common mutation found in patients with MELAS syndrome is a heteroplasmic A-to-G point mutation (m.3243A > G) in the mtDNA gene MTTL1 encoding mt tRNA, affecting approximately 80% of MELAS patients. Other mitochondrial DNA mutations are observed including the m.3244G > A, m.3258 T > C, m.3271 T > C [93].

Mutations in MELAS affect mitochondrial tRNA function, resulting into disruption of the global process of intramitochondrial protein synthesis. Measurements of respiratory enzyme activities revealed that more than one half of the patients with MELAS syndrome may have complex I or complex I + IV deficiency. A close relationship is apparent between MELAS and complex I deficiency. The decreased protein synthesis may ultimately lead to the observed decrease in respiratory chain activity by reduced translation of UUG-rich genes such as *ND6* (component of complex I) [94].

In addition, studies revealed that the 3243 A $\rightarrow$ G mutation produces a severe combined respiratory chain defect in myoblasts, with almost complete lack of assembly of complex I, IV, and V, and a slight decrease of assembled complex III. Selim & Mehaney in 2013 reported the clinical, radiologic and molecular results of a 10 years old Japanese boy with MELAS disease. The patient presented with recurrent episodes of headache, nausea and vomiting of 5 years duration. These episodes were associated with motor weakness on the right side, with difficulties in language and memory and visual disturbance, mostly right sided homonymous hemianopia. Neurological examination revealed generalized muscle weakness, with mild right sided hemiparesis. Magnetic resonance imaging (MRI)

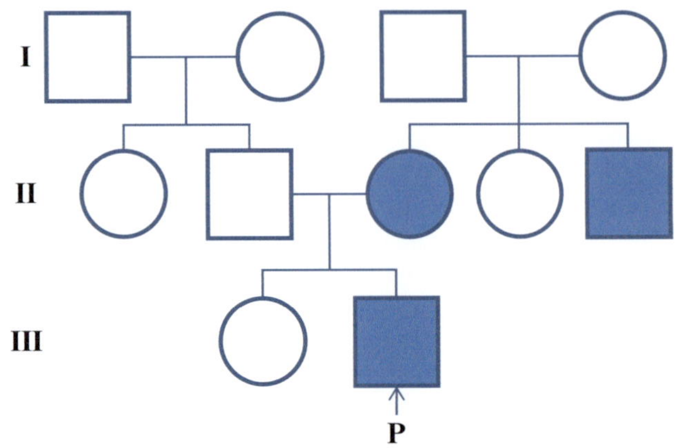

Fig. 8.13 Family Pedigree of the MELAS patient [95]

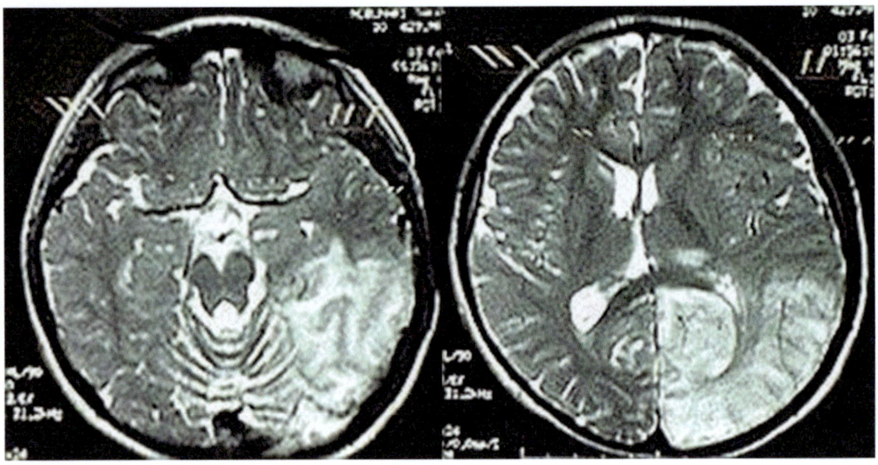

Fig. 8.14 Left parieto-occiptal infarction [95]

showed infarction of left temporo- parieto-occiptal regions without visible vascular abnormality at the Magnetic resonance angiography (MRA) (Fig. 8.14). Laboratory investigations revealed hyper lactic acidemia (lactic acid was increased tenfolds during the metabolic crisis) and a discrete increase in hepatic transaminases with normal creatine Kinase level. The mother reported that her brother (the proband uncle) suffered from the same clinical picture and died by the age of 19 years undiagnosed (Fig. 8.13). The mitochondrial DNA mutations A3243G, T3271C and G13513A were tested using Polymerase Chain Reaction-Restriction Fragment Length Polymorphism analysis and direct sequencing. The heteroplasmic A3243G mutation was detected in the blood of the patient and his mother [95].

We report here in the clinical, neuroimaging and molecular diagnosis of an Egyptian 12 years old male diagnosed with MELAS disease (unpublished).

The proband, fourth child of negative consanguineous parents, was admitted in the intensive care unit for the first time with the chief complaint of generalized tonic clonic seizures and disturbed conscious level. He was delivered by CS, full term pregnancy, had an uneventful perinatal history and had normal neurodevelopmental milestones.

His neurologic problem started 4 years ago, at the age of 8 years, with gradual progressive hearing loss culminating to deafness, an ABR was performed and showed bilateral sensory neural hearing loss and the patient is dependent on hearing devices. Concomitant with the hearing loss patient complained of recurrent episodes of headache.

At 10 years of age, the patient suffered from progressive visual loss resulting in almost blindness with fluorescein angiography and ERG demonstrating retinitis pigmentosa. Upon admission, he had recurrent generalized tonic clonic seizures, received diphenylhydantoin IV with no improvement, followed by depakene with worsening of the seizures associated with loss of speech and the power of ambulation.

Clinical examination revealed a wheel chair bound teenager, with inability to walk, cranial nerve examination revealed deafness, blindness with absent visual fixation and visual following movements, weakness and hypotonia of both upper and lower limbs with preserved reflexes, no speech and coordination could not be assessed at this stage due to marked weakness Sensory examination was normal as well as electromyography which was unremarkable. Chest and heart were clinically free with normal echocardiogram.

Basic laboratory investigations were all normal, lactic acid was increased at 5 mg/dl (normal up to 2,2 mg/dl). Expanded metabolic screen and urine organic acid were normal as well as very long chain fatty acids. Brain MRI revealed abnormal signal intensity in the basal ganglia (Fig. 8.15).

With the introduction of leviteracetam 500 mg twice daily, the seizures were controlled with improvement of his clinical examination which revealed: a well oriented child, with staccato speech and mild volational and truncal ataxia, with muscle power grade 4 in both upper and lower limbs, deafness and marked decrease in visual acuity due to retinitis pigmentosa. Whole exome sequencing revealed the common DNA mutation A3243G.

8.6.8 Mitochondrial Neurogastrointestinal Encephalopathy (MNGIE)

Among the Mendelian-inherited mitochondrial diseases are defects of intergenomic communication i.e. disorders due to nDNA mutations that cause depletion and multiple deletions of mtDNA. Mitochondrial neurogastrointestinal encephalopathy (MNGIE) represents the prototype of such disorders.

Mitochondrial neurogastrointestinal encephalopathy (MNGIE) is a rare multisystem autosomal recessive mitochondrial disorder. The major features of MNGIE disease can appear anytime from infancy to adulthood, but signs and symptoms most often begin in the second decade of life [96].

Abnormalities of the digestive system are among the most common and severe features of MNGIE disease. Most Patients suffer from severe gastrointestinal dysmotility characterized by

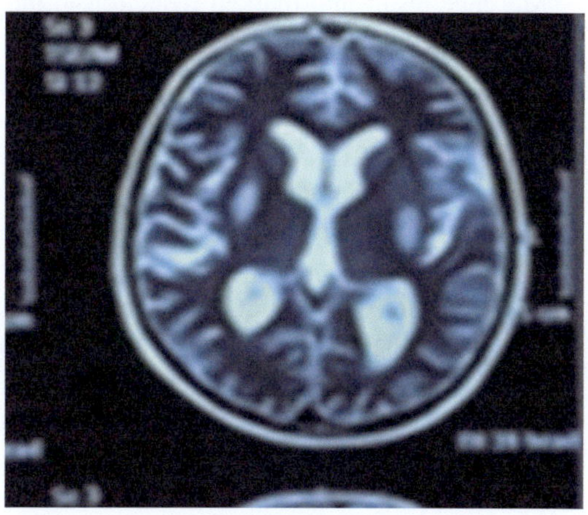

Fig. 8.15 T2 W Brain MRI showing bilateral and symmetrical high signal intensity lesion in both Putamina (Courtesy Prof. Laila Selim)

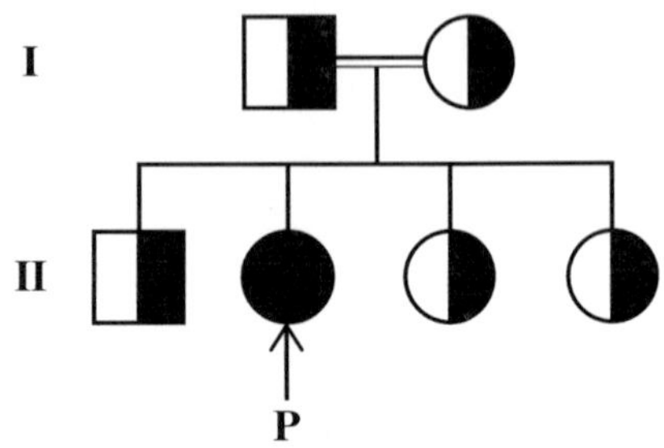

Fig. 8.16 Family pedigree of Case one with MNGIE [101]

early satiety, dysphagia, nausea, vomiting, episodes of diarrhea alternating with constipation, severe abdominal pain mimicking surgical abdomen. These Gastrointestinal problems lead to extreme weight loss and severe cachexia [97].

Abnormalities in both central and peripheral the nervous system are commonly associated with MNGIE. Affected individuals usually experience tingling, numbness and weakness in both hands and feet due to demyelinating peripheral neuropathy, which can be misdiagnosed as Charcot Marie Tooth disease (CMTD) or Chronic demyelinating poly neuropathy [98]. Ocular manifestations, mainly bilateral ptosis and external ophthalmoplegia, as well as sensory neural hearing loss may be present in MNGIE patients [99]. Brain MRI demonstrating leukoencephalopathy is a hallmark of MNGIE disease.

MNGIE disease is caused by mutation in the TYMP gene which provides instructions for the production of the thymidine phosphorylase enzyme which breaks down thymidine into smaller molecules helping the regulation of the level of nucleosides in the cell. Mutations in the TYMP gene result into marked reduction in the activity of thymidine phosphorylase gene allowing thymidine to build up to toxic level in the body with the ultimate result of damaging mitochondrial DNA (mtDNA) and disruption of the usual maintenance and repair of mtDNA causing it to become unstable [100].

Selim et al. 2016, reported the clinical, biochemical and molecular findings of three Egyptian patients suffering from MNGIE disease.

The first patient, a 22-year-old female, was the fourth child of first degree consanguineous parents. She presented with the main complaint of gradual and progressive muscle weakness and wasting in both upper and lower limbs. The first symptoms started at 16 years of age in the form of epigastric discomfort, episodes of diarrhea and constipation, anorexia and loss of weight which were followed 1 year later by the gradual appearance of neurologic symptoms. Muscle weakness was followed sensory symptoms in the form of hypoesthesia in all limbs. Cranial nerve examination revealed bilateral ptosis, external ophthalmoplegia, normal hearing and no signs of bulbar involvement. Motor examination showed hypotonia, distal muscular wasting in upper and lower limbs with pes cavus deformity and hammer toes and generalized hyporeflexia. Main laboratory investigations revealed hyperlactic acidemia and hyperuricemia. Nerve conduction velocity (NCV) testing revealed an axonal peripheral neuropathy affecting predominantly both lower limbs. She had 3 normal sibs, one brother and 2 sisters (Fig. 8.16). Histochemical analysis of the muscle biopsy revealed deficient Cytochrome C oxidase and mitochondrial respiratory chain enzyme assay revealed isolated complex I deficiency. Thymidine Phosphorylase enzyme activity revealed complete absence of enzyme activity (Fig. 8.17). Direct sequencing of Thymidine Phosphorylase gene revealed c.3371A > C homozygous mutation.

The second patient was a 22 years old girl, the second child born to first degree cousins who presented with the main complaint of abdominal discomfort, anorexia and failure to gain weight (Fig. 8.18). Her neurodevelopmental history revealed mild delay. At the age of 10 years, she started to suffer from episodes of abdominal pain, discomfort and pseudo-obstruction associated with severe anorexia and weight loss. Neuromuscular weakness developed insidiously followed by gradual progressive decline of visual

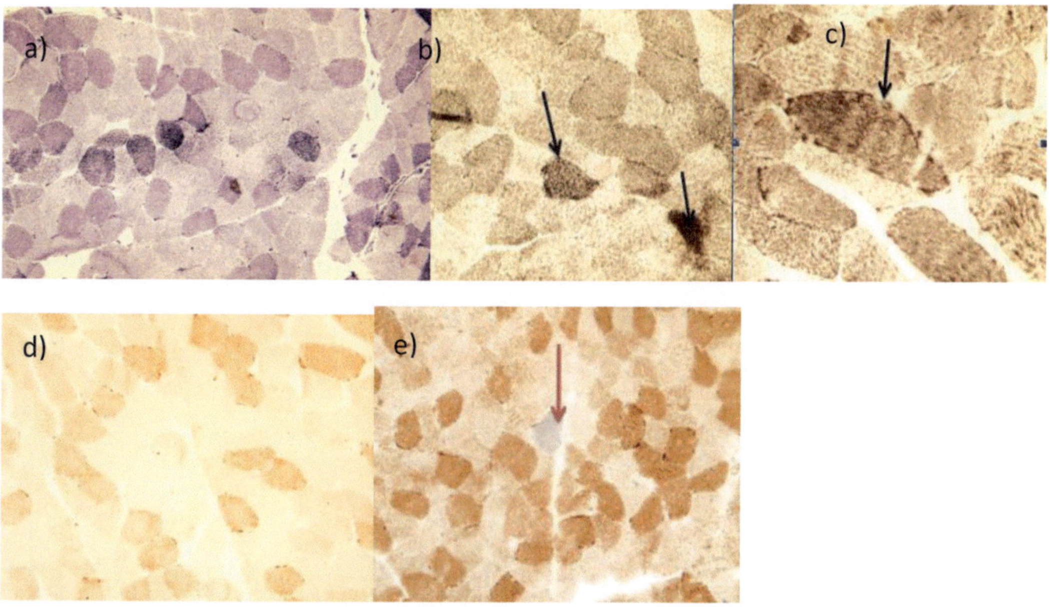

Fig. 8.17 (**a**) NADH-Tr shows occasional very dark fibers. (**b**) SDH showed occasional very dark fibers. (**c**) SDH higher magnification showing dark fibers with subsarcolemmal accumulation of stain. (**d**) COX shows decreased activity in some fibers. (**e**) Combined SDH &COX shows occasional *blue* fibre [101]

NADH-Tr NADH-tetrazolium reductase
SDH succinate dehydrogenase
COX cytochrome C oxidase

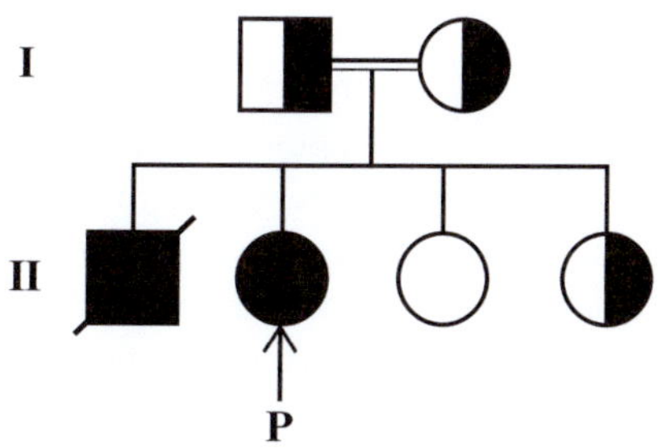

Fig. 8.18 Family pedigree of case 2 with MINGIE syndrome [101]

acuity and progressive hearing loss. Clinical examination revealed a severely emaciated young lady with a weight <3rd centile, walking with high steppage gait.

Inspection of the lower limbs revealed hammer toes, pes cavus, weakness of all four limbs and distal muscular atrophy. Fundus examination detected optic neuritis. Electromyography (EMG) and NCV showed demyelinating radiculoneuropathy with secondary axonal changes. Brain MRI revealed periventricular and subcortical areas of demyelination (Fig. 8.19). The elder brother, 25-year-old male presented by the age of 16 years with the same signs and symptoms. Barium follow through revealed a sluggish flow of barium with hypomotility, prolonged transit time, relatively dilated duodenal loop and two small diverticular outpouchings. Similar EMG/NCV and MRI findings were reported [101].

8.6.9 Mitochondrial Neurodegeneration and Parkinsonism

Parkinson's disease (PD) is the most common neurodegenerative movement disorder charac-

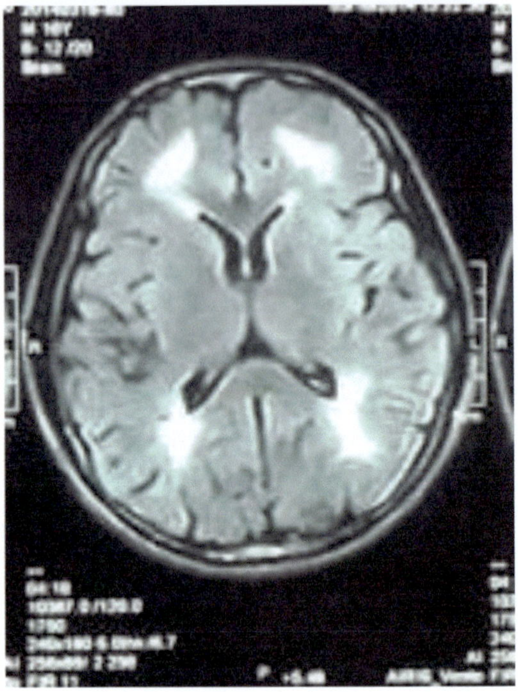

Fig. 8.19 Flair Brain MRI of Case 2 showing periventricular demyelination, the hall mark of MNGIE syndrome [101]

terized by bradykinesia, rigidity, resting tremor, and postural instability in addition to non-motor symptoms including depression and dementia. These clinical manifestations are due to the preferential loss of the dopaminergic neurones of the substantia Nigra, Pars compacta resulting in dopamine depletion [102, 103].

Several observations suggest that dysfunction of Complex I of the mitochondrial respiratory chain is involved in the pathogenesis of Parkinsonian disease (PD) and the degeneration of dopaminergic neurons [104]. It has been observed that point mutations and deletions accumulate in mtDNA of the brain neurons of patient suffering from PD [105]. On the other hand, many genes associated with familial forms of PD are involved in mitochondrial function [106].

Recent studies reveal that α-synuclein contains an amino-terminal mitochondrial targeting sequence and can associate with the inner mitochondrial membrane, interacting with mitochondrial complex I function [107].

It has been observed that overexpression of α-synuclein in transgenic mice impairs mitochondrial function, increases oxidative stress and enhances damage of Substancia Nigra [108]. It has also been suggested that mutant A53T α-synuclein might damage mitochondria directly [109]. Finally, mammalian cell apoptosis can be induced by alpha –synuclein and its mutant form [110]. These observations suggest that α-synuclein plays an important role in regulation of the mitochondrial apoptotic pathway [111].

The mitochondria represent a highly promising target for the development of PD biomarkers. Biochemical detection methods of potential biomarkers in PD are classified as genetic screening, mitochondrial complex I measurement, and α-synuclein levels and isoforms in blood [102, 112].

So far, some compounds with neuroprotective potential, including a few ordinary mitochondrial modulators such as creatine (N-aminoiminomethyl-N-methylglycine) and coenzyme Q10 (CoQ10), have been currently being investigated in clinical trials of PD [113].

8.6.10 Mitochondrial Depletion Syndromes

The mitochondrial DNA depletion syndromes are autosomal recessive disorders characterized by decreased mitochondrial DNA copy number in the clinically affected tissues [114, 115].

A balanced supply of deoxyribonucleoside triphosphates (DNTPs) is required for DNA polymerase c to faithfully replicate the mitochondrial genome, the mitochondrial deoxynucleotide triphosphates (dNTPs) pool is maintained both through the import of cytosolic dNTPs and by salvaging deoxyribonucleosides within the organelle itself [114, 116]. A number of nuclear-encoded enzymes are involved in these processes, including thymidine kinase 1 (TK1) within the cytosol, thymidine kinase 2 (TK2) and deoxyguanosine kinase (dGK) within mitochondria. The last two are key enzymes of the mitochondrial salvage pathway [114, 117]. Selim et al. 2012 described the clinical, histochemical, biochemical and molecular characteristics of one Egyptian pediatric patient with the myopathic form of mitochondrial depletion syndrome.

The proband was a 2.5 years old girl, the 3rd child of negative consanguineous parents who presented with the main complaint of gait unsteadiness (Fig. 8.20). The condition started at the age of 1.5 years with repeated falling and swinging wide base gait. At the age of 2 years, independent walking was completely lost with the appearance of head nodding, nystagmus followed by generalized tonic clonic seizures. Her clinical examination revealed ataxia and generalized truncal and limb hypotonia, bilateral ptosis, external ophthalmoplegia and fine nystagmoid movements. Main laboratory investigations revealed persistent lactic acidemia, 2.8 mmol/L

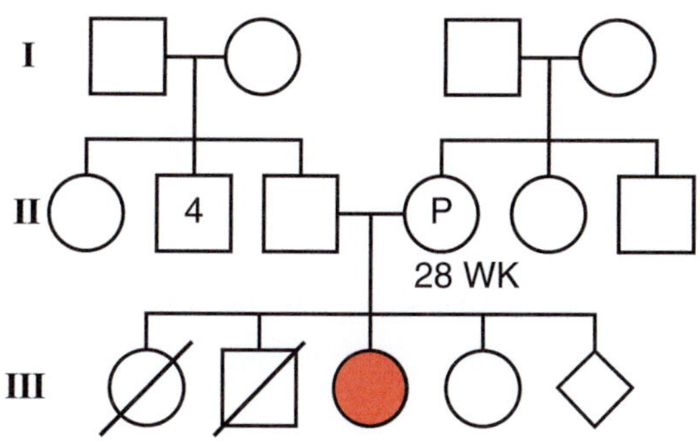

Fig. 8.20 Family pedigree of the studied patient with Mitochondrial depletion [118]

(normal, up to 2.2 mmol/L). Liver and kidney functions, creatine kinase (CK) and plasma ammonia were normal. Brain MRI showed abnormal lesions in the basal ganglia (appearing hypodense in T1 W and hyperintense on T2 W brain MRI, cerebellar demyelination and abnormal signal intensity in the brain stem suggestive of SURF1 gene mutation (Fig. 8.21). EEG showed epileptiform activity. The parents have one healthy daughter (1 year old). They have lost their first child at the age of 8 months undiagnosed, presenting with the same clinical picture and another male boy who died in utero at 32 weeks of gestation.

Histochemical study of muscle biopsy showed Cytochrome Oxidase negative fibers and increased staining for Succinate Dehydrogenase, and biochemical studies of the respiratory chain complexes revealed that complex I was not detected and complex IV activity was about 46% of age matched. Molecular diagnosis was done by quantitative radioactive Southern Blot and sequencing analysis of the whole coding regions of the TK2 gene. Southern blot analysis showed reduction of the mitochondrial /nuclear DNA ratio, the degree of depletion was around 30% of aged-matched controls. Sequencing analysis of the TK2 gene revealed no sequence variation. Targeted molecular diagnosis based on the biochemical analysis of the respiratory chain enzymes makes the molecular evaluation of mitochondrial disorders much easier.

In the following paragraphs, we describe the clinical picture, laboratory and molecular results of a 3 years old male patient who was diagnosed as mitochondrial depletion syndrome by whole exome sequencing.

N.M.R, is a 3 years old male, the 4th child of first degree Syrian cousin, presented with the main complaint of marked global developmental delay, recurrent episodes of metabolic acidosis with severe hyperlactic acidemia. The couple are first degree cousins having 3 previous children who died in the neonatal period. Obstructed delivery, hydrops fetalis, and hydrocephalus were the three consecutive diagnoses.

Clinical examination revealed mild dysmorphic facial features, generalized axial and appen-

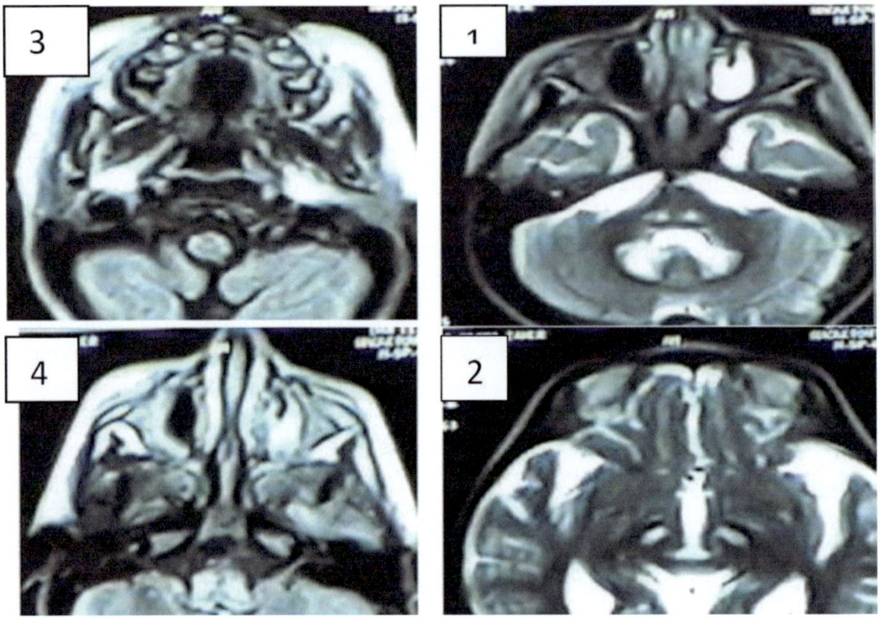

Fig. 8.21 Brain MRI of the proband showing abnormal T2 W and FLAIR; hyperintense signals are noted at: dentate nuclei (*1*), periaqueductal gray matter (*2*), medulla oblongata (*3*) and lower pons (*4*) (*arrows*) [118]

dicular hypotonia, severe intellectual disability. Extended metabolic screen was unremarkable, urine organic acid profile showed very high lactic aciduria in conjunction with extremely elevated plasma lactate (96 mg/dl, normal <20 mg/dl), blood ammonia: 3,7 mg/dl(normal <2 mg/dl). Brain MRI revealed global atrophic changes, bilateral basal ganglia chronic infarcts, periventricular demyelination (Fig. 8.22). Diagnosis by Whole Exome Sequencing revealed a homozygous mutation in the FBXL4 gene(c.292C > T(p. Arg98) diagnostic of mitochondrial depletion syndrome 13, encephalomyopathic type [118].

8.7 Conclusion

It is obvious from the literature that advances in sequencing technology and mitochondrial research unraveled the role of mitochondrial dysfunction in neurodegeneration resulting in a wide spectrum of phenotypically diverse disorders. Although mitochondria as its own genome its proper functioning is dependent upon the coordinated expression of both nuclear and mitochondrial encoded gene products with a major role of the nucleus in mitochondrial DNA repair. Mitochondrial donation though offering a potential cure to maternally inherited mitochondrial diseases further research and follow up of the procedure outcome are required to prove its efficacy and ensure safety.

Being the most common metabolic disorders encountered in the pediatric practice, Mitochondrial disorders are inspiring scientists to perform more advanced research to define more clearly the role of mitochondria in health and disease and to discover new therapeutic options to improve the quality of life of patients suffering from mitochondriopathies.

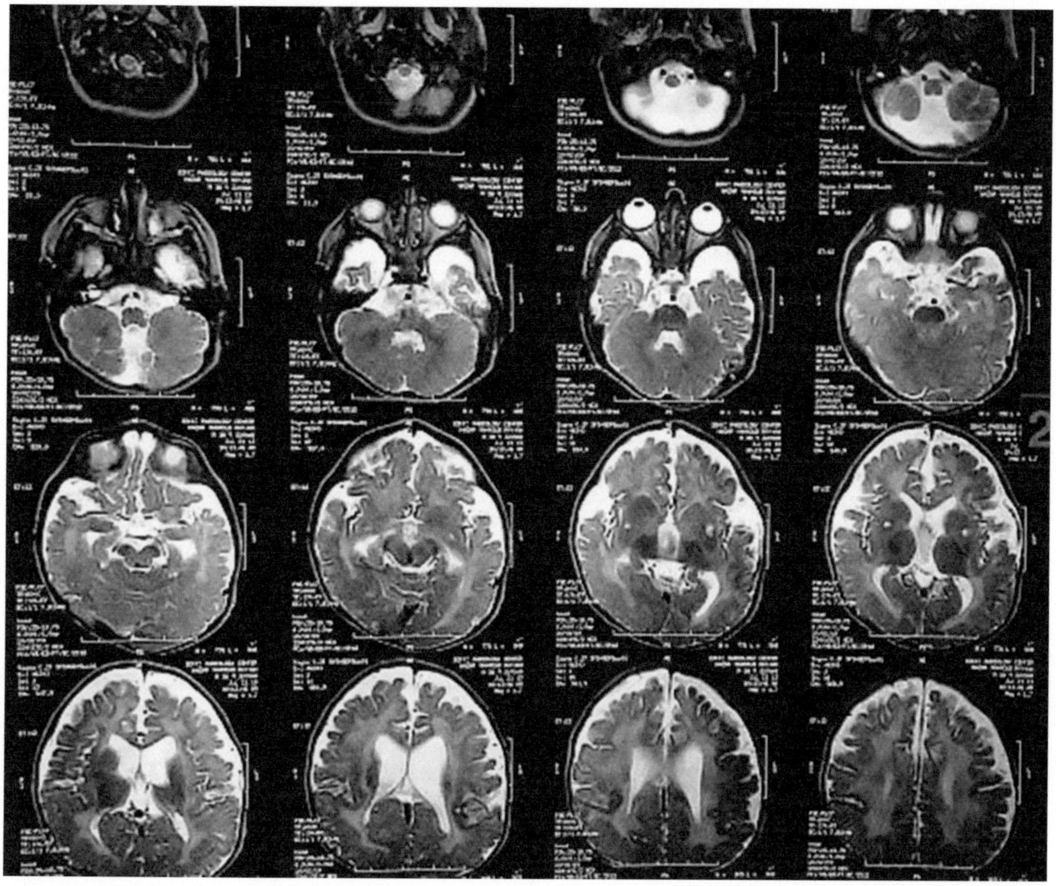

Fig. 8.22 Brain MRI of case 2 with mitochondrial depletion revealing global atrophic changes, bilateral basal ganglia chronic infarcts, and periventricular demyelination [118]

Acknowledgment Centogene, Rostock, Germany for performing whole exome sequencing free of charge.

References

1. "Mitochondria". Online Etymology Dictionary
2. Duchen MR (2004) Mitochondria in health and disease: perspectives on a new mitochondrial biology, Mol Asp Med, vol. 25 (pg. 365–351)
3. Koopman WJH, Willems PHGM, Smeitink JAM (2012) Monogenic mitochondrial disorders. N Engl J Med 366:1132–1141
4. Carroll J, Fearnley IM, Skehel JM, Shannon RJ, Hirst J, Walker JE (2006) Bovine complex I is a complex of 45 different subunits. J Biol Chem 281:32724–32727
5. Kühlbrandt W (2015) Structure and function of mitochondrial membrane protein complexes. BMC Biol 13:89
6. Available at http://cellpics.cimr.cam.ac.uk/mitochondria.html
7. Karbowski M (2010) Mitochondria on guard: role of mitochondrial fusion and fission in the regulation of apoptosis. Adv Exp Med Biol 687:131–142
8. Desler C, Marcker ML, Singh KK, Rasmussen LJ (2011) The importance of mitochondrial DNA in aging and cancer. J Aging Res 2011: 407536-9
9. Chial H, Craig J (2008) mtDNA and mitochondrial diseases. Nat Educ 1(1):217
10. Kudryavtseva AV, Krasnov GS, Dmitriev AA, Alekseev BY, Kardymon OL, Sadritdinova AF, Fedorova MS, Pokrovsky AV, Melnikova NV, Kaprin AD, Moskalev AA, Snezhkina AV (2016) Mitochondrial dysfunction and oxidative stress in aging and cancer. Oncotarget 7(29):44879–44905
11. Mohamed Yusoff AA (2015) Role of mitochondrial DNA mutations in brain tumors: a mini-review. J Cancer Res Ther 11(3):535–544
12. Sazanov LA (2015) Giant molecular proton pump: structure and mechanism of respiratory complex I. Nat Rev Mol Cell Biol 16(6):375–388

13. Koopman WJH, Distelmaier F, Smeitink JAM,Willems PHGM (2013) OXPHOS mutations and neurodegeneration. EMBO J 32(1):9–29
14. Available at https://biochemist01.wordpress.com/tag/electron-transport-chain/
15. Distelmaier F, Koopman WJ, van den Heuvel LP, Rodenburg RJ, Mayatepek E, Willems PH, Smeitink JA (2009) Mitochondrial complex I deficiency: from organelle dysfunction to clinical disease. Brain 132(Pt 4):833–842. doi:10.1093/brain/awp058
16. Alston CL, Compton AG, Formosa LE, Strecker V, Oláhová M, Haack TB, Smet J, Stouffs K, Diakumis P, Ciara E, Cassiman D, Romain N, Yarham JW, He L, De Paepe B, Vanlander AV6, Seneca S, Feichtinger RG, Płoski R, Rokicki D, Pronicka E, Haller RG, Van Hove JL, Bahlo M, Mayr JA, Van Coster R, Prokisch H, Wittig I, Ryan MT, Thorburn DR, Taylor RW (2016) Biallelic mutations in TMEM126B cause severe complex I deficiency with a variable clinical phenotype. Am J Hum Genet 99(1):217–227
17. Belevich I, Verkhovsky MI, Wikström M (2006) Proton-coupled electron transfer drives the proton pump of cytochrome c oxidase. Nature 440: 829–832
18. Mick DU, Fox TD, Rehling P (2011) Inventory control: cytochrome c oxidase assembly regulates mitochondrial translation. Nat Rev Mol Cell Biol 12:14–20
19. Balsa E, Marco R, Perales-Clemente E et al (2012) NDUFA4 is a subunit of complex IV of the mammalian electron transport chain. Cell Metab 16: 378–386
20. Oláhová M, Haack TB, Alston CL, Houghton JA, He L, Morris AA, Brown GK, McFarland R, Chrzanowska-Lightowlers ZM, Lightowlers RN, Prokisch H, Taylor RW (2015) A truncating PET100 variant causing fatal infantile lactic acidosis and isolated cytochrome c oxidase deficiency. Eur J Hum Genet 23(7):935–939
21. Sharma LK, Lu J, Bai Y (2009) Mitochondrial respiratory complex I: structure, function and implication in human diseases. Curr Med Chem 16(10):1266–1277
22. Castellana S, Vicario S, Saccone C (2011) Evolutionary patterns of the mitochondrial genome in Metazoa: exploring the role of mutation and selection in mitochondrial protein–coding genes. Genome Biol Evol 3:1067–1079
23. Chan DC, Schon EA (2012) Eliminating mitochondrial DNA from sperm. Dev Cell 22(3):469–470
24. Pagliarini DJ, Calvo SE, Chang B, Sheth SA, Vafai SB, Ong SE, Walford GA, Sugiana C, Boneh A, Chen WK et al (2008) A mitochondrial protein compendium elucidates complex I disease biology. Cell 134:112–123
25. Kliegman R, Stanton B, Geme JS, Schor NF (2016) Nelson textbook of Pediatrics, 20th edn.1600 John F.Kennedy Blvd, Ste. 1800. Elsevier
26. Available at TutorVista.Com
27. Available at WWW.slide share. Net%2FAmeena1994%2F–mitochondrial-DNA-mutation
28. Nadia R Mitochondrial diseases: the cracked bottleneck of inheritance. J Young Investig. Retrieved from http://www.jyi.org/issue/mitochondrial-diseases-the-cracked-bottleneck-of-inheritance/
29. Amato P, Tachibana M, Sparman M, Mitalipov S (2014) Three-parent in vitro fertilization: gene replacement for the prevention of inherited mitochondrial diseases. Fertil Steril 101(1):31–35
30. Meyers DE, Basha HI, Mary Kay Koenig MK (2013) Mitochondrial cardiomyopathy pathophysiology, diagnosis, and management. Tex Heart Inst J 40(4): 385–394
31. DiMauro S (2011) A history of mitochondrial diseases. J Inherit Metab Dis 34:261–276
32. Debray FG, Lambert M, Mitchell GA (2008) Disorders of mitochondrial function. Curr Opin Pediatr 20:471–482
33. Pitceathly RDS, Smith C, Fratter C, Alston CL, He LP, Craig K, Blakely EL, Evans JC, Taylor J, Shabbir Z et al (2012) Adults with RRM2B-related mitochondrial disease have distinct clinical and molecular characteristics. Brain 135:3392–3403
34. Suomalainen A, Isohanni P (2010) Mitochondrial DNA depletion syndromes—many genes, common mechanisms. Neuromuscul Disord 20:429–437
35. Mayr JA, Haack TB, Freisinger P et al (2015) Spectrum of combined respiratory chain defects. J Inherit Metab Dis 38(4):629–640
36. Chatterjee A, Mambo E, Sidransky D (2006) Mitochondrial DNA mutations in human cancer. Oncogene 25:4663–4674
37. Janssen RJ, Nijtmans LG, van den Heuvel LP, Smeitink JA (2006) Mitochondrial complex I: structure, function and pathology. J Inherit Metab Dis 29:499–515
38. Oláhová M, Thompson K, Hardy SA, Barbosa IA, Besse A, Anagnostou ME, White K, Davey T, Simpson MA, Champion M, Enns G, Schelley S, Lightowlers RN, Chrzanowska-Lightowlers ZM1, McFarland R, Deshpande C, Bonnen PE, Taylor RW (2017) Pathogenic variants in HTRA2 cause an early-onset mitochondrial syndrome associated with 3-methylglutaconic aciduria. J Inherit Metab Dis 40(1):121–130
39. Forster K (2016) Three-person IVF can prevent babies from inheriting deadly genetic diseases. Indepenent. Retrieved from http://www.independent.co.uk/life-style/health-and-families/health-news/three-parent-baby-hfea-allowed-technique-birth-child-ruling-fertility-decision-a7476731.html
40. Palacios-González C (2016) Mitochondrial replacement techniques: egg donation, genealogy and eugenics. 1-Monash Bioeth Rev 34(1):37–51
41. Tibbitts T (2014) Third scientific review of the safety and efficacy of methods to avoid mitochon-

drial disease through assisted conception, human fertilisation and embryology authority
42. Reardon S. Genetic controversial of three parent baby revealed but the child's parents have decided to forego long-term monitoring by researchers. Nat Int Weakly J Sci. Retrieved from https://www.nature.com/news/genetic-details-of-controversial-three--parent-baby-revealed-1.21761
43. Coghlan A (2016) '3-parent' baby method already used for infertility. New scientist. Retrieved from https://www.newscientist.com/article/2108549-exclusive-3-parent-baby-method-already-used-for-infertility/
44. Scutti S (2017) Controversial IVF technique produces a baby girl -- and for some, that's a problem. CNN. Retrieved from http://edition.cnn.com/2017/01/18/health/ivf-three-parent-baby-girl-ukraine-bn/
45. Chiang SC, Meagher M, Kassouf N, Hafezparast M, McKinnon PJ, Haywood R, El-Khamisy SF (2017) Mitochondrial protein-linked DNA breaks perturb mitochondrial gene transcription and trigger free radical-induced DNA damage. Sci Adv 3(4):e1602506. doi: 10.1126/sciadv.1602506. eCollection 2017
46. Bianchi NO, Bianchi MS, Richard SM (2001) Mitochondrial genome instability in human cancers. Mutat Res 488(1):9–23
47. Kazak L, Reyes A, Holt IJ (2012) Minimizing the damage: repair pathways keep mitochondrial DNA intact. Nat Rev Mol Cell Biol 13(10):659–671
48. Richard SM, Bailliet G, Páez GL, Bianchi MS, Peltomäki P, Bianchi NO (2000) Nuclear and mitochondrial genome instability in human breast cancer. Cancer Res 60(15):4231–4237
49. WIand S, Yorek MA (2010) Mitochondrial dysfunction in diabetes: from molecular mechanisms to functional significance and therapeutic opportunities. Antioxid Redox Signal 12(4):537–577
50. Krssak M, Petersen KF, Dresner A et al (1999) Intramyocellular lipid concentrations are correlated with insulin sensitivity in man: a 1H NMR spectroscopy study. Diabetologia 41:113–116
51. Kirches E (2011) LHON: mitochondrial mutations and more. Curr Genomics 12:44–54
52. Chen H, Chan DC (2005) Emerging functions of mammalian mitochondrial fusion and fission. Hum Mol Genet 14:283–289
53. Amati-Bonneau P, Milea D, Bonneau D, Chevrollier A, Ferré M, Guillet V, Gueguen N, Loiseau D, de Crescenzo MA, Verny C, Procaccio V, Lenaers G, Reynier P (2009) OPA1-associated disorders: phenotypes and pathophysiology. Int J Biochem Cell Biol 41(10):1855–1865. doi: 10.1016/j.biocel.2009.04.012. Epub Apr 21. Review
54. Cohn AC, Toomes C, Hewitt AW, Kearns LS, Inglehearn CF, Craig JE, Mackey DA (2007) The natural history of OPA1-related autosomal dominant optic atrophy. Br J Ophthalmol 92(10):1333–1336. doi: 10.1136/bjo.134726
55. Zanna C, Ghelli A, Porcelli AM, Karbowski M, Youle RJ, Schimpf S, Wissinger B, Pinti M, Cossarizza A, Vidoni S, Valentino ML, Rugolo M, Carelli V (2008) OPA1 mutations associated with dominant optic atrophy impair oxidative phosphorylation and mitochondrial fusion. Brain 131(Pt 2):352–367. doi: 10.1093/brain/awm335
56. Available at emedicine.medscape.com/article1217760-overview
57. Federico A, et al (2012) Mitochondria, oxidative stress and neurodegeneration. J Neurol Sci
58. Misko A, Jiang S, Wegorzewska I, Milbrandt J, Baloh RH (2010) Mitofusin 2 is necessary for transport of axonal mitochondria and interacts with the Miro/Milton complex .J Neurosci 30(12):4232–4240
59. Züchner S, Mersiyanova IV, Muglia M, Bissar-Tadmouri N, Rochelle J, Dadali EL, et al. (2004) Mutations in the mitochondrial GTPase mitofusin 2 cause Charcot-Marie-Tooth neuropathy type 2A. Nat Genet 36:449–451
60. Pich S, Bach D, Briones P, Liesa M, Camps M, Testar X, et al. (2005) The Charcot-Marie-Tooth type 2A gene product, Mfn2, up-regulates fuel oxidation through expression of OXPHOS system. Hum Mol Genet 14:1405–1415
61. Funalot B, Magdelaine C, Sturtz F, Ouvrier R, Vallat JM (2009) Ultrastructural lesions of axonal mitochondria in patients with childhood-onset Charcot-Marie-Tooth disease due to MFN2 mutations. Bull Acad Natl Med 193:151–60
62. Rouzier C, Bannwarth S, Chaussenot A, Chevrollier A, Verschueren A, Bonello-Palot N et al (2012) The MFN2 gene is responsible for mitochondrial DNA instability and optic atrophy 'plus' phenotype. Brain 135:23–34
63. Loiseau D, Chevrollier A, Verny C, Guillet V, Gueguen N, Pou de Crescenzo MA et al (2007) Mitochondrial coupling defect in Charcot-Marie-tooth type 2A disease. Ann Neurol 61:315–323
64. Hirano M, DiMauro S (1996) Clinical features of mitochondrial myopathies and encephalomyopathies. In: Lane RJM (ed) Handbook of muscle disease. Marcel Dekker Inc, New York, pp 479–504
65. Wahbi K, Larue S, Jardel C, Meune C, Stojkovic T, Ziegler F, Lombes A, Eymard B, Duboc D, Laforet P (2010) Cardiac involvement is frequent in patients with the m.8344A>G mutation of mitochondrial DNA. Neurology 74:674–677
66. Greaves LC, Reeve AK, Taylor RW, Turnbull DM (2012) Mitochondrial DNA and disease. J Pathol 226:274–286
67. Rommelaere G, Michel S, Malaisse J, Charlier S, Arnould T, Renard P (2012) Hypersensitivity of A8344G MERRF mutated cybrid cells to staurosporine-induced cell death is mediated by calcium-dependent activation of calpains. Int J Biochem Cell Biol 44:139–149
68. Quinzii CM, Hirano M (2011) Primary and secondary CoQ(10) deficiencies in humans. Biofactors 37:361–365

69. Montero R, Pineda M, Aracil A, Vilaseca MA, Briones P, Sánchez-Alcázar JA et al (2007) Clinical, biochemical and molecular aspects of cerebellar ataxia and coenzyme Q10 deficiency. Cerebellum 6:118–122
70. Boitier E, Degoul F, Desguerre I, Charpentier C, François D et al (1998) A case of mitochondrial encephalomyopathy associated with a muscle coenzyme Q10 deficiency. J Neurol Sci 156:41–46
71. Di Giovanni S, Mirabella M, Spinazzola A, Crociani P, Silvestri G et al (2001) Coenzyme Q10 reverses pathological phenotype and reduces apoptosis in familial CoQ10 deficiency. Neurology 57:515–518
72. Dinwiddie DL, Smith LD, Miller NA, Atherton AM, Farrow EG et al (2013) Diagnosis of mitochondrial disorders by concomitant next-generation sequencing of the exome and mitochondrial genome. Genomics 102:148–156
73. Jakobs BS, van den Heuvel LP, Smeets RJ, de Vries MC, Hien S et al (2013) A novel mutation in COQ2 leading to fatal infantile multisystem disease. J Neurol Sci 326:24–28
74. Scalais E, Chafai R, Van Coster R, Bindl L, Nuttin C, et al. (2013) Early myoclonic epilepsy, hypertrophic cardiomyopathy and subsequently a nephrotic syndrome in a patient with CoQ10 deficiency caused by mutations in para-hydroxybenzoate-polyprenyl transferase (COQ2). Eur J Paediatr Neurol 17:625–630
75. Ashraf S, Gee HY, Woerner S, Xie LX, Vega-Warner V et al (2013) ADCK4 mutations promote steroid-resistant nephrotic syndrome through CoQ10 biosynthesis disruption. J Clin Invest 123:5179–5189
76. McCarthy HJ, Bierzynska A, Wherlock M, Ognjanovic M, Kerecuk L et al (2013) Simultaneous sequencing of 24 genes associated with steroid-resistant nephrotic syndrome. Clin J Am Soc Nephrol 8:637–648
77. Heeringa SF, Chernin G, Chaki M, Zhou W, Sloan AJ et al (2011) COQ6 mutations in human patients produce nephrotic syndrome with sensorineural deafness. J Clin Invest 121:2013–2024
78. Horvath R (2012) Update on clinical aspects and treatment of selected vitamin-responsive disorders II (riboflavin and CoQ10). J Inherit Metab Dis 35:679–687
79. Liu YT, Hersheson J, Plagnol V, Fawcett K, Duberley KE et al (2013) Autosomal-recessive cerebellar ataxia caused by a novel ADCK3 mutation that elongates the protein: clinical, genetic and biochemical characterisation. J Neurol Neurosurg Psychiatry
80. Mignot C, Apartis E, Durr A, Marques Lourenço C et al (2013) Phenotypic variability in ARCA2 and identification of a core ataxic phenotype with slow progression. Orphanet J Rare Dis 8:173
81. Horvath R, Schneiderat P, Schoser BG, Gempel K, Neuen-Jacob E et al (2006) Coenzyme Q10 deficiency and isolated myopathy. Neurology 66:253–255
82. Gempel K, Topaloglu H, Talim B, Schneiderat P, Schoser BG et al (2007) The myopathic form of coenzyme Q10 deficiency is caused by mutations in the electron-transferring-flavoprotein dehydrogenase (ETFDH) gene. Brain 130:2037–2044
83. Copeland WC (2008) Inherited mitochondrial diseases of DNA replication. Annu Rev Med 59:131–146. pmid:17892433
84. Nguyen KV, Ostergaard E, Ravn SH, Balslev T, Danielsen ER, Vardag A et al (2005) POLG mutations in Alpers syndrome. Neurology 65:1493–1495
85. Hudson G, Chinnery PF (2006) Mitochondrial DNA polymerase-gamma and human disease. Hum Mol Genet 2:244–252
86. Luoma PT, Eerola J, Ahola S, Hakonen AH, Hellström O, Kivistö KT et al (2007) Mitochondrial DNA polymerase gamma variants in idiopathic sporadic Parkinson disease. Neurology 69:1152–1159
87. Eerola J, Luoma PT, Peuralinna T, Scholz S, Paisan-Ruiz C, Suomalainen A et al (2010) POLG1 polyglutamine tract variants associated with Parkinson's disease. Neurosci Lett 477:1–5
88. Anvret A, Westerlund M, Sydow O, Willows T, Lind C, Galter D et al (2010) Variations of the CAG trinucleotide repeat in DNA polymerase γ (POLG1) is associated with Parkinson's disease in Sweden. Neurosci Lett 485:117–120
89. Mancuso M, Filosto M, Orsucci D, Siciliano G (2008) Mitochondrial DNA sequence variation and neurodegeneration. Hum Genomics 3:71–78
90. Seidowsky A, Hoffmann M, Glowacki F, Dhaenens CM, Devaux JP, Lessore de Sainte Foy C, et al (2012) Renal involvement in MELAS syndrome - a series of 5 cases and review of the literature. Clin Nephrol
91. Meseguer S, Martínez-Zamora A, García-Arumí E, Andreu AL, Armengod ME (2014) The ROS-sensitive microRNA-9/9* controls the expression of mitochondrial tRNA-modifying enzymes and is involved in the molecular mechanism of MELAS syndrome. Hum Mol Genet
92. Testai FD, Gorelick PB (2010) Inherited metabolic disorders and stroke part 1: Fabry disease and mitochondrial myopathy, encephalopathy, lactic acidosis, and strokelike episodes. Arch Neurol 67(1):19–24
93. Liu K, Zhao H, Ji K, Yan C (2014) MERRF/MELAS overlap syndrome due to the m.3291T>C mutation. Metab Brain Dis 29(1):139–144
94. Sasarman F, Antonicka H, Shoubridge EA (2008) The A3243G tRNALeu(UUR) MELAS mutation causes amino acid misincorporation and a combined respiratory chain assembly defect partially suppressed by overexpression of EFTu and EFG2. Hum Mol Genet 17(23):3697–3707
95. Selim L, Mehany D (2013) Mitochondrial encephalopathy with lactic acidosis and stroke-like episodes in a Japanese child: clinical, radiological and molecular genetic analysis. The Egy J Med H Gen 14:317–322

96. Hirano M, MARTI R, Spinazzola A, Nishinol, Nishigaki Y (2004) Thymidine phosphorylase deficiency causes MNGIE: an autosomal recessive mitochondrial disorder. Nucleosides Nucleotides Nucleic Acids 23:1217–1225
97. Garone C, Tadesse S, Hirano M (2011) Clinical and genetic spectrum of mitochondrial neurogastrointestinal encephalomyopathy. Brain 134:3326–3332
98. Said G, Lacroix C, Plante-Bordeneuveu, Messing B, Slama A, Crenn P, Nivelon Chevallier A, Bedenne L, Soichot P, Manceau E, Rigaud D, Guiochon-Mantel A, Matuchansky C (2005) Clinicopathological aspects of the neuropathy of neurogastrointestinal encephalomyopathy (MNGIE) in four patients including two with a Charcot-Marie-Tooth presentation. J Neurol 252:655–662
99. Van Goethem G, Schwartz M, LÖfrena, Dermaut B, Van Van Broeckhoven C, Vissing J (2003) Novel POLG mutations in progressive external ophthalmoplegia mimicking mitochondrial neurogastrointestinal encephalomyopathy. Eur J Hum Genet, 11:547–549
100. Slama A, Lacroix C, Plante-Bordeneuve V, Lombès A, Conti M, Reimund JM, Auxenfants E, Crenn P, Laforêt P, Joannard A, Seguy D, Pillant H, Joly P, Haut S, Messing B, Said G, Legrand A, Guiochon-Mantel A (2005) Thymidine phosphorylase gene mutations in patients with mitochondrial neurogastrointestinal encephalomyopathy syndrome. Mol Genet Meta 84:326–331
101. Selim L, Van Coster R, Mehaney D, Hassan F, Vanlander A, Smet J, De Latter E, VAndemeulebroecke K, Mohamed Abdou D, Nakhla G, Mostafa M, Habets D, Bakker J, Abdel Elbary A (2016) Mitochondrial neurogastrointestinal encephalopathy; clinical, biochemical and molecular study in three Egyptian patients. Genetic Counselling 2:193–205
102. Exner N, Lutz AK, Haass C, Winklhofer KF (2012) Mitochondrial dysfunction in Parkinson's disease: molecular mechanisms and pathophysiological consequences. EMBO J 31:3038–3062
103. Henchcliffe C, Beal MF (2008) Mitochondrial biology and oxidative stress in Parkinson disease pathogenesis. Nat Clin Pract Neurol 4:600–609
104. Swerdlow RH (2009) The neurodegenerative mitochondriopathies. J Alzheimers Dis 17:737–751
105. Kraytsberg Y, Kudryavtseva E, McKee AC, Geula C, Kowall NW, Khrapko K (2006) Mitochondrial DNA deletions are abundant and cause functional impairment in aged human substantia nigra neurons. Nat Genet 38:518–520
106. Winklhofer KF, Haass C (2010) Mitochondrial dysfunction in Parkinson's disease. Biochimica et Biophysica Acta (BBA) – Mol Basis Dis 1802(1):29–44
107. Devi L, Raghavendran V, Prabhu BM, Avadhani NG, Anandatheerthavarada HK (2008) Mitochondrial import and accumulation of α-Synuclein impair complex I in human Dopaminergic neuronal cultures and Parkinson disease brain. J Biol Chem 283(14):9089–9100
108. Song DD, Shults CW, Sisk A, Rockenstein E, Masliah E (2004) Enhanced substantia nigra mitochondrial pathology in human α-synuclein transgenic mice after treatment with MPTP. Exp Neurol 186:158–172
109. Martin LJ, Pan Y, Price AC, Sterling W, Copeland NG, Jenkins NA et al (2006) Parkinson's disease alpha-synuclein transgenic mice develop neuronal mitochondrial degeneration and cell death. J Neurosci 26:41–50
110. Flower TR, Chesnokova LS, Froelich CA, Dixon C, Witt SN (2005) Heat shock prevents alpha-synuclein-induced apoptosis in a yeast model of Parkinson's disease. J Mol Biol 351:1081–1100
111. Battisti C, Formichi P, Radi E, Federico A (2008) Oxidative-stress-induced apoptosis in PBLs of two patients with Parkinson disease secondary to alpha-synuclein mutation. J Neurol Sci 267:120–124
112. Abou-Sleiman PM, Muqit MM, Wood NW (2006) Expanding insights of mitochondrial dysfunction in Parkinson's disease. Nat Rev Neurosci 7:207–219
113. Chaturvedi RK, Beal MF (2013) Mitochondria targeted therapeutic approaches in Parkinson's and Huntington's diseases. Mol Cell Neurosci 55:101–114
114. Blakely E, He L, Gardner JL, Hudson G, Walter J, Hughes I et al (2008) Novel mutations in the TK2 gene associated with fatal mitochondrial DNA depletion myopathy. Neuromuscul Disord 18(7):557–560
115. Moraes CT, Shanske S, Tritschler HJ, Aprille JR, Andreetta F, Bonilla E et al (1991) MtDNA depletion with variable tissue expression: a novel genetic abnormality in mitochondrial diseases. Am J Hum Genet 48(3):492–501
116. Mancuso M, Salviati L, Sacconi S, Otaegui D, Camano P, Marana A et al (2002) Mitochondrial DNA depletion: mutations in thymidine kinase gene with myopathy and SMA. Neurology 59:1197–1202
117. Johansson K, Ramaswamy S, Ljungcrantz C, Knecht W, Piskur J, Munch-Petersen B et al (2001) Structural basis for substrate specificities of cellular deoxyribonucleoside kinases. Nat Struct Biol 8:616–620
118. Selim L, Mehaney D, Hassan F, Sabry R, Zeyada R, Hassan S, Gamal Eldin I, Bertini E (2012) Mitochondrial DNA depletion syndrome presenting with ataxia and external ophthalmoplegia: case report Egy J Med H n13:351–357

9 Personalised Medicine: Genome Maintenance Lessons Learned from Studies in Yeast as a Model Organism

Arwa A. Abugable, Dahlia A. Awwad, Dalia Fleifel, Mohamed M. Ali, Sherif El-Khamisy, and Menattallah Elserafy

Abstract

Yeast research has been tremendously contributing to the understanding of a variety of molecular pathways due to the ease of its genetic manipulation, fast doubling time as well as being cost-effective. The understanding of these pathways did not only help scientists learn more about the cellular functions but also assisted in deciphering the genetic and cellular defects behind multiple diseases. Hence, yeast research not only opened the doors for transforming basic research into applied research, but also paved the roads for improving diagnosis and innovating personalized therapy of different diseases. In this chapter, we discuss how yeast research has contributed to understanding major genome maintenance pathways such as the S-phase checkpoint activation pathways, repair via homologous recombination and non-homologous end joining as well as topoisomerases-induced protein linked DNA breaks repair. Defects in these pathways lead to neurodegenerative diseases and cancer. Thus, the understanding of the exact genetic defects underlying these diseases allowed the development of personalized medicine, improving the diagnosis and treatment and overcoming the detriments of current conventional therapies such as the side effects, toxicity as well as drug resistance.

A.A. Abugable
Center for Genomics, Helmy Institute for Medical Sciences, Zewail City of Science and Technology, Giza, Egypt

Center for Materials Science, Zewail City of Science and Technology, Giza, Egypt

D.A. Awwad
University of Science and Technology, Zewail City of Science and Technology, Giza, Egypt

D. Fleifel • M. Elserafy (✉)
Center for Genomics, Helmy Institute for Medical Sciences, Zewail City of Science and Technology, Giza, Egypt
e-mail: melserafy@zewailcity.edu.eg

M.M. Ali
University of Science and Technology, Zewail City of Science and Technology, Giza, Egypt

Department of Medical Microbiology and Immunology, Faculty of Medicine, Mansoura University, Mansoura, Egypt

S. El-Khamisy
Krebs Institute and Sheffield Institute for Nucleic Acids, Department of Molecular Biology and Biotechnology, Firth Court, University of Sheffield, Sheffield S10 2TN, UK

Center for Genomics, Helmy Institute for Medical Sciences, Zewail City of Science and Technology, Giza, Egypt

S. El-Khamisy (ed.), *Personalised Medicine*, Advances in Experimental Medicine and Biology 1007,
DOI 10.1007/978-3-319-60733-7_9

Keywords
Personalized medicine • Yeast • DNA repair • Genome maintenance • DNA damage repair • Homologous recombination repair • Non-homologous end joining • TDP1 • TDP2 • DNA damage checkpoint

9.1 Introduction

9.1.1 Yeast: A Powerful Model Organism for Understanding Cellular Processes

Being the first eukaryotic organism to be sequenced in 1996 was a huge step towards satisfying the curiosity of scientists trying to understand all the mysterious processes ongoing inside eukaryotic cells. With only 16 chromosomes carrying 6000 genes [1], the budding yeast has basic cellular processes similar to humans as well as a huge number of human orthologs [2].

Several reasons are behind using yeast as a powerful model organism in research including its conserved cellular pathways, fast doubling time as well as its powerful genetics. Gene deletions, tagging and mutagenesis are easier and faster than in human cells and thus deciphering genes' functions is easily achieved. Furthermore, yeast research is more economic when compared to working with cell lines or animal models [3–5].

9.1.1.1 Yeast as a Model Organism for Studying DNA Repair and Genome Maintenance

Many different DNA repair pathways were better understood via researching on yeast. These pathways include repair via Homologous Recombination (HR) and Non-Homologous End Joining (NHEJ), Protein-linked DNA Breaks (PDBs) repair, Mismatch Repair, Nucleotide Excision Repair, Base Excision Repair, removal of ribonucleotides misincorporated into the genome and resolving R-loops accumulated at undesired loci [6–12]. In addition to its great impact on deciphering the signaling required for activation of the S-phase checkpoint to achieve genome maintenance [13].

In this chapter, we focus on the contribution of yeast research; both performed on *Saccharomyces cerevisiae*/Budding yeast and *Schizosaccharomyces pombe*/Fission yeast, to understanding of several genome maintenance pathways. These pathways include S-phase checkpoint activation, HR, NHEJ and finally repair of Topoisomerases induced PDBs. We then discuss the impact of deciphering the respective molecular pathways on understanding a variety of neurodegenerative diseases and cancers. Finally, we review the advancement in personalized medicine of the discussed diseases after identifying the exact genetic defects.

9.2 Yeast Research Contribution to Understanding of DNA Damage Checkpoints and Associated Diseases

Hartwell was the first to postulate the idea of checkpoints to ensure the correct sequence of cell cycle phases using *Saccharomyces cerevisiae*. He proposed that the cell cycle arrests when DNA is damaged, allowing time for repair before progressing to the next phase. He identified a number of cell division cycle (*CDC*) genes, including *CDC28* that was found later by Paul Nurse in *Schizosaccharomyces pombe* (*CDC2*) in addition to the multiple CDKs in humans controlling cell cycle checkpoints transition [14–17]. The relevance of their work, in addition to the findings of Sir Timothy Hunt who used sea urchin as a model organism, was accentuated by awarding them the Nobel Prize in Physiology and Medicine in 2001. Consequently, yeast has been a valuable model in the dissection of the S-phase checkpoint pathway, which is essential for maintaining genomic integrity [18].

In this section, we discuss the contribution of yeast to deciphering the function of key kinases; ATM, ATR, CHK1 and CHK2 in S-phase checkpoint. We then reflect on neurodegenerative diseases and cancers associated with defects in these players and their potential personalised therapeutic approaches.

9.2.1 ATM/ATR-Mediated Checkpoints

Three types of S-phase checkpoint pathways have been reported according to the type of DNA damage they respond to; replication-dependent checkpoints including *Replication Checkpoint* and *S/M* besides the *Replication-Independent/Intra S-phase Checkpoint* [18].

The Replication Checkpoint is activated in response to replication-related stresses such as depletion of deoxyribonucleotides (dNTPs), chemical inhibition of DNA polymerases and collision of replication forks with aberrant DNA structures. Similarly, the *S/M Checkpoint* ensures precise, error-free duplication of the entire genome before entering the M-phase. The *Intra S-phase Checkpoint* is activated by DNA Double-Strand Breaks (DSBs) resulting from genotoxic agents such as Ionizing Radiation (IR) [18, 19].

Checkpoint responses to DNA damage follow an evolutionary-conserved 'unified' model where ATM and ATR are the main 'sensor kinases' phosphorylating the downstream 'effector kinases'; CHK2 and CHK1, respectively. The ATM-CHK2 pathway responds mainly to DSBs, and the ATR-CHK1 pathway responds to wider stimuli including single strand DNA breaks (SSBs), DSBs and replication blocks. This is done through phosphorylating downstream targets to achieve cell cycle arrest, expression of DNA damage repair genes and stabilization of replication forks [20, 21] (Fig. 9.1).

9.2.1.1 Discovery of *ATM, ATR, CHK1* and *CHK2* in Yeast

ATM, *ATR*, *CHK1* and *CHK2* were all initially discovered in yeast. *MEC1*/*ATR* was primarily identified in 1994 as a gene required for DNA repair, cell cycle progression, cell growth and meiotic recombination in yeast [22, 23]. *TEL1*/*ATM* was initially discovered in a yeast mutant screen for genes involved in telomere maintenance in 1986 [24]. A potential role of *TEL1*/*ATM* in DNA repair and cell cycle checkpoints was later uncovered and *TEL1* was reported to be ATM's homologue and functionally redundant with *MEC1* [25–28]. However, later studies identified Mec1 as a protein kinase that has a key function in both the intra-S and replication checkpoints [29, 30] and is rather homologous to ATR in mammals [31].

In 1993, Chk1 was described in fission yeast as a serine/threonine kinase, regulating the G2/M phase transition, the constitutive expression of which arrests the cell cycle [32]. In 1997, the human ortholog was identified [33]. Rad53/*CHK2* was first identified in yeast in 1974 as its mutation exhibited sensitivity to X-ray radiation [34]. Almost 20 years later, it was reported as an essential nuclear kinase during the S-phase, playing a role in DNA replication and repair [22, 35–37]. In 1998, *CHK2* was identified as the mammalian

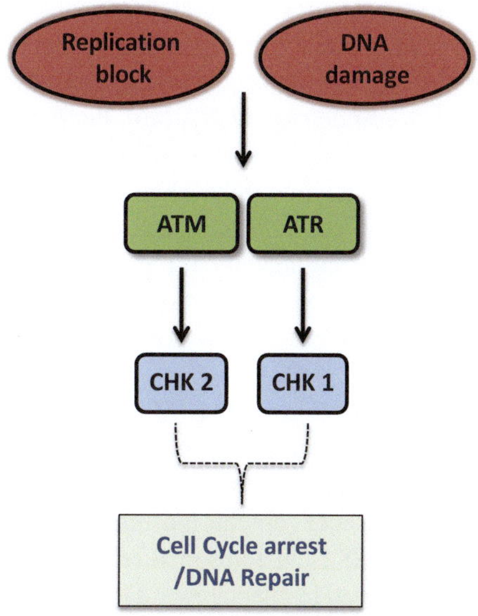

Fig. 9.1 Simplified overview of ATM/CHK2 and ATR/CHK1 pathways: to activate the S-phase checkpoint, the sensor kinases, ATM and ATR phosphorylate downstream effector kinases CHK2 and CHK1, respectively to activate downstream signaling

homologue of yeast *RAD53*, and was linked to the ATM-mediated response to DNA damage [38].

9.2.2 ATM/CHK2 and ATR/CHK1 Pathways, Associated Diseases and Potential Personalized Therapy

9.2.2.1 Ataxia-Telangiectasia (A-T)

A-T is an autosomal recessive disorder, associated with telangiectasia, cerebellar ataxia, immune defects, and increased cancer susceptibility. Patients have mutated *ATM* gene. Thus, the gene was named Ataxia-Telangiectasia Mutated, after the disease [39–41].

ATM-deficient mammalian cells show impaired checkpoint and DSBs repair pathways [42–44]. Impaired intra-S-phase checkpoint response leads to radio-resistant DNA synthesis (RDS) where cells are unable to slow down DNA replication when irradiated [41, 44, 45].

The therapeutic field for this disease is still quite immature. The most recent approaches involve induced pluripotent stem cells to create an in vitro A-T model in 2013. Using this model, researchers identified potential therapeutic compounds, called Small Molecule Read-Through that increased ATM protein activity and improved the ability to repair damaged DNA [46]. Furthermore, a Spanish team is currently trying to introduce ATM mini-genes into cells obtained from A-T patients to express ATM and enhancing their delivery system, giving hope to A-T patients that one day gene therapy would be possible (http://www.atsociety.org.uk/gene-therapy-project-in-granada).

9.2.2.2 Seckel Syndrome (SS)

ATR mutations increase susceptibility to DNA damage, impair checkpoint functions and increase incidence of chromosomal breakages [22, 23, 47]. SS is an autosomal recessive disorder characterized by mental retardation, impaired growth and microcephaly [48]. The first identified genetic cause, c.2101A>G mutation in *ATR*, results in skipping of exon 9. This mutation reinforces a splicing silencer (ESS) and weakens a splicing enhancer (ESE). Elucidating the molecular mechanism of this mutation gave rise to two potential RNA-based therapies: using an antisense oligonucleotide (AON^{ATR}) that targets c.2101A position recovering the exon inclusion as well as using a U1snRNA which base-pairs with the weak 5′ splice sites, rescuing exon inclusion in the ATR^{SS}-allele [48, 49].

9.2.2.3 Cancer

The ATR/CHK1 pathway is seldom mutated or lost, with rare exceptions of some malignancies [50]. In addition, siRNA inhibition of *CHK1* enhanced the sensitization of ovarian, breast cancer and neuroblastoma to chemo-and radio therapeutic agents [51–53]. Therefore, it is an attractive strategy in cancer therapy to combine the depletion of DNA damage response players with conventional chemotherapy, creating the so-called ‘synthetic lethality’ [54].

Along these lines, ablation of the ATR-CHK1 axis has been found to have anti-tumor activity by exacerbating the replication stress on cells [55]. In addition, treating melanomas exhibiting high levels of DNA damage with CHK1 inhibitors, AR323 and AR678, demonstrated significant lethality [56]. Furthermore, several trials identified chemotherapy-enhancing CHK1 inhibitors [57, 58].

Mutations and epigenetic modifications in components of the ATM/CHK2 axis were shown to be associated with malignancy [59–70]. However, some human cancers exhibit overexpression of ATM and/or Chk2 or other components of the ATM-Chk2 pathway [71–74].

Multiple studies have shown that administration of ATM, ATR or CHK1 inhibitors as well as silencing them have an anti-cancer effect, in addition to sensitizing several cancer types to radio- and chemotherapy [56, 75–103]. For example, ATM was found to be activated upon the inhibition of Poly (ADP-Ribose) Polymerase (PARP-1), probably due to replication fork collapse and subsequent activation of repair by HR. [104] Along these lines, inhibiting ATM was found to have a sensitizing effect to PARP inhibitors in mantle cell lymphoma cells and breast cancer cells [105, 106]. Similarly, inhibiting CHK2 in combination with PARP inhibitors elicited a synergistic lethal response in lymphoma cells overexpressing MYC [107]. Nonetheless, definitive results regarding the chemo- and radio-sensitizing effect of ATM/CHK2 inhibition are still lacking. CHK2 inactivation, for instance, was reported to confer a radio-protective effect in some malignant cells [108, 109]. In addition, some of the sensitizing drugs have shown poor bioavailability making them not suitable for clinical administration. Thus, further experimentations, validating drugs action in vivo and on patients in clinical trials are needed [110].

It is also worth mentioning that induced mutations in CHK1 leads to its constitutive activation in the absence of DNA damage thus inhibiting cancer cells' proliferation [111]. This notion leads to the intriguing idea that over-activating CHK1 in the absence of DNA damaging agents would kill cancer cells. This method would entail minimal side effects since it does not involve using other chemotoxic agents [54].

In spite of promising preclinical results, few inhibitors only have entered clinical trials so far. Some CHK1 or CHK1/2 inhibitors (e.g. LY2603618, MK-8776, UCN-01 and CBP501) were tolerated by advanced solid tumors or lymphoma patients [112–117]. However, adverse side effects were evident in studies of other CHK1 inhibitors (e.g. AZD7762 and UCN-01), most notably cardiotoxicity [97, 112]. Further elaboration on the clinical trials are reviewed in [97]. However, it is clear that further clinical investigations of CHK1 inhibitors are required to improve efficacy, bioavailability and decrease undesirable effects to develop them into bedside treatments.

9.3 Yeast Research Contribution to Understanding DNA DSBs Repair via HR and Associated Diseases

Homologous Recombination (HR) is conserved across all three domains of life [118]. Thus, a huge amount of what we currently know about HR both in meiosis and mitosis is learned from yeast studies [119]. In this chapter, we focus on HR in DSBs repair and explain how yeast work took research on DSBs repair via HR to a whole new level. Finally, we elaborate on the contribution of these findings to understanding different neurodegenerative diseases and cancers and innovation of personalised medicine to treat them.

9.3.1 HR Molecular Mechanism

When a DSB happens, the MRN complex or MRX in yeast, comprising Mre11, Rad50 and Xrs2/human NBS1, recognizes it and resects the 3′-DNA broken ends. RPA proteins then bind to the ssDNA to stabilize it till Rad52 together with mediators relieve RPA and recruit Rad51. This is slightly different in humans as BRCA2 along with DSS1 promote RPA-RAD51 exchange [120, 121]. However, RAD52 takes over BRCA2 function if it is mutated; but with lower efficiency [122].

Rad55-Rad57 dimer then binds, protecting and stabilizing Rad51 nucleofilament so that the homology search could start [123–126]. Rad54 ATPase then interacts with Rad51 stimulating its strand exchange activity. RAD54 translocation activity is thought to efficiently deliver dsDNA to the site of homology search causing base pairing disruption. Thus, facilitating the interaction with ssDNA filament, forming a Holliday Junction which is later resolved by Resolvase [125, 127] (Fig. 9.2).

9.3.2 Discovery of HR Key Players in Yeast

It is remarkable that the discovery, identification of functions and interactions of the majority of HR key players was first accomplished in yeast. The story begins as follows. In 1974, deletion of the majority of HR players in yeast exhibited meiotic defects, susceptibility to IR and inadequate vegetative growth [34]. Afterwards, in 1975 and 1976, Rad52 protein was found necessary for DSBs repair [128, 129]. In 1979, it was reported that Rad51 plays a similar role as Rad52

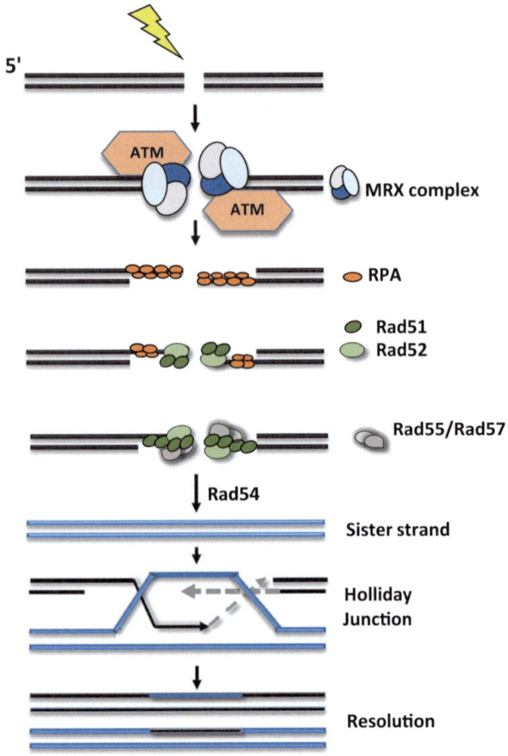

Fig. 9.2 The molecular mechanism of HR: the MRX complex senses the DSB and resects the 3′-DNA broken ends. RPA proteins then bind to the ssDNA to stabilize it. Rad52 together with mediators relieve RPA and recruit Rad51. Rad55-Rad57 dimer then binds to protect and stabilize Rad51 nucleofilaments and Rad54 ATPase helps Rad51 interact with the homologous strand. Holliday Junction form to achieve repair then it gets resolved by Resolvase

[130]. In 1980 and 1981, it was then shown that Rad52 is required for meiotic and mitotic recombination [131, 132].

The 1990s were a great time for scientists interested in HR. In 1992, Rad51 was found to be similar to the bacterial homologue RecA and an interaction with Rad52; crucial for recombination was reported [133]. Around the same time, proteins comprising the MRX complex were also identified to be important for HR and repair [134, 135]. Great progress was then made when *RAD51* human and mouse homologues were identified in 1993 and that of *RAD52* were identified in 1994 [136, 137]. The signaling of HR got more clear when a two-hybrid screen showed in vivo direct interaction between Rad51 and both Rad54 and Rad55 and between Rad55 and Rad57 in addition to Mre11 and Rad50 to achieve their role in meiotic and mitotic HR. [138–140] MRX complex identification in yeast triggered scientists to look for homologues. In 1995, the human MRE11 was found in a two-hybrid screen [141]. In 1996 and 1998, human RAD50 and NBS1 were discovered, respectively [142, 143]. It is worth mentioning that the MRX complex function in different pathways other than HR Mitotic DSB repair [144, 145].

More mechanistic data were available again through yeast studies. In 1997, Rad52 was found to be a mediator between RPA and Rad51 [146] and Rad55 and Rad57 heterodimer were reported to function together with RPA to promote Rad51 DNA strand exchange [147]. It was then possible to show that RAD52 in human stimulates RAD51 homologous pairing [148]. More secrets about the HR are still revealed through yeast studies. For example, it was shown in 2015 that yeast mitochondrial HR and DSBs repair are also dependent on Rad51 and Rad52 [149].

9.3.3 HR Associated Diseases and Potential Therapy

Mutations in the MRN complex genes are associated with several human diseases such as Nijmegen Breakage Syndrome (NBS) and an NBS-like disorder [143, 150]. In addition, they are implicated in several tumors [151–154]. In this chapter, we focus however on diseases associated with *RAD51* and *RAD52* genes.

9.3.3.1 *RAD51* Associated Diseases

Mutations in *RAD51* have been associated with neurological disorders and cancers. Moreover, mutations and overexpression of other *RAD51* paralogues, known to have a role in HR and DNA repair, were found to be associated with diseases such as Fanconi Anemia and cancers [155–157]. However, here we focus on *RAD51* and not its paralogues.

Congenital Mirror Movements (CMM) Neurological Disorder

CMM is a hereditary disorder where movements on one body side are mirrored involuntarily on the other. A significant down-regulation of *RAD51* mRNA levels in CMM patients was found as a consequence of exon 9 mutation, resulting in a premature stop codon and mRNA nonsense-mediated decay. Lack of therapeutic attempts result from an unclear disease mechanism; explaining how *RAD51* mutations and subsequent protein deficiency cause CMM [158].

Cancer

RAD51 expression is elevated in multiple cancers contributing to tumor cells chemo-resistance. Thus, RAD51 represents a good diagnostic and therapeutic target for cancer [159–163]. It is imperative to note that being an essential gene, selectivity of the different therapeutic options to cancer cells is essential to avoid its toxicity on normal cells [164].

Several therapeutic approaches have been proposed. For instance, combining RAD51 small molecule inhibitors with chemotherapeutic agents such as doxorubicin and cisplatin sensitizes cancer cells and mice xenografts to chemotherapy [165–167]. Moreover, inhibiting histone deacetylases in acute myelogenous leukemia induced miR-182, targeting RAD51 which sensitizes cells to sapacitabine [168].

In addition, indirect inhibition via Gleevec, which inhibits c-Abl that plays a role in RAD51 regulation, rendered glioma cell lines radiosensitive, indicating differential regulation and selectivity between normal and cancerous cells [169]. Furthermore, combining RAD51 siRNA knockdown with Gemcitabine, a pyrimidine analog, increased tumor cell sensitivity [170]. The use of siRNA against both RAD51 and BRCA2 sensitized brain glioma cells to alkylating agents as well [171].

Interestingly, modestly elevated RAD51 levels leads to increased HR activity in some cancer types, however, very high levels lead to lower HR efficiency and decreased cell fitness [172]. Thus, RS-1, a RAD51 stimulatory compound which stimulates its DNA binding activity was used to increase RAD51 to very high levels in immortalized cell lines and mice models to kill tumor cells [173].

9.3.3.2 *RAD52* Associated Diseases

RAD52 polymorphisms have been linked to some cancer types [174–176]. It has been also hypothesized that before breast cancer onset, SNPs in the 3′-UTR of *RAD52* mRNA interferes with the binding site for the miRNA let-7, causing increased RAD52 expression. Consequently, enhancing DSB repair and contributing to breast cancer development [177]. Likewise, targeting RAD52 with a short hairpin RNA (shRNA) decreased its levels and induced senescence in mouse bronchial epithelial cells [176]. Depletion of RAD52 also led to decreased cell proliferation in BRCA2-deficient breast cancer cells [178]. Moreover, High-throughput screening approaches identified various small molecules as RAD52 activity inhibitors that showed lethality in BRCA1 and BRCA2-deficient cancer cells [179–181].

Despite the numerous approaches aiming at achieving anti-tumor effects through the inhibition of RAD51 and RAD52, it is evident that further experimentations are still needed. The ultimate goal would be shifting these lab or preclinical trials into clinical trials testing the applicability of the drugs as personalized cancer therapies for humans.

9.4 Yeast Research Contribution to Understanding NHEJ and Associated Diseases

NHEJ plays a pivotal role in DSB repair. In contrast to HR, it does not need a homologous template to ligate the broken ends rendering it error-prone. Proteins involved in NHEJ in mammalian cells include the KU70/80 heterodimer, Artemis, XRCC4, DNA-dependent protein kinase (DNA-PK), DNA ligase IV and XRCC-like factor (XLF) [182–185].

9.4.1 NHEJ Molecular Mechanism

KU70/80 heterodimer detects DSBs in a sequence-independent manner, serving as a scaffold to recruit other proteins including DNA-PK which gets activated upon interaction with the DNA and KU70/80 [186, 187]. This interaction plays a role in forming a complex that holds the broken ends of the DNA together [188]. The XRCC4-DNA ligase IV complex is then assembled and XRCC4 serves as a second scaffold. Then, several processing enzymes are recruited to the DNA damaged site [186] (Fig. 9.3). In complex DNA damage, when base damages exist close to the DSBs such as DNA overhangs and non-ligatable termini, more players get involved to repair the break [189–192].

Although yeast lacks DNA-PK, it contributed significantly to the discovery and understanding of NHEJ ligases. Here, we discuss yeast contribution to understanding NHEJ and focus on diseases associated with defects in DNA ligase IV and potential personalized therapies.

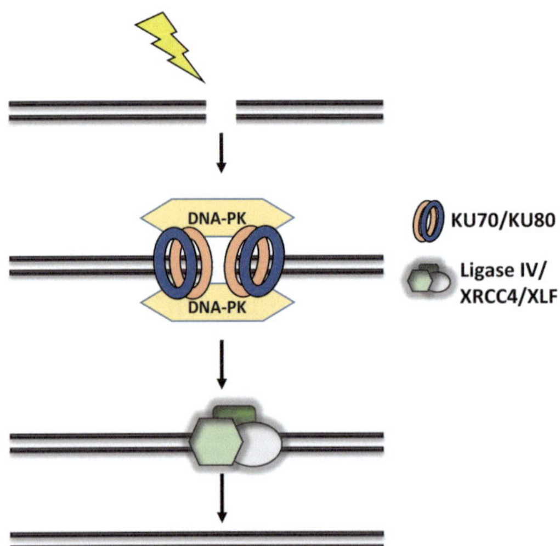

Fig. 9.3 NHEJ in higher eukaryotes. Ku70/80 heterodimer recognizes the break and helps recruits DNA-PK. Finally, XRCC4-Ligase IV complex mediates strands sealing. Other players are not shown

9.4.2 Yeast Research Contribution to Understanding NHEJ

DNA ligases have an essential role in joining DNA strands together after IR or other agents that induce breaks. Earlier studies have reported only one DNA ligase in *S. cerevisiae* [193]. On the other hand, four DNA ligases with different biochemical activities have been identified in mammalian cells [194–196]. The function of three of which was known, however, the physiological function of ligase IV remained unknown [194]. In 1997, yeast research helped identify Ligase IV function. Researchers found an increase in radio-sensitivity in *Δlig4Δrad52* strains when compared to *Δrad52* strains. Thus, reflecting that *LIG4* is involved in DSBs repair in a *RAD52*-independent manner [197].

To study whether Lig4 operates in the same pathway as Ku, the radio sensitivity of *Δlig4Δrad52Δyku70* strains was assessed and found to be indifferent from that of *Δlig4Δrad52* or *Δrad52Δyku70* indicating that Ku and Lig4 work in the same repair pathway. Moreover, it was found that *LIG4* yeast mutants have severe defects in NHEJ that cannot be compensated for by DNA ligase I in yeast, confirming Lig4's crucial role in NHEJ. Due to LIG4's sequence homology to human DNA ligase IV, the function of the human homologue was better understood [197].

DNA ligase IV end-joining activity comes last in the NHEJ process. This was revealed through a yeast-two hybrid screen performed in 1997 that showed that XRCC4 co-immunoprecipitates with DNA ligase IV only, indicating that DNA ligase IV-XRCC4 interaction is specific. DNA-ligase IV activity was compared in the presence and absence of XRCC4 and it was found that co-expression of XRCC4 increased the ligase activity seven to eightfolds. This proved that XRCC4 is needed to induce the ligase activity of DNA ligase IV, mainly through direct structural interaction [198].

In 2006, a yeast-two-hybrid screen was performed using human XRCC4 as bait to test for its interaction with all human coding genes represented by a brain cDNA library. A novel gene was identified to interact with XRCC4 and was referred to as Cernunnos or XRCC4-like factor (XLF) due to its structure sequence similarity to XRCC4. Protein interaction studies confirmed that XLF functions with XRCC4-DNA Ligase IV complex. To assess whether XLF was implicated in the NHEJ pathway, it was knocked down and interestingly, these cells showed increased radio sensitivity. In addition, the degree of radio sensitivity in XLF-depleted cells was the same as that of XRCC4-depleted cells, proving its involvement with XRCC4 in DSB repair [199].

It is now known that cells use two mechanistically distinct NHEJ pathways: Classic-NHEJ (C-NHEJ) leading to minimal alterations at the nick sites and alternative NHEJ (alt-NHEJ) causing extensive insertions and deletions, hence, disrupting normal sequences at repair sites. C-NHEJ, as previously explained, includes the function of KU70/80, LIG4, DNA-PK and XRCC4. On the other hand, alt-NHEJ depends on PARP1 signaling and 5′ to 3′ DNA resection at injury site by Ct Interacting Protein (CtIP) and MRN proteins. DNA ends are annealed through base pairing and are subject to fill-in synthesis by DNA polymerase θ where end-joining is promoted by LIG3 [200].

9.4.3 NHEJ Associated Diseases and Potential Personalized Therapy

Multiple diseases are associated with NHEJ defects. Here, we focus on neurological defects and cancers associated with DNA ligase IV defects.

9.4.3.1 Neurological Diseases

DNA ligase IV deficiency, named as LIG4 syndrome, is a rare hereditary autosomal disease caused by a hypomorphic missense or deletion mutation in the *LIG4* gene, reducing enzyme functionality. Some mutations directly disrupt the ligase domain while others impair the interaction between LIG4 and XRCC4 [201]. Patients suffer mainly from microcephaly, developmental delays, radio sensitivity and immune abnormalities [202]. These phenotypes overlap with other DNA-repair deficient syndromes such as Nijmegen Breakage Syndrome [201]. The first reported case of LIG4 syndrome caused by a missense mutation (R278H) lying within the active site was evident in a patient with T cell acute lymphoblastic leukemia. The mutation impairs the DSB rejoining through compromising the nick ligation activity of the mutant LIG4 without affecting the interaction between LIG4 and XRCC4 [201, 203–205]. The prevalence of LIG4 syndrome is not well studied as only 28 cases have been globally reported and current treatment involves haematopoietic stem cell transplantation, immunoglobulin administration as well as chemoprophylaxis to support the patients [206].

In neurons, NHEJ is the predominant repair pathway to DSBs. It has long been hypothesized that there is a positive correlation between aging and increased DNA damage. Reduced DNA repair was reported in Alzheimer's Disease (AD), however, with no specific mutations in NHEJ-involved genes. Nevertheless, it has been shown that DNA-PK levels are significantly lower in brains of AD patients [207]. These results were supported by a study where KU80 and DNA-PK levels were reduced in AD brains. A hallmark of AD is the accumulation of extracellular amyloid plaques caused by disruption in somostatin signaling pathway. Since Ku80 is a somostatin receptor, its deficiency can elicit the previously mentioned response, which induces DNA-PKc degradation [208] Since the end-joining activity is correlated with the expression of the DNA-PK and their catalytic activity, the NHEJ repair pathway might be deficient in AD.

Finally, defects in XLF, has been implicated in neurological diseases too. Patients with Cernunnos/XLF deficiency are symptomatic with microcephaly, growth retardation, and immunodeficiency due to defect in V(D)J recombination. Prospective treatment for immunodeficiency in such patients includes temporarily administering Intravenous Immunoglobulin (IVIG) and bone marrow transplantation [209].

Therapeutics for neurodegenerative diseases aim at correcting the function of mutated NHEJ players to regain normal cell response to DNA damage. The availability of personalised therapeutics for the diseases we have mentioned is still challenging as more research should be done to understand the exact contribution of the mentioned genetic defects to the development of the respective diseases.

9.4.3.2 Cancers

It seems that NHEJ involvement in cancer is complex as its over-activity or under-activity can lead to repair aberrations in neoplastic tissues [210]. Recent studies show that DNA-PK is upregulated in hepatocellular carcinoma and other cancer types, with a positive correlation to low differentiation levels and high metastatic ability. DNA-PK protects tumor cells against DNA damage induced by chemotherapy, rendering the cells resistant [211]. The up-regulation is hypothesized to be due to genomic aberrations, where DNA-PK gene locus (8q11.21) was found to be amplified [212]. Accordingly, small inhibitors are recently developed targeting the DNA-PK but pre-clinical studies in mice models are needed to further understand their effectiveness and side effects [211, 213, 214].

Similar results were found in cervical carcinoma surviving radiotherapy where DNA-PK, KU70 and KU80 were overexpressed [215]. However, DNA ligase IV was reported to be down regulated in chronic myeloid leukemia cancer cells [216] proposing that the expression levels of DNA ligases could be useful biomarkers of abnormal DNA repair in some cancer types [217]. Moreover, Leong et al. have shown that there is no difference in the expression levels of key NHEJ players such as Ku70/80, XRCC4 or DNA Ligase IV between radiosensitive and control lymphoblastoid cells. This shows that differential expression levels or abnormalities in these NHEJ proteins might not underlie the cause for clinical radiation sensitivity [218]. Therefore, determining the exact personalized therapies should depend on the cancer type and the specific expression of NHEJ genes in the cells of every patient.

Several studies aimed at identifying specific Ligase IV inhibitors. In 2008, in silico modeling of DNA Ligase inhibitors was conducted. Out of the identified hits, none were specific to Ligase IV only, however, they could be utilized as lead compounds for future development of more specific inhibitors [219]. In 2012, SCR7, DNA Ligase IV inhibitor, was found to reduce cancer cell proliferation in a DNA Ligase IV-dependent manner. Moreover, it reduced the growth of tumor cells formed in mice xenografts and elevated the tumor-inhibitory effects of DSB-inducing agents [220]. Results of these preclinical studies show that DNA ligase inhibitors could be developed as potential anti-cancer drugs.

9.5 Yeast Research Contribution to Understanding Topoisomerase-Induced PDBs Repair and Diseases Caused by Their Defects

DNA topoisomerases (TOPs) are vital enzymes known to resolve DNA entanglements and torsional stresses resulting from DNA processes such as gene transcription, replication, recombination as well as chromatin compaction [221, 222]. Six human genes code for TOPs, however, we shall focus on TOP1 and TOP2 [223], the neurodegenerative diseases and cancers associated with their defects and how personalized therapy is developing after revealing their molecular function.

TOP1 and TOP2 cleave and reseal one and two DNA strands, respectively via the nucleophilic tyrosine residue (Tyr) in their active site. This results in a transient break and covalent phosphotyrosyl bond formation between Tyr and the 3′ or 5′ end, forming the topoisomerase cleavage complex; TOP1cc and TOP2cc, respectively [221, 224]. PDBs form when the TOPs fail to complete their catalytic cycle and remain trapped on the DNA [225, 226]. Upon collision with RNA or DNA polymerases, the cleavage complex is converted to a DSB that requires DNA repair machinery to remove it [227–229].

Cells are equipped with Tyrosyl-DNA phosphodiesterases (TDPs) that hydrolyze the phosphodiester bond between the Tyr and the DNA strand. TOP1 and TOP2 are removed with TDP1 and TDP2, respectively [230, 231]. It is necessary that the TOP1 and TOP2 get proteolytically degraded before TDPs can act on the TOPcc [232–235]. The exact signaling pathways are illustrated in (Fig. 9.4). When TDP activity is deficient, other error-prone or error-free repair pathways takeover depending on the nature of the break (SSB or DSB) and the pathways the cells follow [236–246].

9.5.1 Discovery of TDP1 in Yeast

TDP1 was discovered in chemically mutagenized yeast, based on its ability to hydrolyse the phosphotyrosyl bonds between the 3′-DNA strand and TOP1, restoring the 3′-phosphate terminus at the TOP1-induced SSBs [230, 247]. Phosphotyrosine oligonucleotides bearing a phosphodiester bond at the 3′-end and a radiolabelled 5′-end were subjected to crude yeast enzymes extract. Then chromatography was performed to assess the ability to release tyrosine from the radiolabelled oligonucleotides. A partially purified enzyme was found to convert the tyrosine-oligonucleotide into a unique product reporting the first TDP activity in yeast in 1996 [247]. In 1999, the gene coding for TDP1 responsible for the TDP activity in yeast was identified and the existence of a human homologue was reported [230].

9.5.2 TDP1 Associated Diseases

9.5.2.1 Spinocerebellar Ataxia with Axonal Neuropathy (SCAN1)

A homozygous H493R mutation in *TDP1* was identified in a Saudi Arabian family with autosomal recessive SCAN1 resulting in loss of TDP1 activity. They suffered from peripheral axonal

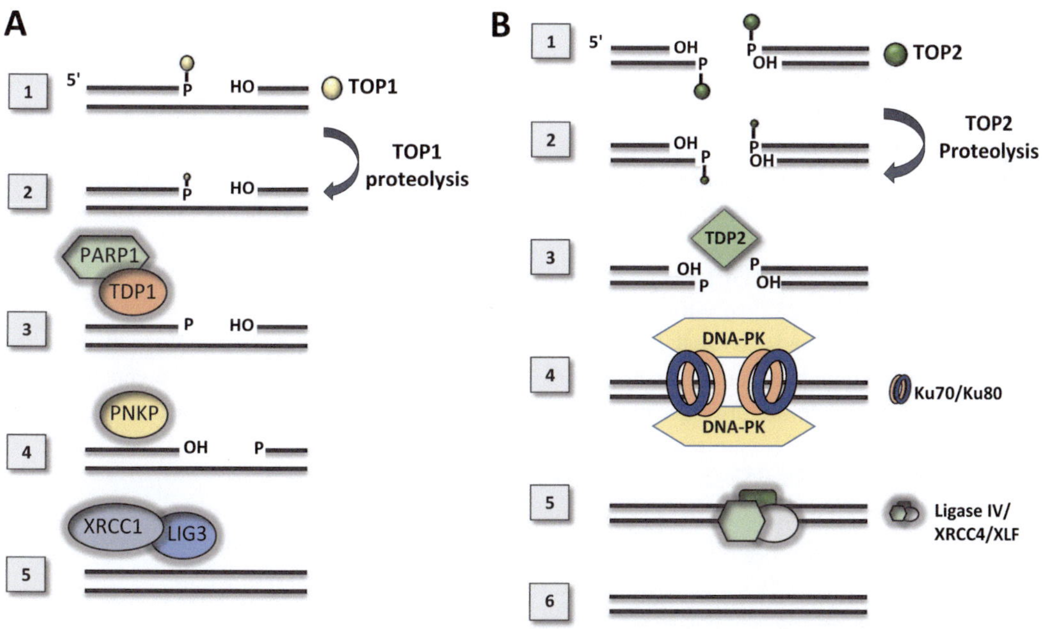

Fig. 9.4 Topoisomerases-induced PDBs repair: (**a**) TDP1 removes the TOP1 to liberate the 3′-Phosphate which is then converted to 3′-OH by PNKP, so DNA polymerase can complete the synthesis of the DNA strand and LIG3 can seal the nick formed. (**b**) TDP2 removes TOP2 enzyme restoring the 5′-phosphate, followed by error-free NHEJ (Adapted from Ref. [11])

motor and sensory neuropathy, distal muscular atrophy, *pes cavus* and steppage gait. Some family members had cerebellar ataxia and axonal neuropathy, one of which had seizures while two had mild brain atrophy [248].

TDP1 inactivity may contribute to SCAN1's complex etiology [249]. Therefore, identification of the mutated *TDP1* through sequencing is necessary for establishing a personalized treatment plan [248]. Current therapy involves using prostheses and walking aids to enhance patients' mobility. However, there are no approved drugs yet for the treatment of SCAN1 based on the *TDP1* mutation. Nevertheless, since SCAN1 patients can be TDP1 deficient, exposure to TOP1 poisons and IR should be avoided due to increased hypersensitivity and delayed rate of removal of IR-induced SSBs, respectively [249, 250]. Notably, these early studies on Tdp1 in yeast led to the conceptual idea that protein-linked DNA breaks are pathogenic, which has now been shown in a number of neurological disorders, most recently in frontotemporal dementia and ALS, in a study came out this month in Nature Neuroscience [251].

9.5.2.2 Cancers

Discovering TDP1 and understanding its role in cancer makes it a promising target for the development of small molecule inhibitors. Studies have shown that TDP1-deficient patients are viable and hence, TDP1 inhibitors are less likely to be toxic [248]. Moreover, TDP1's crystal structure has been resolved [252] so virtual screening of libraries of compounds as well as in silico studies of interactions between different ligands and TDP1 can facilitate the drug discovery process. Furthermore, TDP1 can resolve various 3′-DNA ends [240, 250, 253–255] and hence, TDP1 inhibitors are thought to have a significant effect on current therapies that involve inducing PDBs such as TOP1 poisons.

Overexpression of TDP1 was detected in CPT-resistant non-small cell lung cancer cells, giving rise to the possibility of developing TDP1 inhibitors for such patients to overcome CPT's resistance [256]. On the other hand, a study in 2014 revealed that TDP1 is completely inactivated in two out of eight lung cancer cell lines, suggesting that TDP1 expression level does not completely correlate with sensitivity to the TOP1 poison, topotecan and hence, can be considered as a partial pharmacodynamics biomarker to determine the cellular sensitivity of patients to TOP1-targeted drugs [257].

Glioblastoma-resistant cancer cells treated with Temozolomide (TMZ), showed higher cellular sensitivity to TMZ when TDP1 is depleted, opening the door to combination therapy involving TDP1 inhibitors [240]. Moreover, depletion of TDP1 was found to cause irinotecan hypersensitivity in a TOP1-dependent manner while TDP1 over-expression was found to protect the colorectal cancer cells from irinotecan-mediated cell death. This highlights the possibility of combining irinotecan and a TDP1 inhibitor. However, it is imperative that TOP1 and TDP1 levels of patients are assayed as TOP1 activity is a prerequisite for TDP1-based therapeutics [258].

Several TDP1 inhibitors have been discovered over the past few years that can serve as lead compounds for developing highly potent and specific TDP1 inhibitors. These include aminoglycosides [259], furamidine [260], suramin, methyl-3,4-dephostatin, aurintricarboxylic acid [261], benzopentathiepine [262] and fluoroquinolone derivatives [263]. In addition, JBIR-21 isolated from anamorphic fungus was found to inhibit TDP1 activity [264]. Among the most recent developments was usnic acid enamine derivatives, demonstrating high potency, low toxicity as well as improved CPT's cytotoxicity [265].

The above-mentioned examples reflect on the importance of identification of the genetic defect to personalize the medications patients receive in order to maximize their benefit.

9.5.3 Research in Yeast Allowed *TDP2* Discovery

Although lacking a yeast homologue, TDP2 was discovered through a yeast genetic screen [231]. A strain lacking *TDP1* and *RAD1-RAD10* nuclease; the human endonuclease XPF-ERCC1 ortholog [266] playing a similar role in yeast, were transformed with a human cDNA library and the resulting populations were screened for resistance to CPT [231]. The CPT resistant transformants contained TDP1, TTRAP (TRAF and TNF receptor associated protein) [267] and APEX1 (a close relative to Apurinic/apyrimidinic endonuclease-1) [268]. TTRAP hydrolyzes the 5′-phosphotyrosyl bonds, restoring the 5′-phosphate terminus. This activity is complementary to that of TDP1, and hence, the enzyme was later referred to as TDP2 [231].

9.5.4 Discovery of TDP2 Led to Understanding of Diseases Associated with Gene Defects

9.5.4.1 Neurological Diseases

TDP2 is known to be necessary for induction of transcription of genes whose expression is TOP2-dependent and are associated with normal neurological development [269–272]. Consequently, its depletion or mutagenesis is reported to cause neurological diseases [273].

Three Irish siblings had intellectual impairment, seizures and progressive ataxia. Two siblings who had developed seizures at the age of 2 years and 6 months underwent electroencephalography to confirme their diagnosis with epileptic encephalopathy. The three started walking at a normal age however, they required support or wheelchair later. Their exome sequencing showed a putative splice-site mutation in *TDP2* resulting in a premature stop codon and deletion of conserved domains, critical for TDP2 activity. Furthermore, the mutant mRNA was truncated and labile to nonsense-mediated decay. A different homozygous *TDP2* mutation resulting in the introduction of a premature stop codon and a truncated TDP2 was also identified in Egyptian siblings with intellectual impairment, fits and ataxia [273].

9.5.4.2 Cancer

Overexpression of TDP2 in small-cell lung cancer, rendering the cells resistant to therapy, opens doors for developing TDP2 inhibitors to increase the cellular sensitivity to TOP2 poisons [274]. In 2013, the first TDP2 small molecule inhibitors, Toxoflavins and Deazaflavins, were reported as a novel approach to increase the sensitivity to TOP2 poisons [275]. Their mode of action as competitive ligands and the crystal structures when bound to TDP2 were resolved in 2016 [276].

Finally, in 2016, a high-throughput screening for TDP2 inhibitors was conducted and the researchers identified NSC111041 that prevents TDP2 from binding to DNA without being intercalated. Upon combination with etoposide in TDP2-expressing cells, it had a synergistic effect, enhancing its efficacy and minimizing the dose, side effects and non-specific toxicity [277]. In addition, isoquinoline-1,3-dione analogs were reported as specific TDP2 inhibitors, however, they were not synergistic with etoposide and hence can serve as a scaffold for future drug developments [278]. Finally, In 2016, a potential lead compound for TDP2 inhibitors, called isoeugenol, was reported to enhance CPT's cytotoxicity in TDP1-deficient cells, through inhibiting TDP2 [279].

9.6 Future Perspectives

We have discussed several therapeutic approaches targeting specific disease-causing mutations. However, to achieve better personalised therapy, future diagnostic techniques should determine the exact mutations in a rapid and cost-efficient manner. Stem cell therapy is currently approaching clinical trials for the treatment of Parkinson's disease (PD). Scientists aim to depend on parthenogenetic pluripotent stem cells and differentiate them into neural cells that can secrete dopamine, the neurotransmitter whose depletion results in PD [280]. This gives hope for patients suffering from different neurodegenerative disorders. A possible suggestion for the treatment of patients carrying mutations causing the discussed neurological diseases is to use stem cells and differentiate them into neural tissues that can express normal levels of the defective proteins. In addition, CRISPR/Cas9 has recently emerged as a promising technique for genome editing, especially with the first human trial launched in 2016 [281]. This raises the potential to use it as a therapy for patients suffering from neurodegenerative diseases and cancers arising from specific mutations. The challenging aspect regarding genome editing is the delivery of the Cas proteins across the blood brain barrier. Current studies are focusing on optimizing the delivery process through the use of different carriers, which will eventually have a great impact on the development of personalized medicine [282–284].

9.7 Conclusion

Considering genetic variations between individuals as a guide to making decisions on prevention, diagnosis and treatment of diseases paved the way to developing personalized medicine. In this chapter, we discussed how yeast research has contributed to the discovery of several genes and their functions. Malfunctioning of such genes in human cells was found to result in different neurological diseases and cancers. Unleashing the exact genetic defect behind the disease has a significant impact on improving the diagnosis and treatment plans. It is bound to replace conventional therapy to overcome its side effects, toxicity and resistance. Since most cancers have an over-expression of the implicated protein, development of inhibitors seems promising unlike in the neurological diseases where the genes are silenced or mutated, making its treatment more challenging.

Acknowledgement This work is funded by a grant from Zewail City to Sherif El-Khamisy. The authors would like to thank members of the Center of Genomics at Zewail City for help and useful discussions.

References

1. Goffeau A et al (1996) Life with 6000 genes. Science 274:546–567
2. Mohammadi S, Saberidokht B, Subramaniam S, Grama A (2015) Scope and limitations of yeast as a model organism for studying human tissue-specific pathways. BMC Syst Biol 9:96
3. Stearns T, Ma H, Botstein D (1990) Manipulating yeast genome using plasmid vectors. Methods Enzymol 185:280–297
4. Gardner JM, Jaspersen SL (2014) Manipulating the yeast genome: deletion, mutation, and tagging by PCR. Methods Mol Biol 1205:45–78
5. Janke C et al (2004) A versatile toolbox for PCR-based tagging of yeast genes: new fluorescent proteins, more markers and promoter substitution cassettes. Yeast 21:947–962
6. Dudášová Z, Dudáš A, Chovanec M (2004) Non-homologous end-joining factors of *Saccharomyces cerevisiae*. FEMS Microbiol Rev 28:581–601
7. Aylon Y, Kupiec M (2004) DSB repair: the yeast paradigm. DNA Repair 3:797–815
8. Prakash S, Prakash L (2000) Nucleotide excision repair in yeast. Mutat Res 451:13–24
9. Hamperl S, Cimprich KA (2014) The contribution of co-transcriptional RNA:DNA hybrid structures to DNA damage and genome instability. DNA Repair (Amst) 19:84–94
10. Bonner JN, Zhao X (2016) Replication-associated recombinational repair: lessons from budding yeast. Genes 7
11. Ashour ME, Atteya R, El-Khamisy SF (2015) Topoisomerase-mediated chromosomal break repair: an emerging player in many games. Nat Rev Cancer 15:137–151
12. Boiteux S, Jinks-Robertson S (2013) DNA repair mechanisms and the bypass of DNA damage in *Saccharomyces cerevisiae*. Genetics 193:1025–1064
13. Labib K, De Piccoli G (2011) Surviving chromosome replication: the many roles of the S-phase checkpoint pathway. Philos Trans R Soc B Biol Sci 366:3554–3561
14. Beach D, Durkacz B, Nurse P (1982) Functionally homologous cell cycle control genes in budding and fission yeast. Nature 300:706–709
15. Nurse P (2002) Cyclin dependent kinases and cell cycle control (nobel lecture). Chembiochem 3:596–603
16. Lee MG, Nurse P (1987) Complementation used to clone a human homologue of the fission yeast cell cycle control gene cdc2. Nature 327:31–35
17. Nurse P (1990) Universal control mechanism regulating onset of M-phase. Nature 344:503–508
18. Bartek J, Lukas C, Lukas J (2004) Checking on DNA damage in S phase. Nat Rev Mol Cell Biol 5:792–804
19. Merrick CJ, Jackson D, Diffley JF (2004) Visualization of altered replication dynamics after DNA damage in human cells. J Biol Chem 279:20067–20075
20. Melo J, Toczyski D (2002) A unified view of the DNA-damage checkpoint. Curr Opin Cell Biol 14:237–245
21. Maréchal A, Zou L (2013) DNA damage sensing by the ATM and ATR kinases. Cold Spring Harb Perspect Biol 5
22. Weinert TA, Kiser GL, Hartwell LH (1994) Mitotic checkpoint genes in budding yeast and the dependence of mitosis on DNA replication and repair. Genes Dev 8:652–665
23. Kato R, Ogawa H (1994) An essential gene, ESR1, is required for mitotic cell growth, DNA repair and meiotic recombination in *Saccharomyces cerevisiae*. Nucleic Acids Res 22:3104–3112

24. Lustig AJ, Petes TD (1986) Identification of yeast mutants with altered telomere structure. Proc Natl Acad Sci U S A 83:1398–1402
25. Keith CT, Schreiber SL (1995) PIK-related kinases: DNA repair, recombination, and cell cycle checkpoints. Science 270:50–51
26. Jackson SP (1996) The recognition of DNA damage. Curr Opin Genet Dev 6:19–25
27. Greenwell PW et al (1995) TEL1, a gene involved in controlling telomere length in *S. cerevisiae*, is homologous to the human ataxia telangiectasia gene. Cell 82:823–829
28. Morrow DM, Tagle DA, Shiloh Y, Collins FS, Hieter P (1995) TEL1, an *S. cerevisiae* homolog of the human gene mutated in ataxia telangiectasia, is functionally related to the yeast checkpoint gene MEC1. Cell 82:831–840
29. Foiani M et al (2000) DNA damage checkpoints and DNA replication controls in *Saccharomyces cerevisiae*. Mutat Res 451:187–196
30. Elledge SJ (1996) Cell cycle checkpoints: preventing an identity crisis. Science 274:1664–1672
31. Cimprich KA, Shin TB, Keith CT, Schreiber SL (1996) cDNA cloning and gene mapping of a candidate human cell cycle checkpoint protein. Proc Natl Acad Sci U S A 93:2850–2855
32. Walworth N, Davey S, Beach D (1993) Fission yeast chk1 protein kinase links the rad checkpoint pathway to cdc2. Nature 363:368–371
33. Sanchez Y et al (1997) Conservation of the Chk1 checkpoint pathway in mammals: linkage of DNA damage to Cdk regulation through Cdc25. Science 277:1497–1501
34. Game JC, Mortimer RK (1974) A genetic study of X-ray sensitive mutants in yeast. Mutat Res Fundam Mol Mech Mutagen 24:281–292
35. Zheng P et al (1993) SPK1 is an essential S-phase-specific gene of *Saccharomyces cerevisiae* that encodes a nuclear serine/threonine/tyrosine kinase. Mol Cell Biol 13:5829–5842
36. Allen JB, Zhou Z, Siede W, Friedberg EC, Elledge SJ (1994) The SAD1/RAD53 protein kinase controls multiple checkpoints and DNA damage-induced transcription in yeast. Genes Dev 8:2401–2415
37. Lopes M et al (2001) The DNA replication checkpoint response stabilizes stalled replication forks. Nature 412:557–561
38. Matsuoka S, Huang M, Elledge SJ (1998) Linkage of ATM to cell cycle regulation by the Chk2 protein kinase. Science 282:1893–1897
39. Savitsky K et al (1995) A single ataxia telangiectasia gene with a product similar to PI-3 kinase. Science 268:1749–1753
40. Shiloh Y (2003) ATM: ready, set, go. Cell Cycle 2:116–117
41. Shiloh Y (2003) ATM and related protein kinases: safeguarding genome integrity. Nat Rev Cancer 3:155–168
42. Kastan MB et al (1992) A mammalian cell cycle checkpoint pathway utilizing p53 and GADD45 is defective in ataxia-telangiectasia. Cell 71:587–597
43. Kuhne M et al (2004) A double-strand break repair defect in ATM-deficient cells contributes to radiosensitivity. Cancer Res 64:500–508
44. Painter RB, Young BR (1980) Radiosensitivity in ataxia-telangiectasia: a new explanation. Proc Natl Acad Sci U S A 77:7315–7317
45. Shiloh Y, Kastan MB (2001) ATM: genome stability, neuronal development, and cancer cross paths. Adv Cancer Res 83:209–254
46. Lee P et al (2013) SMRT compounds abrogate cellular phenotypes of ataxia telangiectasia in neural derivatives of patient-specific hiPSCs. Nat Commun 4:1824
47. Cha RS, Kleckner N (2002) ATR homolog Mec1 promotes fork progression, thus averting breaks in replication slow zones. Science 297:602–606
48. O'Driscoll M, Ruiz-Perez VL, Woods CG, Jeggo PA, Goodship JA (2003) A splicing mutation affecting expression of ataxia-telangiectasia and Rad3-related protein (ATR) results in Seckel syndrome. Nat Genet 33:497–501
49. Scalet D et al (2017) Exploring splicing-switching molecules for Seckel Syndrome Therapy. Biochim Biophys Acta Mol basis Dis 1863:15–20
50. Mu K et al (2011) Detection of CHK1 and CCND1 gene copy number changes in breast cancer with dual-colour fluorescence in-situ hybridization. Histopathology 58:601–607
51. Arora S et al (2010) RNAi screening of the kinome identifies modulators of cisplatin response in ovarian cancer cells. Gynecol Oncol 118:220–227
52. Bennett CN et al (2012) Cross-species genomic and functional analyses identify a combination therapy using a CHK1 inhibitor and a ribonucleotide reductase inhibitor to treat triple-negative breast cancer. Breast Cancer Res 14:R109
53. Cole KA et al (2011) RNAi screen of the protein kinome identifies checkpoint kinase 1 (CHK1) as a therapeutic target in neuroblastoma. Proc Natl Acad Sci U S A 108:3336–3341
54. Zhang Y, Hunter T (2014) Roles of Chk1 in cell biology and cancer therapy. Int J Cancer 134:1013–1023
55. Lecona E, Fernández-Capetillo O (2014) Replication stress and cancer: it takes two to tango. Exp Cell Res 329:26–34
56. Brooks K et al (2012) A potent Chk1 inhibitor is selectively cytotoxic in melanomas with high levels of replicative stress. Oncogene 32:1–9
57. Carrassa L, Damia G (2011) Unleashing Chk1 in cancer therapy. Cell Cycle 10:2121–2128
58. Maugeri-Sacca M, Bartucci M, De Maria R (2013) Checkpoint kinase 1 inhibitors for potentiating systemic anticancer therapy. Cancer Treat Rev 39:525–533
59. Antoni L, Sodha N, Collins I, Garrett MD (2007) CHK2 kinase: cancer susceptibility and cancer therapy – two sides of the same coin? Nat Rev Cancer 7:925–936
60. Ding L et al (2008) Somatic mutations affect key pathways in lung adenocarcinoma. Nature 455:1069–1075

61. Jiang H et al (2009) The combined status of ATM and p53 link tumor development with therapeutic response. Genes Dev 23:1895–1909
62. Salimi M, Mozdarani H, Majidzadeh K (2012) Expression pattern of ATM and cyclin D1 in ductal carcinoma, normal adjacent and normal breast tissues of Iranian breast cancer patients. Med Oncol 29:1502–1509
63. Haidar MA et al (2000) ATM gene deletion in patients with adult acute lymphoblastic leukemia. Cancer 88:1057–1062
64. Biankin AV et al (2012) Pancreatic cancer genomes reveal aberrations in axon guidance pathway genes. Nature 491:399–405
65. Ripolles L et al (2006) Genetic abnormalities and clinical outcome in chronic lymphocytic leukemia. Cancer Genet Cytogenet 171:57–64
66. Kim DS et al (2009) Epigenetic inactivation of checkpoint kinase 2 gene in non-small cell lung cancer and its relationship with clinicopathological features. Lung Cancer 65:247–250
67. Zhang P et al (2004) CHK2 kinase expression is down-regulated due to promoter methylation in non-small cell lung cancer. Mol Cancer 3:14
68. Ertych N et al (2014) Increased microtubule assembly rates influence chromosomal instability in colorectal cancer cells. Nat Cell Biol 16:779–791
69. Bell DW et al (1999) Heterozygous germ line hCHK2 mutations in Li-Fraumeni syndrome. Science 286:2528–2531
70. Shaag A et al (2005) Functional and genomic approaches reveal an ancient CHEK2 allele associated with breast cancer in the Ashkenazi Jewish population. Hum Mol Genet 14:555–563
71. Bartkova J et al (2005) DNA damage response as a candidate anti-cancer barrier in early human tumorigenesis. Nature 434:864–870
72. Mahajan K et al (2012) Ack1-mediated androgen receptor phosphorylation modulates radiation resistance in castration-resistant prostate cancer. J Biol Chem 287:22112–22122
73. Alkema NG et al (2014) Checkpoint kinase 2 (Chk2) supports sensitivity to platinum-based treatment in high grade serous ovarian cancer. Gynecol Oncol 133:591–598
74. DiTullio RA et al (2002) 53BP1 functions in an ATM-dependent checkpoint pathway that is constitutively activated in human cancer. Nat Cell Biol 4:998–1002
75. Lainchbury M et al (2012) Discovery of 3-alkoxyamino-5-(pyridin-2-ylamino)pyrazine-2-carbonitriles as selective, orally bioavailable CHK1 inhibitors. J Med Chem 55:10229–10240
76. Wang F-Z et al (2014) The checkpoint 1 kinase inhibitor LY2603618 induces cell cycle arrest, DNA damage response and autophagy in cancer cells. Apoptosis 19:1389–1398
77. Davies KD et al (2011) Single-agent inhibition of Chk1 is antiproliferative in human cancer cell lines in vitro and inhibits tumor xenograft growth in vivo. Oncol Res Featuring Preclinical Clin Cancer Ther 19:349–363
78. Foote KM et al (2013) Discovery of 4-{4-[(3 R)-3-Methylmorpholin-4-yl]-6-[1-(methylsulfonyl)cyclopropyl]pyrimidin-2-yl}-1 H -indole (AZ20): a potent and selective inhibitor of ATR protein kinase with monotherapy in vivo antitumor activity. J Med Chem 56:2125–2138
79. Golding SE et al (2009) Improved ATM kinase inhibitor KU-60019 radiosensitizes glioma cells, compromises insulin, AKT and ERK prosurvival signaling, and inhibits migration and invasion. Mol Cancer Ther 8:2894–2902
80. Golding SE et al (2012) Dynamic inhibition of ATM kinase provides a strategy for glioblastoma multiforme radiosensitization and growth control. Cell Cycle 11:1167–1173
81. Biddlestone-Thorpe L et al (2013) ATM kinase inhibition preferentially sensitizes p53-mutant glioma to ionizing radiation. Clin Cancer Res 19:3189–3200
82. Roossink F et al (2011) The role of ATM and 53BP1 as predictive markers and therapeutic targets in cervical cancer. Int J Gynecol Cancer 21:S196
83. Hickson I et al (2004) Identification and characterization of a novel and specific inhibitor of the ataxia-telangiectasia mutated kinase ATM. Cancer Res 64:9152–9159
84. Vecchio D et al (2015) Pharmacokinetics, pharmacodynamics and efficacy on pediatric tumors of the glioma radiosensitizer KU60019. Int J Cancer 136:1445–1457
85. Pires IM et al (2012) Targeting radiation-resistant hypoxic tumour cells through ATR inhibition. Br J Cancer 107:291–299
86. Fokas E et al (2012) Targeting ATR in vivo using the novel inhibitor VE-822 results in selective sensitization of pancreatic tumors to radiation. Cell Death Dis 3:e441
87. Charrier JD et al (2011) Discovery of potent and selective inhibitors of ataxia telangiectasia mutated and Rad3 related (ATR) protein kinase as potential anticancer agents. J Med Chem 54:2320–2330
88. Yang H et al (2011) Inhibition of checkpoint kinase 1 sensitizes lung cancer brain metastases to radiotherapy. Biochem Biophys Res Commun 406:53–58
89. Jobson AG et al (2009) Cellular inhibition of checkpoint kinase 2 (Chk2) and potentiation of camptothecins and radiation by the novel Chk2 inhibitor PV1019 [7-nitro-1H-indole-2-carboxylic acid {4-[1-(guanidinohydrazone)-ethyl]-phenyl}-amide]. J Pharmacol Exp Ther 331:816–826
90. Kleiman LB, Krebs AM, Kim SY, Hong TS, Haigis KM (2013) Comparative analysis of radiosensitizers for K-RAS mutant rectal cancers. PLoS One 8
91. Riesterer O et al (2011) A novel Chk inhibitor, XL-844, increases human cancer cell radiosensitivity through promotion of mitotic catastrophe. Investig New Drugs 29:514–522
92. Mitchell JB et al (2010) In vitro and in vivo radiation sensitization of human tumor cells by a novel

checkpoint kinase inhibitor, AZD7762. Clin Cancer Res 16:2076–2084
93. Morgan MA et al (2010) Mechanism of radiosensitization by the Chk1/2 inhibitor AZD7762 involves abrogation of the G2 checkpoint and inhibition of homologous recombinational DNA repair. Cancer Res 70:4972–4981
94. Borst GR et al (2013) Targeted radiosensitization by the Chk1 inhibitor SAR-020106. Int J Radiat Oncol Biol Phys 85:1110–1118
95. Rawlinson R, Massey AJ (2014) γH2AX and Chk1 phosphorylation as predictive pharmacodynamic biomarkers of Chk1 inhibitor-chemotherapy combination treatments. BMC Cancer 14:483
96. Höglund A et al (2011) Therapeutic implications for the induced levels of Chk1 in Myc-expressing cancer cells. Clin Cancer Res 17:7067–7079
97. Manic G, Obrist F, Sistigu A, Vitale I (2015) Trial watch: targeting ATM-CHK2 and ATR-CHK1 pathways for anticancer therapy. Mol Cell Oncol 2:e1012976
98. Krajewska M et al (2015) ATR inhibition preferentially targets homologous recombination-deficient tumor cells. Oncogene 34:3474–3481
99. Rainey MD, Charlton ME, Stanton RV, Kastan MB (2008) Transient inhibition of ATM kinase is sufficient to enhance cellular sensitivity to ionizing radiation. Cancer Res 68:7466–7474
100. Hall AB et al (2014) Potentiation of tumor responses to DNA damaging therapy by the selective ATR inhibitor VX-970. Oncotarget 5:5674–5685
101. Kwok M et al (2016) ATR inhibition induces synthetic lethality and overcomes chemoresistance in TP53- or ATM-defective chronic lymphocytic leukemia cells. Blood 127:582–595
102. Patel R et al (2017) An orally bioavailable Chk1 inhibitor, CCT244747, sensitizes bladder and head and neck cancer cell lines to radiation. Radiother Oncol 400:2–7
103. Liu R et al (2017) The depletion of ATM inhibits colon cancer proliferation and migration via B56γ2-mediated Chk1/p53/CD44 cascades. Cancer Lett 390:48–57
104. Bryant HE, Helleday T (2006) Inhibition of poly (ADP-ribose) polymerase activates ATM which is required for subsequent homologous recombination repair. Nucleic Acids Res 34:1685–1691
105. Gilardini Montani MS et al (2013) ATM-depletion in breast cancer cells confers sensitivity to PARP inhibition. J Exp Clin Cancer Res 32:95
106. Williamson CT et al (2010) ATM deficiency sensitizes mantle cell lymphoma cells to poly(ADP-ribose) polymerase-1 inhibitors. Mol Cancer Ther 9:347–357
107. Höglund A, Strömvall K, Li Y, Forshell LP, Nilsson JA (2011) Chk2 deficiency in Myc overexpressing lymphoma cells elicits a synergistic lethal response in combination with PARP inhibition. Cell Cycle 10:3598–3607
108. Nguyen TNT et al (2012) Radioprotection by hymenialdisine-derived checkpoint kinase 2 inhibitors. ACS Chem Biol 7:172–184
109. Arienti KL et al (2005) Checkpoint kinase inhibitors: SAR and radioprotective properties of a series of 2-arylbenzimidazoles. J Med Chem 48:1873–1885
110. Benada J, Macurek L, Heyer W-D, Helleday T, Hanaoka F (2015) Targeting the checkpoint to kill cancer cells. Biomol Ther 5:1912–1937
111. Wang J, Han X, Zhang Y (2012) Autoregulatory mechanisms of phosphorylation of checkpoint kinase 1. Cancer Res 72:3786–3794
112. Daud AI et al (2015) Phase I dose-escalation trial of checkpoint kinase 1 inhibitor MK-8776 as monotherapy and in combination with gemcitabine in patients with advanced solid tumors. J Clin Oncol 33:1060–1066
113. Dees EC et al (2005) A phase I and pharmacokinetic study of short infusions of UCN-01 in patients with refractory solid tumors. Clin Cancer Res 11:664–671
114. Shapiro G et al (2011) Phase I studies of CBP501, a G2 checkpoint abrogator, as monotherapy and in combination with cisplatin in patients with advanced solid tumors. Clin Cancer Res 17:3431–3442
115. Wickremsinhe ER et al (2014) Disposition and metabolism of LY2603618, a Chk-1 inhibitor following intravenous administration in patients with advanced and/or metastatic solid tumors. Xenobiotica 44:827–841
116. Hynes SM et al (2015) Evaluation of the likelihood of a selective CHK1 inhibitor (LY2603618) to inhibit CYP2D6 with desipramine as a probe substrate in cancer patients. Biopharm Drug Dispos 36:49–63
117. Sausville E et al (2014) Phase I dose-escalation study of AZD7762, a checkpoint kinase inhibitor, in combination with gemcitabine in US patients with advanced solid tumors. Cancer Chemother Pharmacol 73:539–549
118. Pâques F, Haber JE (1999) Multiple pathways of recombination induced by double-strand breaks in *Saccharomyces cerevisiae*. Microbiol Mol Biol Rev 63:349–404
119. Andersen SL, Sekelsky J (2010) Meiotic versus mitotic recombination: two different routes for double-strand break repair. BioEssays 32:1058–1066
120. Jensen RB, Carreira A, Kowalczykowski SC (2010) Purified human BRCA2 stimulates RAD51-mediated recombination. Nature 467:678–683
121. Liu J, Doty T, Gibson B, Heyer W-D (2010) Human BRCA2 protein promotes RAD51 filament formation on RPA-covered single-stranded DNA. Nat Struct Mol Biol 17:1260–1262
122. Feng Z et al (2011) Rad52 inactivation is synthetically lethal with BRCA2 deficiency. Proc Natl Acad Sci U S A 108:686–691
123. Krejci L, Altmannova V, Spirek M, Zhao X (2012) Homologous recombination and its regulation. Nucleic Acids Res 40:5795–5818

124. San Filippo J, Sung P, Klein H (2008) Mechanism of eukaryotic homologous recombination. Annu Rev Biochem 77:229–257
125. Symington LS (2002) Role of RAD52 epistasis group genes in homologous recombination and double-strand break repair. Microbiol Mol Biol Rev 66:630–670., table of contents
126. Zhao W et al (2015) Promotion of BRCA2-dependent homologous recombination by DSS1 via RPA targeting and DNA mimicry. Mol Cell 59:176–187
127. Mazin AV, Mazina OM, Bugreev DV, Rossi MJ (2010) Rad54, the motor of homologous recombination. DNA Repair 9:286–302
128. Resnick MA, Martin P (1976) The repair of double-strand breaks in the nuclear DNA of *Saccharomyces cerevisiae* and its genetic control. MGG Mol Gen Genet 143:119–129
129. Ho KS (1975) Induction of DNA double-strand breaks by X-rays in a radiosensitive strain of the yeast *Saccharomyces cerevisiae*. Mutat Res 30:327–334
130. Mowat MRA (1979) Repair of γ-ray induced DNA strand breaks in radiation sensitive mutants of yeast. at http://inis.iaea.org/Search/search.aspx?orig_q=RN:14719298
131. Prakash L, Taillon-Miller P (1981) Effects of the rad52 gene on sister chromatid recombination in *Saccharomyces cerevisiae*. Curr Genet 3:247–250
132. Prakash S, Prakash L, Burke W, Montelone BA (1980) Effects of the RAD52 gene on recombination in *Saccharomyces cerevisiae*. Genetics 94:31 LP–31 50
133. Shinohara A, Ogawa H, Ogawa T (1992) Rad51 protein involved in repair and recombination in *S. cerevisiae* is a RecA-like protein. Cell 69:457–470
134. Ivanov EL, Korolev VG, Fabre F (1992) XRS2, a DNA repair gene of *Saccharomyces cerevisiae*, is needed for meiotic recombination. Genetics 132:651–664
135. Ajimura M, Leem S-H, Ogawa H (1993) Identification of new genes required for meiotic recombination in *Saccharomyces cerevisiae*. Genetics 133:51–66
136. Shinohara A et al (1993) Cloning of human, mouse and fission yeast recombination genes homologous to RAD51 and recA. Nat Genet 4:239–243
137. Muris DF et al (1994) Cloning of human and mouse genes homologous to RAD52, a yeast gene involved in DNA repair and recombination. Mutat Res 315:295–305
138. Johzuka K, Ogawa H (1995) Interaction of Mre11 and Rad50: two proteins required for DNA repair and meiosis-specific double-strand break formation in *Saccharomyces cerevisiae*. Genetics 139:1521–1532
139. Hays SL, Firmenich AA, Berg P (1995) Complex formation in yeast double-strand break repair: participation of Rad51, Rad52, Rad55, and Rad57 proteins. Proc Natl Acad Sci U S A 92:6925–6929
140. Jiang H et al (1996) Direct association between the yeast Rad51 and Rad54 recombination proteins. J Biol Chem 271:33181–33186
141. Petrini JHJ et al (1995) Isolation and characterization of the human MRE11 homolog. Genomics 29:80–86
142. Dolganov GM et al (1996) Human Rad50 is physically associated with human Mre11: identification of a conserved multiprotein complex implicated in recombinational DNA repair. Mol Cell Biol 16:4832–4841
143. Varon R et al (1998) Nibrin, a novel DNA double-strand break repair protein, is mutated in Nijmegen breakage syndrome. Cell 93:467–476
144. Borde V (2007) The multiple roles of the Mre11 complex for meiotic recombination. Chromosom Res 15:551–563
145. Rass E et al (2009) Role of Mre11 in chromosomal nonhomologous end joining in mammalian cells. Nat Struct Mol Biol 16:819–824
146. Sung P (1997) Communications: function of yeast Rad52 protein as a function of yeast Rad52 protein as a mediator between. 1–5. doi:10.1074/jbc.272.45.28194
147. Sung P (1997) Yeast Rad55 and Rad57 proteins form a heterodimer that functions with replication protein A to promote DNA strand exchange by Rad51 recombinase. Genes Dev 11:1111–1121
148. Benson FE, Baumann P, West SC (1998) Synergistic actions of Rad51 and Rad52 in recombination and DNA repair. Nature 391:401–404
149. Stein A, Kalifa L, Sia EA (2015) Members of the RAD52 epistasis group contribute to mitochondrial homologous recombination and double-strand break repair in *Saccharomyces cerevisiae*. PLoS Genet 11:1–20
150. Waltes R et al (2009) Human RAD50 deficiency in a Nijmegen breakage syndrome-like disorder. Am J Hum Genet 84:605–616
151. Damiola F et al (2014) Rare key functional domain missense substitutions in MRE11A, RAD50, and NBN contribute to breast cancer susceptibility: results from a Breast Cancer Family Registry case-control mutation-screening study. Breast Cancer Res 16:R58
152. Heikkinen K (2003) Mutation screening of Mre11 complex genes: indication of RAD50 involvement in breast and ovarian cancer susceptibility. J Med Genet 40:131e–1131
153. Heikkinen K et al (2006) RAD50 and NBS1 are breast cancer susceptibility genes associated with genomic instability. Carcinogenesis 27:1593–1599
154. Zheng J et al (2011) Functional NBS1 polymorphism is associated with occurrence and advanced disease status of nasopharyngeal carcinoma. Mol Carcinog 50:689–696
155. Loveday C et al (2011) Germline mutations in RAD51D confer susceptibility to ovarian cancer. Nat Genet 43:879–882
156. Meindl A et al (2010) Germline mutations in breast and ovarian cancer pedigrees establish RAD51C as a human cancer susceptibility gene. Nat Genet 42:410–414
157. Kalvala A et al (2014) Overexpression of Rad51C splice variants in colorectal tumors. Oncotarget 6:1–11

158. Depienne C et al (2012) RAD51 haploinsufficiency causes congenital mirror movements in humans. Am J Hum Genet 90:301–307
159. Han H et al (2002) Identification of differentially expressed genes in pancreatic cancer cells using cDNA microarray. Cancer Res 62:2890–2896
160. Nagathihalli NS, Nagaraju G (2011) RAD51 as a potential biomarker and therapeutic target for pancreatic cancer. Biochim Biophys Acta – Rev Cancer 1816:209–218
161. Tennstedt P et al (2013) RAD51 overexpression is a negative prognostic marker for colorectal adenocarcinoma. Int J Cancer 132:2118–2126
162. Qiao G-B et al (2005) High-level expression of Rad51 is an independent prognostic marker of survival in non-small-cell lung cancer patients. Br J Cancer 93:137–143
163. Hannay JAF et al (2007) Rad51 overexpression contributes to chemoresistance in human soft tissue sarcoma cells: a role for p53/activator protein 2 transcriptional regulation. Mol Cancer Ther 6:1650–1660
164. Lim DS, Hasty P (1996) A mutation in mouse rad51 results in an early embryonic lethal that is suppressed by a mutation in p53. Mol Cell Biol 16:7133–7143
165. Alagpulinsa DA, Ayyadevara S, Shmookler Reis RJ (2014) A small-molecule inhibitor of RAD51 reduces homologous recombination and sensitizes multiple myeloma cells to doxorubicin. Front Oncol 4:289
166. Huang F, Mazin AV (2014) A small molecule inhibitor of human RAD51 potentiates breast cancer cell killing by therapeutic agents in mouse xenografts. PLoS One 9
167. Ito M et al (2005) Rad51 siRNA delivered by HVJ envelope vector enhances the anti-cancer effect of cisplatin. J Gene Med 7:1044–1052
168. Lai T-H et al (2016) HDAC inhibition induces MicroRNA-182, which targets RAD51 and impairs HR tepair to sensitize cells to sapacitabine in acute myelogenous leukemia. Clin Cancer Res 22:3537–3549
169. Russell JS et al (2003) Gleevec-mediated inhibition of Rad51 expression and enhancement of tumor cell radiosensitivity. Cancer Res 63:7377–7383
170. Tsai M-S, Kuo Y-H, Chiu Y-F, Su Y-C, Lin Y-W (2010) Down-regulation of Rad51 expression overcomes drug resistance to gemcitabine in human non-small-cell lung cancer cells. J Pharmacol Exp Ther 335:830–840
171. Quiros S, Roos WP, Kaina B (2011) Rad51 and BRCA2-New molecular targets for sensitizing glioma cells to alkylating anticancer drugs. PLoS One 6:e27183
172. Kim PM, Allen C, Wagener BM, Shen Z, Nickoloff JA (2001) Overexpression of human RAD51 and RAD52 reduces double-strand break-induced homologous recombination in mammalian cells. Nucleic Acids Res 29:4352–4360
173. Mason JM et al (2014) The rad51-stimulatory compound rs-1 can exploit the rad51 overexpression that exists in cancer cells and tumors. Cancer Res 74:3546–3555
174. Siraj AK et al (2008) RAD52 polymorphisms contribute to the development of papillary thyroid cancer susceptibility in Middle Eastern population. J Endocrinol Investig 31:893–899
175. Gonzalez R et al (1999) Detection of loss of heterozygosity at RAD51, RAD52, RAD54 and BRCA1 and BRCA2 loci in breast cancer: pathological correlations. Br J Cancer 81:503
176. Lieberman R et al (2015) Functional characterization of RAD52 as a lung cancer susceptibility gene in the 12p13. 33 locus. Mol Carcinog
177. Jiang Y et al (2013) Genetic variation in a hsa-let-7 binding site in RAD52 is associated with breast cancer susceptibility. Carcinogenesis 34:689–693
178. Feng Z et al (2011) Rad52 inactivation is synthetically lethal with BRCA2 deficiency. Proc Natl Acad Sci 108:686–691
179. Sullivan K et al (2016) Identification of a Small Molecule Inhibitor of RAD52 by Structure-Based Selection. PLoS One 11:e0147230
180. Huang F et al (2016) Targeting BRCA1- and BRCA2-deficient cells with RAD52 small molecule inhibitors. Nucleic Acids Res 44:gkw087
181. Sullivan K et al (2015) Identification of a Small Molecule Inhibitor of RAD52 to Induce Synthetic Lethality in BRCA-Deficient Leukemias. Blood 126:4434
182. Zha S et al (2011) ATM damage response and XLF repair factor are functionally redundant in joining DNA breaks. Nature 469:250–254
183. Woodbine L et al (2013) PRKDC mutations in a SCID patient with profound neurological abnormalities. J Clin Invest 123:2969–2980
184. Helmink BA, Sleckman BP (2012) The response to and repair of RAG-mediated DNA double-strand breaks. Annu Rev Immunol 30:175–202
185. Hefferin ML, Tomkinson AE (2005) Mechanism of DNA double-strand break repair by non-homologous end joining. DNA Repair 4:639–648
186. Davis AJ, Chen DJ (2013) DNA double strand break repair via non-homologous end-joining. Transl Cancer Res 2:130–143
187. Zhang Z et al (2004) Solution structure of the C-terminal domain of Ku80 suggests important sites for protein-protein interactions. Structure 12:495–502
188. Weterings E, Van Gent DC (2004) The mechanism of non-homologous end-joining: a synopsis of synapsis. DNA Repair 3:1425–1435
189. Bernstein NK et al (2005) The molecular architecture of the mammalian DNA repair enzyme, polynucleotide kinase. Mol Cell 17:657–670
190. Ma Y, Pannicke U, Schwarz K, Lieber MR (2002) Hairpin opening and overhang processing by an Artemis/DNA-dependent protein kinase complex in nonhomologous end joining and V(D)J recombination. Cell 108:781–794

191. Perry JJP et al (2006) WRN exonuclease structure and molecular mechanism imply an editing role in DNA end processing. Nat Struct Mol Biol 13:414–422
192. Wang C, Lees-Miller SP (2013) Detection and repair of ionizing radiation-induced dna double strand breaks: new developments in nonhomologous end joining. Int J Radiat Oncol Biol Phys 86:440–449
193. Johnston LH, Nasmyth KIMA (1978) *Saccharomyces cerevisiae* cell cycle mutant cdc9 is defective in DNA ligase. Nature 274:891–893
194. Robins P, Lindahl T (1996) DNA ligase IV from HeLa cell nuclei. J Biol Chem 271:24257–24261
195. Wei YF et al (1995) Molecular cloning and expression of human cDNAs encoding a novel DNA ligase IV and DNA ligase III, an enzyme active in DNA repair and recombination. Mol Cell Biol 15:3206–3216
196. Tomkinson AE, Roberts E, Daly G, Totty NF, Lindahl T (1991) Three distinct DNA ligases in mammalian cells. J Biol Chem 266:21728–21735
197. Teo S, Jackson SP (1997) Identification of *Saccharomyces cerevisiae* DNA ligase IV: involvement in DNA double-strand break repair. EMBO J. 16:4788 LP–4784795
198. Grawunder U et al (1997) Activity of DNA ligase IV stimulated by complex formation with XRCC4 protein in mammalian cells. Nature 388:492–495
199. Ahnesorg P, Smith P, Jackson SP (2006) XLF interacts with the XRCC4-DNA Ligase IV complex to promote DNA nonhomologous end-joining. Cell 124:301–313
200. Lazzerini-Denchi E, Sfeir A (2016) Stop pulling my strings-what telomeres taught us about the DNA damage response. Nat Rev Mol Cell Biol 17
201. O'Driscoll M et al (2001) DNA ligase IV mutations identified in patients exhibiting developmental delay and immunodeficiency. Mol Cell 8:1175–1185
202. Chistiakov D, Ligase A (2010) IV syndrome. Adv Exp Med Biol 685:175–185
203. Riballo E et al (1999) Identification of a defect in DNA ligase IV in a radiosensitive leukaemia patient. Curr Biol 9:699–702
204. Riballo E et al (2001) Cellular and biochemical impact of a mutation in DNA ligase IV conferring clinical radiosensitivity. J Biol Chem 276:31124–31132
205. Bryans M, Valenzano MC, Stamato TD (1999) Absence of DNA ligase IV protein in XR-1 cells: evidence for stabilization by XRCC4. Mutat Res – DNA Repair 433:53–58
206. Altmann T, Gennery AR (2016) DNA ligase IV syndrome; a review. Orphanet J Rare Dis 11:137
207. Shackelford DA (2006) DNA end joining activity is reduced in Alzheimer's disease. Neurobiol Aging 27:596–605
208. Kanungo J (2016) DNA-PK deficiency in Alzheimer's disease. J Neurol Neuromedicine 1:17–22
209. Cipe FE et al (2014) Cernunnos/XLF deficiency: a syndromic primary immunodeficiency. Case Rep Pediatr 2014:614238
210. Brady N, Gaymes TJ, Cheung M, Mufti GJ, Rassool FV (2003) Increased error-prone NHEJ activity in myeloid leukemias is associated with DNA damage at sites that recruit key nonhomologous end-joining proteins. Cancer Res 63:1798–1805
211. Pascale RM et al (2016) DNA-PKcs: a promising therapeutic target in human hepatocellular carcinoma? DNA Repair 47:12–20
212. Cornell L et al (2015) DNA-PK- A candidate driver of hepatocarcinogenesis and tissue biomarker that predicts response to treatment and survival. Clin Cancer Res 21:925–933
213. Munck JM et al (2012) Chemosensitization of cancer cells by KU-0060648, a dual inhibitor of DNA-PK and PI-3K. Mol Cancer Ther 11:1789–1798
214. Velic D et al (2015) DNA damage signalling and repair inhibitors: the long-sought-after Achilles' heel of cancer. Biomol Ther 5:3204–3259
215. Beskow C et al (2009) Radioresistant cervical cancer shows upregulation of the NHEJ proteins DNA-PKcs, Ku70 and Ku86. Br J Cancer 101:816–821
216. Sallmyr A, Tomkinson AE, Rassool FV (2008) Up-regulation of WRN and DNA ligase IIIalpha in chronic myeloid leukemia: consequences for the repair of DNA double-strand breaks. Blood 112:1413–1423
217. Tomkinson AE, Howes TRL, Wiest NE (2013) DNA ligases as therapeutic targets. Transl Cancer Res 2:203–214
218. Leong T, Chao M, Bassal S, McKay M (2003) Radiation-hypersensitive cancer patients do not manifest protein expression abnormalities in components of the nonhomologous end-joining (NHEJ) pathway. Br J Cancer 88:1251–1255
219. Zhong S et al (2008) Identification and validation of human DNA ligase inhibitors using computer-aided drug design. J Med Chem 51:4553–4562
220. Srivastava M et al (2012) An inhibitor of nonhomologous end-joining abrogates double-strand break repair and impedes cancer progression. Cell 151:1474–1487
221. Wang JC (1971) Interaction between DNA and an *Escherichia coli* protein omega. J Mol Biol 55:523–533
222. Champoux JJ, Dulbecco R (1972) An activity from mammalian cells that untwists superhelical DNA – a possible swivel for DNA replication (polyoma-ethidium bromide-mouse-embryo cells-dye binding assay). Proc Natl Acad Sci U S A 69:143–146
223. Pommier Y (2013) Drugging topoisomerases: lessons and challenges. ACS Chem Biol. doi:10.1021/cb300648v
224. Wang JC (2002) Cellular roles of DNA topoisomerases: a molecular perspective. Nat Rev Mol Cell Biol 3:430–440
225. Nitiss JL, Wang JC (1996) Mechanisms of cell killing by drugs that trap covalent complexes between

DNA topoisomerases and DNA. Mol Pharmacol 50:1095–1102
226. Pommier Y et al (2006) Repair of topoisomerase I-mediated DNA damage. Prog Nucleic Acid Res Mol Biol 81:179–229
227. Liu LF, Duann P, Lin CT, D'Arpa P, Wu J (1996) Mechanism of action of camptothecin. Ann N Y Acad Sci 803:44–49
228. Pommier, Y. et al (2008) Repair of topoisomerase I-mediated DNA damage. October 6603, 1–37
229. Pommier Y, Leo E, Zhang H, Marchand C (2010) DNA topoisomerases and their poisoning by anticancer and antibacterial drugs. Chem Biol 17:421–433
230. Pouliot JJ et al (1999) Yeast gene for a Tyr-DNA phosphodiesterase that repairs topoisomerase I complexes. Science 286:552–555
231. Ledesma FC, El Khamisy SF, Zuma MC, Osborn K, Caldecott KW (2009) A human 5′-tyrosyl DNA phosphodiesterase that repairs topoisomerase-mediated DNA damage. Nature 461:674–678
232. Gao R et al (2014) Proteolytic degradation of topoisomerase II (Top2) enables the processing of Top2·DNA and Top2·RNA covalent complexes by tyrosyl-DNA-phosphodiesterase 2 (TDP2). J Biol Chem 289:17960–17969
233. Alagoz M, Chiang SC, Sharma A, El-Khamisy SF (2013) ATM deficiency results in accumulation of DNA-topoisomerase I covalent intermediates in neural cells. PLoS One 8
234. Stingele J, Schwarz MS, Bloemeke N, Wolf PG, Jentsch S (2014) A DNA-dependent protease involved in DNA-protein crosslink repair. Cell 158:327–338
235. Katyal S et al (2014) Aberrant topoisomerase-1 DNA lesions are pathogenic in neurodegenerative genome instability syndromes. Nat Neurosci 17:813–821
236. Reczek CR, Szabolcs M, Stark JM, Ludwig T, Baer R (2013) The interaction between CtIP and BRCA1 is not essential for resection-mediated DNA repair or tumor suppression. J Cell Biol 201:693–707
237. Nakamura K et al (2010) Collaborative action of Brca1 and CtIP in elimination of covalent modifications from double-strand breaks to facilitate subsequent break repair. PLoS Genet 6
238. Kim Y et al (2013) Regulation of multiple DNA repair pathways by the Fanconi anemia protein. Blood J 121:54–63
239. Makharashvili N et al (2014) Catalytic and noncatalytic roles of the CtIP endonuclease in double-strand break end resection. Mol Cell 54:1022–1033
240. Alagoz M, Wells OS, El-Khamisy SF (2014) TDP1 deficiency sensitizes human cells to base damage via distinct topoisomerase I and PARP mechanisms with potential applications for cancer therapy. Nucleic Acids Res 42:3089–3103
241. Das BB et al (2014) PARP1-TDP1 coupling for the repair of topoisomerase I-induced DNA damage. Nucleic Acids Res 42:4435–4449
242. Berti M et al (2013) Human RECQ1 promotes restart of replication forks reversed by DNA topoisomerase I inhibition. Nat Struct Mol Biol 20:347–354
243. Caldecott K, Tyrosyl W (2012) DNA phosphodiesterase 2, an enzyme fit for purpose. Nat Struct Mol Biol 19:1212–1213
244. Quennet V, Beucher A, Barton O, Takeda S, Löbrich M (2011) CtIP and MRN promote non-homologous end-joining of etoposide-induced DNA double-strand breaks in G1. Nucleic Acids Res 39:2144–2152
245. Sartori AA et al (2007) Human CtIP promotes DNA end resection. Nature 450:509–514
246. Heo J et al (2015) TDP1 promotes assembly of non-homologous end joining protein complexes on DNA. DNA Repair (Amst) 30(28–37)
247. Yang SW et al (1996) A eukaryotic enzyme that can disjoin dead-end covalent complexes between DNA and type I topoisomerases. Proc Natl Acad Sci U S A 93:11534–11539
248. Takashima H et al (2002) Mutation of TDP1, encoding a topoisomerase I-dependent DNA damage repair enzyme, in spinocerebellar ataxia with axonal neuropathy. Nat Genet 32:267–272
249. Hirano R et al (2007) Spinocerebellar ataxia with axonal neuropathy: consequence of a Tdp1 recessive neomorphic mutation? EMBO J 26:4732–4743
250. El-Khamisy SF, Hartsuiker E, Caldecott KW (2007) TDP1 facilitates repair of ionizing radiation-induced DNA single-strand breaks. DNA Repair (Amst) 6:1485–1495
251. Walker C, Herranz-Martin S, Karyka E, Liao C, Lewis K, Elsayed W, Lukashchuk V, Chiang SC, Ray S, Mulcahy PJ, Jurga M, Tsagakis I, Iannitti T, Chandran J, Coldicott I, De Vos KJ, Hassan MK, Higginbottom A, Shaw PJ, Hautbergue GM, Azzouz M, El-Khamisy SF (2017) C9orf72 expansion disrupts ATM-mediated chromosomal break repair. Nat Neurosci. doi:10.1038/nn.4604. [Epub ahead of print]. https://www.ncbi.nlm.nih.gov/pubmed/28714954
252. Davies DR, Interthal H, Champoux JJ, Hol WGJ (2002) The crystal structure of human tyrosyl-DNA phosphodiesterase, Tdp1. Structure 10:237–248
253. Inamdar KV et al (2002) Conversion of phosphoglycolate to phosphate termini on 3??? overhangs of DNA double strand breaks by the human tyrosyl-DNA phosphodiesterase hTdp1. J Biol Chem 277:27162–27168
254. Nilsen L, Forstrøm RJ, Bjørs M, Alseth I (2012) AP endonuclease independent repair of abasic sites in Schizosaccharomyces pombe. Nucleic Acids Res 40:2000–2009
255. Huang SYN et al (2013) TDP1 repairs nuclear and mitochondrial DNA damage induced by chain-terminating anticancer and antiviral nucleoside analogs. Nucleic Acids Res 41:7793–7803
256. Liu C et al (2007) Increased expression and activity of repair genes TDP1 and XPF in non-small cell lung cancer. Lung Cancer 55:303–311
257. Gao R et al (2014) Epigenetic and genetic inactivation of tyrosyl-DNA-phosphodiesterase 1 (TDP1)

in human lung cancer cells from the NCI-60 panel. DNA Repair (Amst) 13:1–9
258. Meisenberg C et al (2015) Clinical and cellular roles for TDP1 and TOP1 in modulating colorectal cancer response to irinotecan. Mol Cancer Ther 14:575–585
259. Liao Z, Thibaut L, Jobson A, Pommier Y (2006) Inhibition of human tyrosyl-DNA phosphodiesterase by aminoglycoside antibiotics and ribosome inhibitors. Mol Pharmacol 70:366–372
260. Antony S et al (2007) Novel high-throughput electrochemiluminescent assay for identification of human tyrosyl-DNA phosphodiesterase (Tdp1) inhibitors and characterization of furamidine (NSC 305831) as an inhibitor of Tdp1. Nucleic Acids Res 35:4474–4484
261. Marchand C et al (2009) Identification of phosphotyrosine mimetic inhibitors of human tyrosyl-DNA phosphodiesterase I by a novel AlphaScreen high-throughput assay. Mol Cancer Ther 8:240–248
262. Zakharenko A et al (2015) Synthesis and biological evaluation of novel tyrosyl-DNA phosphodiesterase 1 inhibitors with a benzopentathiepine moiety. Bioorg Med Chem 23:2044–2052
263. Pommier Y, Marchand C, Selvam P, Dexheimer T, Maddali K (2014) Fluoroquinolone derivatives or sulfonamide moiety-containing compounds as inhibitors of tyrosyl-dnaphosphodiesterase (TDP1)
264. Takagi M et al (2012) Tyrosyl-DNA phosphodiesterase 1 inhibitor from an anamorphic fungus. J Nat Prod 75:764–767
265. Zakharenko A et al (2016) Tyrosyl-DNA phosphodiesterase 1 inhibitors: usnic acid enamines enhance the cytotoxic effect of camptothecin. J Nat Prod 79:2961–2967
266. Ciccia A, McDonald N, West SC (2008) Structural and functional relationships of the XPF/MUS81 family of proteins. Annu Rev Biochem 77:259–287
267. Pype S et al (2000) TTRAP, a novel protein that associates with CD40, tumor necrosis factor (TNF) receptor-75 and TNF receptor-associated factors (TRAFs), and that inhibits nuclear factor-??B activation. J Biol Chem 275:18586–18593
268. Rodrigues-Lima F, Josephs M, Katan M, Cassinat B (2001) Sequence analysis identifies TTRAP, a protein that associates with CD40 and TNF receptor-associated factors, as a member of a superfamily of divalent cation-dependent phosphodiesterases. Biochem Biophys Res Commun 285:1274–1279
269. Ju B (2006) A topoisomerase II beta-mediated dsDNA break required for regulated transcription. Science 312:1798–1802
270. King IF et al (2013) Topoisomerases facilitate transcription of long genes linked to autism. Nature 501:58–62
271. Nitiss JL (2009) DNA topoisomerase II and its growing repertoire of biological functions. Nat Rev Cancer 9:327–337
272. Tiwari VK et al (2012) Target genes of Topoisomerase IIβ regulate neuronal survival and are defined by their chromatin state. Proc Natl Acad Sci 109:E934–E943
273. Gómez-Herreros F et al (2014) TDP2 protects transcription from abortive topoisomerase activity and is required for normal neural function. Nat Genet 46:516–521
274. Do PM et al (2012) Mutant p53 cooperates with ETS2 to promote etoposide resistance. Genes Dev 26:830–845
275. Raoof A et al (2013) Toxoflavins and deazaflavins as the first reported selective small 2 molecule inhibitors of tyrosyl-DNA phosphodiesterase II 1. 54–70
276. Hornyak P et al (2016) Mode of action of DNA-competitive small molecule inhibitors of tyrosyl DNA phosphodiesterase 2. Biochem J 473: 1869–1879
277. Kont YS et al (2016) Depletion of tyrosyl DNA phosphodiesterase 2 activity enhances etoposide-mediated double-strand break formation and cell killing. DNA Repair (Amst) 43:38–47
278. Kankanala J et al (2016) Isoquinoline-1,3-diones as selective inhibitors of Tyrosyl DNA Phosphodiesterase II (TDP2). J Med Chem 59:2734–2746
279. Elsayed W, El-Shafie L, Hassan MK, Farag MA, El-Khamisy SF (2016) Isoeugenol is a selective potentiator of camptothecin cytotoxicity in vertebrate cells lacking TDP1. Sci Rep 6:26626
280. Palmer C, Coronel R, Liste I (2016) Treatment of Parkinson ' s disease using human stem cells. 1:71–77
281. Cyranoski D (2016) CRISPR gene editing tested in a person. Nature 539:479
282. Burger C, Nash K, Mandel RJ (2005) Recombinant adeno-associated viral vectors in the nervous system. Hum Gene Ther 16:781–791
283. Taymans J-M et al (2007) Comparative analysis of adeno-associated viral vector serotypes 1, 2, 5, 7, and 8 in mouse brain. Hum Gene Ther 18:195–206
284. Ran FA et al (2015) In vivo genome editing using *Staphylococcus aureus* Cas9. Nature 520:186–190

The Power of Zebrafish in Personalised Medicine

10

Sarah Baxendale, Freek van Eeden, and Robert Wilkinson

Abstract

The goal of personalised medicine is to develop tailor-made therapies for patients in whom currently available therapeutics fail. This approach requires correlating individual patient genotype data to specific disease phenotype data and using these stratified data sets to identify bespoke therapeutics. Applications for personalised medicine include common complex diseases which may have multiple targets, as well as rare monogenic disorders, for which the target may be unknown. In both cases, whole genome sequence analysis (WGS) is discovering large numbers of disease associated mutations in new candidate genes and potential modifier genes. Currently, the main limiting factor is the determination of which mutated genes are important for disease progression and therefore represent potential targets for drug discovery. Zebrafish have gained popularity as a model organism for understanding developmental processes, disease mechanisms and more recently for drug discovery and toxicity testing. In this chapter, we will examine the diverse roles that zebrafish can make in the expanding field of personalised medicine, from generating humanised disease models to xenograft screening of different cancer cell lines, through to finding new drugs via in vivo phenotypic screens. We will discuss the tools available for zebrafish research and recent advances in techniques, highlighting the advantages and potential of using zebrafish for high throughput disease modeling and precision drug discovery.

S. Baxendale (✉) • F. van Eeden
The Bateson Centre, Department of Biomedical Science, University of Sheffield, Sheffield S10 2TN, UK
e-mail: s.baxendale@sheffield.ac.uk; f.j.vaneeden@sheffield.ac.uk

R. Wilkinson
The Bateson Centre, Department of Biomedical Science, University of Sheffield, Sheffield S10 2TN, UK

Department of Infection, Immunity and Cardiovascular Disease, Medical School, Beech Hill Rd, University of Sheffield, Sheffield S10 2RX, UK
e-mail: robert.wilkinson@sheffield.ac.uk

S. El-Khamisy (ed.), *Personalised Medicine*, Advances in Experimental Medicine and Biology 1007,
DOI 10.1007/978-3-319-60733-7_10

Keywords
Zebrafish • Personalised medicine • CRISPR • Xenograft • Chemical screen • Cancer • Neurological disorder • Transgenic

10.1 Introduction

Zebrafish have swum a long way from the shallow pools of the Ganges Delta from where they originate; they can be found in fish tanks and aquaria around the globe, where they thrive due to their hardiness and ease of breeding. This small fresh-water fish is also found widely in research labs, where it has become an ideal model species for many experimental biologists. The reasons behind its attractiveness as a research subject are many: the embryos are transparent and develop rapidly, enabling the imaging of internal cells and structures in real time under the microscope; the embryos develop externally, with a pair of fish able to spawn several hundred embryos in a single clutch and they are relatively cheap to maintain compared to mammals.

Over the past 30 years, zebrafish have been used to study developmental mechanisms and disease models through the comparative analysis of wild-type and mutant lines. The wealth of data generated has highlighted the high degree of conservation, at the genetic, cellular and physiological level between zebrafish and other vertebrates, including ourselves. Many experimental techniques have been developed to generate disease models in zebrafish as highlighted in Table 10.1. Along with genetic models of disease, zebrafish are amenable to the experimental study of many different types of biological process, including tissue regeneration, infectious disease progression, cancer metastasis, and pharmacologically induced neurological disorders. Moreover, combining these features with fluorescent reporter transgenes enables live imaging across the scales, from the whole organism to cellular and subcellular events in vivo.

All this puts zebrafish at a unique advantage – it is a vertebrate model with a complex physiology, a conserved genome, a wide range of disease models and the free-swimming larvae can fit easily in to a multiwell plate, enabling it to be combined with high-throughput methodologies. In addition, larvae are also permeable to small molecules added directly to their aqueous environment, making them an ideal model for drug discovery. This chapter will focus on how zebrafish models of human disorders can assist in the development of personalized therapies, highlighting the value of genetic models of disease, xenograft models and phenotypic drug screening approaches.

10.2 Generating Accurate Models of Human Disease in Zebrafish

A fundamental tenet of personalised medicine, or genomic medicine, is that patients can be stratified according to their predicted response to treatment or risk of disease. This approach to customisation of healthcare recognises that inherent variability in disease progression and outcome is intimately linked with variation between patient genomes, in addition to environmental contributions. While this variability may reflect different pathogenic mutations within the same gene or within different genes, it may also reflect wider variation in additional genetic modifiers of disease pathology. Human disease susceptibility is therefore a consequence of rare genetic variants with high penetrance in addition to common genomic variants with low penetrance. One approach to understand the relative contributions of this variability in vivo is to generate exact models of human disease in non-human organisms, by faithfully recreating disease causing mutations in orthologous genes and by characterising genetic modifiers of disease pathology [1]. When conducted in parallel with clinical studies, this approach has the potential to generate novel insights into the relative functions of pathogenic

Table 10.1 Tools and resources for zebrafish research

Tool	Model	Remarks	References
Gene knock down/out	ENU mutagenesis	Generated large numbers of mutants at random sites in the genome; high through-put sequencing (TILLING) has identified many mutation sites	[30, 31, 146]
	Proviral insertion	Mutagenesis at random insertion sites	[147]
	Morpholino	Transient knock-down with antisense oligo; high through-put; can produce off target and toxic effects	[63, 148, 149]
	TALENs	Site specific mutation using TALE nuclease to generate double stranded breaks	[8, 9]
	CRISPR/Cas9	Site specific mutation with higher efficiency than TALENs	[10, 11]
	CRISPRi	Use of a non-functional Cas9 for transcriptional knock-down	[150, 151]
Transgenesis	Stable lines	Gateway cloning; high efficiency transgenesis with Tol2; PhiC31 landing site for site directed transgenesis	[48, 152]
	Inducible expression	Stage and spatial specific expression using Heatshock; Gal4/UAS; Cre LoxP	[153, 154]
	Zebrabow	Clonal fate mapping with heritable colour bar-coding	[155, 156]
	Reporter lines signalling pathways	Imaging individual cells and tissues or signaling pathway readout in vivo	[157, 158]
Expression analysis	In situ hybridisation	Detailed temporal and spatial analysis of gene expression	[159, 160]
	Antibody staining		www.zfin.org
Chemical biology	Small molecule screening	Drug treatment by addition of compounds to aqueous environment	[100]
		Gavage in fish to determine the amount of drug administer	[161]
Functional analysis	Behaviour	Catalogue of zebrafish quantifiable behaviours	[117]
	Electrophysiology	In vivo recording of neurons, e.g. lateral line	[162]

(continued)

Table 10.1 (continued)

Tool	Model	Remarks	References
Live imaging	Timelapse	Fluorescent imaging in real time	[163]
	High speed	Dynamic imaging, including circulation, C startle flight response, calcium dynamics	[164–166]
Xenograft	Cancer/iPS cells	Injection of cells into zebrafish host	[84]
Infection	Bacteria/funghi/viral	Injection of cells/virus into zebrafish host	[167, 168]
Molecular analysis	Sequence profiling	Transcriptomics in zebrafish	[169, 170]
Bioinformatics	zfin	In silico mining of data and resources previously generated	www.zfin.org

A list of techniques used for disease modeling and phenotypic analysis in zebrafish. The type of analysis, the method used, remarks about the technique and key and recent references are included

mutations and their interactions with genetic modifiers. Moreover, by utilising appropriate experimental models such as the zebrafish, it is now possible to rapidly identify genes that contribute to disease phenotypes and directly visualise the biological consequence of mutations, while also being able to screen for therapeutics in the context of a whole organism (Fig. 10.1).

The utility of an animal model of disease is only as good as its degree of shared physiology and its amenability to genetic manipulation. While the common ancestor between zebrafish and humans diverged 450 million years ago, 82% of known human disease-related genes and 76% of human genes implicated in genome-wide association studies have orthologues in zebrafish [2]. Furthermore, the genetic tractability of this model, and thus our ability to generate accurate zebrafish models of human disease, has been greatly facilitated by the advent of genome editing.

10.2.1 Genome Editing in Zebrafish

Genome editing utilises programmable nucleases to engineer heritable alterations in DNA. Nucleases are targeted to a specific region of DNA where they induce double-strand breaks which are subsequently repaired by the host cell via non-homologous end joining or homologous recombination, which frequently results in targeted mutation. Genome editing has transformed the study of gene function in the laboratory, and while we are still in the early days of its clinical application [3], its potential to directly modify the genome of a patients' somatic cells has already exemplified its usefulness for treating diseases such as acute lymphoblastic leukaemia [4].

The zebrafish community has played a central role in development and application of genome editing technology from its inception, initially during in vivo application of zinc finger nucleases (ZFN) [5–7], through to the increased efficiency and flexibility provided by transcription activator-like effector nucleases (TALENs) [8, 9] and more recently, development of the bacterial antiviral defence mechanism, the clustered regularly interspaced short palindromic repeat (CRISPR)/Cas9 system [10, 11]. While all three approaches induce double-strand breaks in target DNA molecules, ZFNs and TALENs achieve sequence specificity via protein-DNA interactions, whereas CRISPR-Cas9, relies on sgRNA-guided Cas9 nucleases to target specific recognition or PAM (protospacer adjacent motif) sequences in DNA, reviewed in [12]. Much of the early focus in zebrafish genome engineering was centred on improving the efficiency of these technologies to

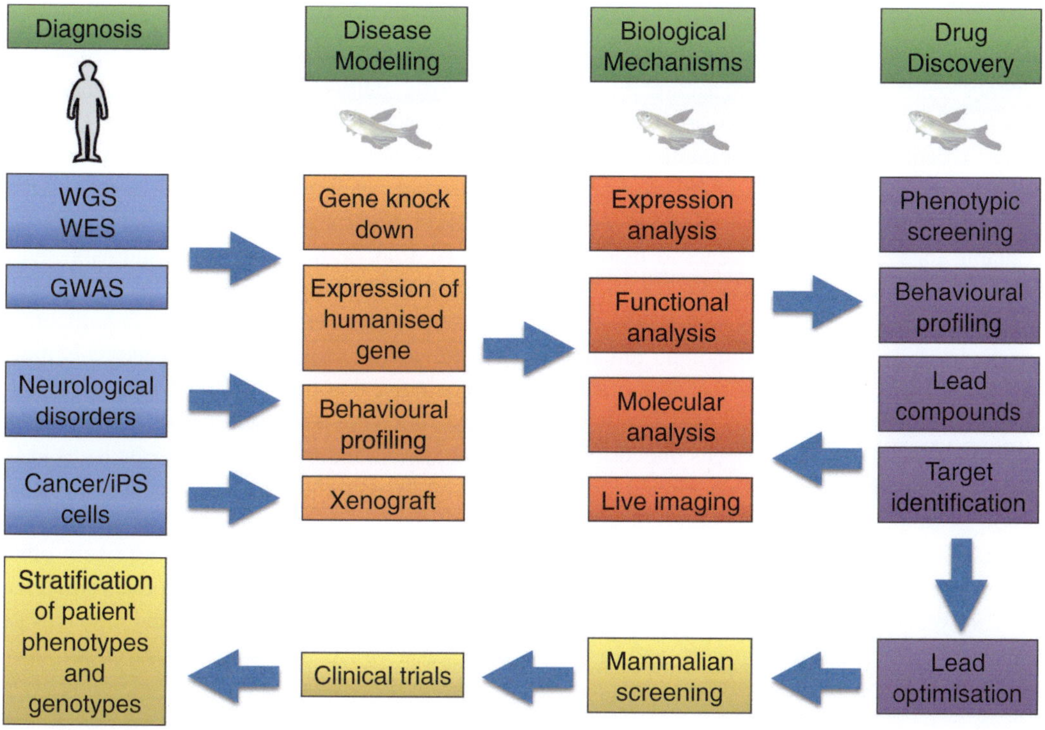

Fig. 10.1 Overview of the role of Zebrafish Research in Personalised Medicine. A work plan for using zebrafish models in personalised medicine strategies. Following disease diagnosis in patients, zebrafish can be used to develop disease models; to understand the biological mechanisms of diseases and to design phenotypic assays for drug discovery. Lead compounds taken forward to clinical trials can be tested on patient groups, stratified by genotype and/or phenotype to optimize drug specificity for individual therapies. The blue column lists the data types suitable for this approach that are discussed in this chapter. WGS/WES/GWAS data can be used to identify genetic lesions that cause a disease or are modifiers of the disease phenotype. Genetic disease models (*orange column*) are generated in zebrafish using methods such as gene knock-down and overexpression, and analysed for phenocopy of the disease (see Table 10.1). Note that information about zebrafish orthologues can be found at the ZFIN website (www.zfin.org) and mutant models that already exists can be ordered from ZIRC (www.zebrafish.org/) or EZRC (www.ezrc.kit.edu/). Complex neurological disorders and cancer/iPS cells can also be analysed in zebrafish using behavioural profiling and xenografts, respectively. The disease model phenotype is analysed at the cellular, molecular and functional level (*red column*) and can be used to develop in vivo phenotypic screens (*purple column*) to identify compounds and suitable targets for the drug discovery pipeline
Abbreviations: *WGS* whole genome sequencing, *WES* whole exome sequencing, *GWAS* genome-wide association study, *iPS* induced pluripotent stem cell, *ZIRC* Zebrafish International Resource Centre, *EZRC* European Zebrafish Resource Centre

inactivate genes by generating small insertions or deletions. This has allowed the generation of numerous disease models carrying homozygous pathogenic mutations and can be readily achieved in just two generations or less. Amongst many others, the diseases which have been modelled in this way using zebrafish range from blood disorders [13, 14] cardiac and vascular diseases, reviewed in [15, 16], through to neurodegeneration, reviewed in [17, 18].

While in zebrafish, non-homologous end joining is the predominant DNA repair mechanism induced following double strand breaks, precise genome editing via targeted induction of homology-directed repair is also possible. Several studies have reported knock-ins mediated via genome editing in zebrafish and these have incorporated single nucleotide, single codon, reporter tags, *loxP* sites and *Gal4* promoters [11, 19–26]. The mechanism by which these integrations occur remains undetermined and can result in imprecise integrations, however, the potential to generate mutations which more accurately reflect those occurring in patients is clear. The application of recent advances in programmable nuclease technology which allow single base editing [27], will further extend the molecular toolbox available for zebrafish researchers to model the effects of human genomic variants.

One of the key advantages of the zebrafish is its amenability for high throughput functional genetic screens [28–31]. The recent application of CRISPR-Cas9 to systematically test gene function in zebrafish [32] opens the door for large-scale testing of candidate human disease genes in addition to identification of genetic modifiers of disease in existing zebrafish disease models [33]. Whole genome CRISPR screens have not yet been reported in zebrafish, although these have been performed in vitro and in other animal models, reviewed in [34].

10.2.2 Potential Limitations and Solutions

The genome editing field is still in its relative infancy, yet it is constantly adapting to overcome several technical limitations which include off target effects and limitations in target DNA recognition, reviewed in Tsai and Joung, 2016 [35]. Some recent advances with respect to the widely used CRISPR-Cas9 system have focused on limiting off target effects by engineering high-fidelity versions of Cas9 [36]. These hurdles are especially important to overcome if we are to translate these powerful tools into effective clinical applications in patient cells. However, in zebrafish, it is relatively simple to outcross carriers to reduce the impact of unlinked off-target effects. The range of DNA target sequences available for targeting using CRISPR-Cas9 is continually expanding through the development of engineered Cas9 nucleases with altered PAM specificities and also by utilisation of Cas9 molecules isolated from different bacterial species [36–38].

It is important to note that in several cases, targeted zebrafish mutants have failed to recapitulate previously published phenotypes generated by morpholino-induced gene knockdown [39–41]. This was originally hypothesised to be a consequence of well-established off-target effects induced by morpholinos, and in many cases this may be true [39]. However, a landmark study recently identified the presence of unexpected transcriptional adaptation in zebrafish harbouring genetic mutations induced by genome-editing. Surprisingly, this transcriptional adaptation was absent following both transcriptional and translational knockdown of the same genetic locus [42]. Put simply, current evidence supports the existence of an as yet unidentified mechanism whereby the zebrafish genome, and likely other genomes, is able to interpret genetic lesions, leading to loss of protein function, and can activate compensatory pathways to overcome this. However, the genome is unable to similarly compensate for loss of protein function when the same gene has been subjected to morpholino knockdown. The zebrafish has undergone a partial genome duplication which could be expected to increase the likelihood of compensatory mechanisms, however, gene duplication has been demonstrated to impart both fragility on protein interaction networks and robustness [43]. It therefore remains to be seen whether transcriptional adaptation may be more prevalent in zebrafish than other organisms. Collectively, genome editing has substantially improved our ability to generate precise zebrafish models of human disease and interrogate genetic contributions to disease pathology. Genome editing has undoubtedly revolutionised genetic engineering and may have a comparable impact on personalised medicine.

10.2.3 Generation of Transgenic or Humanised Zebrafish Disease Models

To date, genome editing has largely been employed as a loss-of-function approach to generate zebrafish models of human disease, however, a distinctive strategy in the application of zebrafish in personalised medicine is the generation of transgenic or "humanised" disease models. Generally, these tend to be gain-of-function approaches and several strategies can be employed in the generation of such models. The simplest approach is the use of transient overexpression studies to link the biological function of human mutations to disease pathology. For example, transient mRNA overexpression studies in zebrafish embryos have implicated human gain-of-function mutations in *NRAS* as contributing to craniofacial defects underlying Noonan syndrome [44]. Similar studies demonstrated that gain-of-function mutations within the phosphatidylserine synthase 1 (*PTDSS1*) gene, which cause Lenz-Majewski syndrome, also result in craniofacial abnormalities when overexpressed in zebrafish embryos [45]. While constitutive overexpression studies can demonstrate conservation of gene function, care must be taken when interpreting results provided by ectopic expression at non-physiological levels.

An alternative approach to transient overexpression is the generation of stable transgenic zebrafish models, where DNA is integrated into the host genome to provide spatiotemporal control of transgene expression. Historically, transgenesis has been conducted such that transgene integration occurs randomly within the genome, either by DNA injection alone, via meganuclease-mediated integration [46], and now more commonly, transposon-mediated integration [47]. Random integration can create variability in transgene expression due to position-specific effects, however, targeted integration of transgenes using site specific recombination or 'landing-pads' such as PhiC31-based integration can overcome this [48, 49].

Amongst the first transgenic disease models established in zebrafish, and the first transgenic zebrafish cancer model, was a model of T-Cell leukaemia or acute lymphoblastic leukaemia (T-ALL) [50], a common childhood cancer caused by distinct chromosomal translocations. The mouse c-Myc gene fused to GFP was driven by a zebrafish *rag2* promoter to facilitate visualisation of leukaemic T-cells and monitor disease progression. Subsequently, more sophisticated T-ALL models were developed to allow temporal control over transgene activation using Cre-Lox-mediated recombination [51]. Modifier screens have also been performed in zebrafish using different T-ALL models, which revealed genetic interactions between *bcl-2* mediated apoptosis and Notch signalling during T-ALL progression [52, 53]. Solid tumours, including melanoma, have also been successfully modelled in zebrafish [54]. Since the majority of melanoma tumour samples contain the activating $BRAF^{V600E}$ mutation [55], this mutant allele was placed under the control of the zebrafish *mitfa* promoter, which is active in melanocytes [54]. Under normal circumstances, *mitfa*: $BRAFV^{600E}$ induced nevus formation in zebrafish, which did not progress to melanoma. However, in a *p53* mutant background, the transgene induced malignant melanomas, which when transplanted induced melanoma formation in recipient fish [54].

10.2.4 Zebrafish Models of Neurodegeneration

Humanised transgenic zebrafish have also been developed to study neurodegeneration. An elegant example of this is the use of zebrafish as a model to study human α-synculein (aSyn) toxicity during neurodegenerative processes including Parkinson's disease [56]. Accumulation of neuronal aSyn is associated with multiple neurodegenerative diseases, however the mechanism by which it contributes to neuronal degeneration is not fully understood. O'Donnell et al. employed the GAL4/UAS system to overexpress human aSyn in zebrafish neurons, a strategy which induced subsequent toxicity and abnormal mitochondrial function, suggesting axonopathy is an early consequence of aSyn accumulation. Similar gain-of-function approaches have also been employed to study nucleotide repeat expansions in *C9orf72*, an underlying cause of amyotrophic lateral sclerosis [57]. An important caveat to studies applying similar approaches is that the level of overexpression achieved using amplification via GAL4/UAS is unlikely to represent physiologically relevant levels of pathogenic protein accumulation. It is therefore advisable wherever possible to use transgene-specific regulatory regions to drive transgene expression.

10.2.5 Evaluating Genetic Mutations in Zebrafish

Dominant human disease mutations can also be tested in zebrafish to compare the effects of different mutations on the level of disease penetrance [58, 59]. Spinal Cerebellar Ataxia type 13 is associated with locomotor impairment and neuronal death in the cerebellum and is caused by mutations in Kv3.3, a voltage-gated K+ channel [60]. The infantile and adult forms of the disease are associated with different mutations and overexpression of these different alleles in zebrafish produces different phenotypes. While the severe infant form causes path-finding defects in the developing motor neurons, the adult mutation leads to a later, weaker effect on axon arborisation; both being consistent with the disease symptoms seen in patients [61].

For many disorders the disease-causing mutation is not known. WGS/WES sequence data is identifying many rare mutations in patients that can potentially cause or modify disease progression. Gonzaga-Jauregui et al. used WES analysis of 40 individuals from 37 different families with Charcot-Marie Tooth syndrome to identify three new candidate genes, PMP2, SPTLC3 and DNAJB5 [62]. Interestingly, they also noted a significant increase of mutations in a group of 58 neuropathy-associated genes, when compared to a matched control group. To test if any of these mutations might contribute to the neuropathy phenotype they used a morpholino screening approach and found combinations of genes that interacted genetically and exacerbated suppression by a single gene. Why the disease associated genome accumulates neuropathy relevant mutations is not known. It will be of interest to see if this is a general feature of other neurological diseases. Zebrafish knockdown screening approaches can also be used with GWAS data to test potential susceptibility loci for complex disorders. Using morpholinos to screen many candidate genes can provide a quick high throughput test of gene function, however care must be taken, since they can produce off target effects [63]. An alternative approach maybe to use the multiplex transient CRISPR method, as described in Shah et al. [32].

10.3 Xenotransplantation

10.3.1 Zebrafish Avatars

How can xenotransplantation contribute to personalised treatment? Instead of modifying the genome of a model organism to precisely mimic the genotype of a patient, xenotransplanting patient cells into a model organism could be a faster alternative [64, 65]. If such cells display disease-relevant characteristics, these could be used as a read-out to find the best treatment. The advantage of using a vertebrate organism to culture those cells are clear, it includes a functional vascular system, drug metabolising organs, and innate immune cells, which contribute to providing a more realistic microenvironment than a culture dish.

Currently, however, there are few published examples of the use of zebrafish xenografts to tailor patient treatment. Even in mice, where these approaches were pioneered, this strategy is still highly experimental [66].

In zebrafish, one could envisage two main possibilities; cancer studies or patient derived (stem) cell transplants. The creation of fish "avatars" of human cancers could indeed be attractive, as they could significantly reduce cost and increase throughput as compared to e.g. nude mice. Hundreds of xenotransplanted embryos can be created in days, once tumour cells are available, whereas mouse xenografts tend to take much longer to establish. Importantly, since only hundreds of cells are required per transplant into fish, resulting chimeric embryos could therefore be screened to find the most effective therapy for that particular cancer.

10.3.2 Physiological Considerations in Xenotransplantation

Although highly attractive at first sight, the physiological differences between fish and human cells need careful consideration. Firstly, cells can be xenotransplanted because fish embryos still lack an adaptive immune system, which could attack foreign cells. The adaptive immune system matures around 4 weeks post fertilisation [67]. Therefore, drug/adaptive immunity interactions cannot be modelled in embryos.

Secondly, although the small size of the fish embryos offers an advantage in terms of handling, cost and imaging, it also means that tumours that are being generated by xenografting are generally very small (<100 μm). Therefore normal diffusion will suffice to supply cancer cells with oxygen [68]. As a result, hypoxia, an important modulator of tumour and immune cell behaviour, will be absent, unless applied globally [69].

Thirdly, there is a large difference in optimal temperature that needs to be bridged: 28 vs. 37 °C. Therefore, transplanted cells, host, or both may be under some form of temperature stress that may affect outcomes. Early embryos are sensitive to temperatures above 32 °C and temperatures above 34 °C are lethal [70]. Fortunately, older embryos (2dpf) and adults may be more resistant, the former appear normal for several days at 35 °C [71], and in the wild, adult zebrafish have been observed in water at 38 °C [72].

Finally, although signalling pathways are conserved in vertebrates, mis- or poor communication between tumour and host is certainly possible. For instance for CXCR4/CXCL12, Nodal, FGF, VEGF and TGF-β, fish-to-human and/or human-to-fish crosstalk was clearly established. However, where tested, differences in fish and human ligand efficiencies were observed [73–76].

Despite these potential issues, numerous cell lines have been transplanted successfully, and tumour cells show behaviours that are very reminiscent of their expected behaviour. When injected into the circulation (Duct of Cuvier) or into the yolk, or in the perivitelline space, many cell lines were shown to leave the site of injection or extravasate and invade tissues (often into the caudal haematopoietic tissue) and form micrometastases within a week [71, 74, 77, 78]. Furthermore, transplant-derived cell masses are often able to attract blood vessels from the host embryo [76].

10.3.3 Adult Models

Xenografts are most frequently established using host embryos for reason of convenience, and the opportunity to perform detailed imaging of cancer cell behaviour in an intact organism. Nevertheless, adult stages are useful for longer-term studies of cancer development, especially if larger tumours with more extensive vascularisation and a hypoxic microenvironment are needed. Such models will still have significant cost and space advantages over mouse xenotransplant models. Generation of immunodeficient animals similar to rodent models has been achieved by X-ray treatment [79] or by employing immunosuppressants [80], but when reverse genetics became feasible, more stable genetic models were developed to study long-term behaviour of tumours [81, 82]. In an interesting report, it was shown that cell-line specific "xenotolerance" could be achieved in adults, by an embryonic transplant of irradiated cells of the same line [83]. In this way, animals with a native immune system can be used as hosts, thereby avoiding the need for complex "pathogen-free" conditions and providing an even better replica of a normal tumour environment. This is an exciting avenue that could be explored for patient-specific cellular xenografts.

10.3.4 Current Zebrafish Xenotransplant Cancer Models

By now, more than 100 reports have been published that exploit zebrafish xenografts. Usually transplants of 100–300 cells are performed at 32–35 °C, either in the perivitelline space or in the Duct of Cuvier at 48hpf. Mostly well-established tumour cell lines are used to assay the role of candidate signalling pathways such as TGF-β, CXCR4, Wnt, KRAS and Nodal, with cells labelled via transfection of fluorescent protein, or by CM-DiI labelling. Often, xenografted larvae are used to test therapeutic potential of compounds or enhanced delivery systems, or simply to gain basic understanding of tumour cell behaviours.

Several reports successfully use the fish as a direct recipient for patient cells [75, 84–90]. There exists a single report where transplants were performed with the direct aim of tailoring patient treatment [84]. This study used T-cell acute lymphoblastic leukaemia (T-ALL) cells derived from two patients, and transplanted approximately 500 CM-DiI labeled cells into the yolk of 48hpf zebrafish. Embryos were then treated with three different inhibitors that target commonly mutated pathways in T-ALL. In one patient, a strong response was found to a γ-secretase inhibitor. The subsequent identification of an activating Notch mutation provided a clear explanation for this response. Another report demonstrated that multiple myeloma cells directly transplanted from patients established themselves rapidly in fish embryos, and their responses to drugs conformed with predictions [89]. Overall, these studies show that using zebrafish as patient avatars is a promising area of future research.

10.3.5 Non-cancer Models

Xenografting of non-cancerous cells has been less well studied. Two reports describe transplanting human CD34+ haematopoietic stem cells [75, 91]. CD34+ hematopoietic cells sorted from umbilical cord blood were labelled with CM-Dil or PKH26, and injected into the circulation. Cells were detected in injected larvae at 1 days post injection in both studies but longer-term survival and homing to haematopoietic tissues was only reported in one study [91]. The reasons for differences between the two studies is currently unclear. Three reports describe transplantation of adipocyte-derived and mesenchymal stem cells and show cell survival [92–94]. Melanocytes and fibroblasts have also been transplanted into blastoderm embryos and were shown to survive for several days [71, 94–96]. The possibility to integrate human iPS cells in the zebrafish could hold great promise. Two groups describe transplant of early vascular cells derived from human induced pluripotent stem (iPS) cell lines. Although high-resolution analysis and long term follow-up was not performed, cells appeared to integrate in the embryonic vasculature and expressed an endothelial marker. Interestingly these iPS-derived cells outperformed commonly used HUVECs in this assay [97–99]. Thus, at least in some cases, it may be possible to xenograft human cells in order to recreate and study aspects of genetic diseases, and test potential treatments. However, it will require significant optimisation of cell differentiation and transplantation protocols in order to get cells in the correct state of differentiation at the right place and time in the embryo such that they will properly participate in development.

10.4 Zebrafish Drug Discovery

10.4.1 Advantages of Phenotypic Screening

The goal of personalised medicine is to predict how individual patients will respond to therapies before their treatment begins, taking in to account their background genetic variation. To produce bespoke therapies, there is a need for high-throughput testing of drugs in disease models that can reliably reproduce the human conditions [1].

Zebrafish research is ideally placed to benefit from a recent resurgence in phenotypic drug screening, aided by the increasing number of disease models available [100, 101]. For over 30 years, target based drug discovery has been the predominant approach to finding new therapeutics, however the yield of new 'first in the class' drugs brought to market through this approach has been disappointing. Whereas in the same time frame, phenotypic drug screening has had more successes, despite the relatively small number of screens performed using this approach [102]. Phenotypic screening methods are widely applicable to the full range of disease models available in zebrafish. From rare monogenic disorders where a single target – single drug scenario, – a prerequisite for target driven drug discovery, is appropriate, to complex multifactoral disorders where multiple gene mutations and modifiers may also play a role and drugs are required that can potentially hit multiple targets in different pathways. Phenotypic in vivo screens have the advantage that no prior knowledge of the target is necessary and in the case of whole organism assays, all available targets are present in one assay, increasing to the likelihood of identifying novel important targets. In addition, with whole organism screens there is the possibility to assess multiple endpoints in the primary assay and include counter-screens for many drug characteristics that are usually only tested much later in the drug discovery pipeline; such as the ability for the drug to reach the desired tissue and the testing of off target effects and toxicity.

10.4.2 Screening Applications

Since the first chemical screen using zebrafish in multiwell plates in 2000 [103] the number of screens has increased rapidly [104]. Many different approaches that have been taken; from simple gene expression screens [105, 106], fluorescent reporter [107, 108] and behavioural screens [109, 110] to therapeutic screens for rescue of many different disease phenotypes [111–113]. But with the number of zebrafish drug screens rising, are any drugs making it through to the clinic and proving this is a successful strategy to take? Although the numbers of lead compounds being taken on by companies is still quite small [100], there are a few examples that are progressing to clinical trials. PROTO-1 (Oricula Therapeutics), is a compound that protects against the ototoxic side effects caused by other therapeutics, including chemotherapeutics and some aminoglycoside antibiotics. Ototoxic side effects can cause long term damage to the hair cells of the inner ear and lead to permanent deafness. The zebrafish lateral line sensory system is an excellent model system for studying hair cell toxicity and regeneration and PROTO-1, a benzothiophene carboxamide, was identified in a screen for compounds that blocked aminoglycoside induced hair cell death [114]. Zebrafish can also be used to find new uses for existing drugs, as is the case with leflunomide, a current treatment for arthritis that is now in clinical trials as an adjuvant therapy for melanoma. White et al. used a simple gene expression screen to identify drugs that inhibit neural crest cell derivatives in the zebrafish embryo [115]. Neural crest progenitor genes are found to be activated in melanoma [116] and using a combination of zebrafish, xenopus and mouse xenograft studies leflunomide was found to inhibit neural crest gene transcriptional elongation and melanoma growth.

10.4.3 Screens for New CNS Therapeutics

The search for new drugs to treat CNS disorders is extremely challenging and very few new drugs make it to the market. One reason for this is the multifactorial nature of many neurological diseases, which requires complex polypharmacology and can often result in toxic side effects. Target-based drug discovery platforms designed to find a single drug for a single target are not suitable for multigenic disorders, where there are complex biological mechanisms. The genetic basis of these diseases is often unclear; with few familial cases and potentially hundreds of susceptibility genes. Using phenotypic screening, to identify drugs with multiple targets or multiple pathways in one assay, is more appropriate. However, modelling neurological disorders is difficult, particularly where there is a late onset of symptoms diagnosed by changes in behavior that cannot be analysed in cell or tissue based assays.

10.4.3.1 Behavioural Assays

Zebrafish have a number of advantages over other models for neuropharmacological research. Firstly, for neurological disorders, the most informative readouts are behavioural assays, and although zebrafish have a simplified brain structure compared to our own, they have a wide repertoire of behaviours in response to different stimuli and environments, which are reproducible and can be quantified [117]. Secondly, the small size and aquatic nature of zebrafish make them amenable to high throughput behavioural profiling in ways that other vertebrate models of neurological disorders are not [109]. Zebrafish larvae can be screened at high throughput in multiwell plates, while the adult fish, although at lower throughput, can be screened simultaneously in different arenas, with appropriate commercial (Viewpoint, France, Ethovision) and custom-built equipment. Recent studies have defined specific phenotypic signatures for complex behavioral responses to sensory or pharmacological stimuli in larvae and adults, and improvements in signature clustering and analysis, are making huge advances in this field [118, 119].

Profiling zebrafish behaviour in response to different drugs and drug combinations enables clustering of compounds that have similar or related behavioural signatures. Signatures associated with neurological disorders can be compared to profiles of known psychotic and antipsychotic drugs in order to identify correlations between particular compounds and behaviours. An elegant example is the work of Rennekamp et al. who used a simple photomotor response assay to measure freezing in fish over alternating light-dark cycles [120]. This highly conserved response mediated by the limbic system is often impaired in psychiatric disorders such as schizophrenia. Using phenotypic clustering of compounds that disrupt freezing behaviour, followed by chemical structure mining, they identified finazines as a new class of anti-psychotic drugs and sigma-1 as a functional target of the fight or flight response pathway. In a complementary study, finazines were also identified in a screen for compounds that mirrored the behavioural signatures of a known anti-psychotic drug, haloperidol. In this screen of 24,760 compounds, movement of zebrafish larvae was monitored as a quantifiable response to a series of light and sound stimuli, and the resulting compound profiles were compared using phenoBLAST, which enables identification of the best match to a chosen signature [121]. Bruni et al. then demonstrated that finazine suppressed drug-induced hyperactivity in mice, further validating this approach.

10.4.3.2 Screens for Anti-convulsants

An example where it is hoped the use of zebrafish in precision medicine can make a real difference is in the identification of compounds targeting pathology underlying epilepsy. Although there are a number of anti-convulsant drugs currently available, many have severe side effects or are not effective, with up to a third of sufferers having no available treatment. Zebrafish have been widely used to model epilepsy for drug discovery and for understanding disease onset and progression [122]. Initial approaches used drug-induced zebrafish models of epilepsy, using the convulsant pentylenetetrazol, PTZ, and screened for rescue of the behavioural phenotype [123, 124] or for reduction of PTZ-induced expression of *cfos* [105]; both with success. Different genetic defects that can cause seizures, along with the environmental and experience related triggers have also been studied in zebrafish. Dravet syndrome is an inherited childhood epilepsy syndrome caused by mutations in the SCN1a protein [125]. Phenotypic screening in a zebrafish model of Dravet syndrome identified clemizole as a potential treatment [126]. Further analysis found clemizole acts as a serotonin receptor agonist to suppress seizures, and FDA approved compounds with similar activities have been tested in Dravet syndrome patients, with initial results showing a reduction in seizure frequency [127]. These findings demonstrate the power of high-throughput chemical screens in zebrafish as a means of repurposing existing drugs to rapidly move from tank to bedside.

10.4.4 Future Developments for Drug Discovery

For zebrafish to be a viable screening tool for precision medicine, new therapeutics need to be easily transferable to the clinic, accurately predicting the correct drug response. How well this works depends on a number of factors, including the accuracy of the disease model and how the drug is metabolized. Some doubt has been cast on using animal models [128, 129] particularly for diseases such as multiple sclerosis, where some induced mouse models of MS have been unreliable at accurately predicting new therapeutics [130]. However, growing evidence from multiple zebrafish screens, in particular those that have gone on to confirm potential 'hit' compounds in other species, suggest zebrafish have comparable drug responses. In the case of neurological disorders, compounds must also be able to cross the blood brain barrier and studies have shown that the blood brain barrier is conserved in zebrafish and develops between 3 and 10 days of development [131–133], therefore it is important to test if compounds are effective after this stage.

One potential way to increase the accuracy of the drug response between fish and man is by humanizing the zebrafish metabolism and pharmacological responses to drugs. Zebrafish have a full range of cytochrome P450 genes [134], however, the levels of some CYP genes are low during early development [135] which could lead to some metabolites not being detected in early zebrafish screens. In addition, CYP3A4 is responsible for metabolising 50% of drugs [136], and the zebrafish homologous gene is quite divergent from the human gene at the DNA sequence level. To overcome any metabolic differences this may produce, a zebrafish transgenic line has been generated which expresses the human version of CYP3A4 under the control of the zebrafish liver specific *lfabp* promoter, and these transgenic fish were found to have a higher level of metabolism of CYP3A4 substrates, than wild-type fish [137], thus highlighting the potential to humanize the zebrafish liver by gene delivery. In addition to metabolism by the liver, drugs are also metabolised by the microbes in the gut. Studies that compare different microbiomes and transfer microbes between different models [138, 139] will be useful to determine how much of a role in personalising therapeutic responses to drugs different microbiomes can make.

A major obstacle to systems biology approaches to drug discovery with zebrafish, is the difficulty in comparative imaging of multiple embryos for precise quantification. Many drug screening approaches use larvae imaged in multiwell plates to determine morphological, fluorescent or stained differences that result from the effects of the drugs added. The embryo and larvae have complex 3D shapes that lie at different angles of orientation without manipulation; this is compounded if there are multiple larvae which may overlay each other, thereby obscuring the area that needs to be analysed. In addition, aliquoting embryos into multiwell plates can be time consuming. Many methods to overcome these issues have been developed, including moulds to orientate the larvae [140], the VAST system (Union Biometrica) which is also able to aspirate individual larvae from multiwell plates and deliver them into a capillary that can be rotated to any angle with precision imaging [141, 142] and the ARQiv-HTS platform for automated reporter quantification [143]. These improvements in automation and image analysis will facilitate higher throughput methods and more accurate quantification of zebrafish larval data.

10.5 Conclusions

The need for precision medicine is increasing [144] with an aging population. Common multifactorial diseases including cancer, neurodegeneration and cardiovascular disease are set to rise and there is a need to find personalised therapies that work for particular cohorts of patients, thus maximising treatment specificity and efficacy. In addition, there are at least 7000 known rare diseases, with over half having genetic linkage, however 95% of these diseases do not yet have a single approved drug to target them [145]. As the quantity of sequencing data from patient WES/WGS and GWAS studies increases, the need for functional analysis of new genetic variants will also increase.

Zebrafish have the potential to contribute to advances in human genomic medicine at multiple levels. As shown in Fig. 10.1 different stages of the personalised medicine pipeline for different disease types can all benefit from zebrafish approaches; from testing genes of unknown function, right through to drug discovery. The zebrafish is the only high-throughput vertebrate disease model, which when combined with advanced molecular tools and genetic tractability, positions this model to make a major contribution to the mammoth task ahead of finding precise cures for all diseases.

Acknowledgements We thank Vincent Cunliffe for comments on the manuscript. SB is funded by a grant from the BBSRC (BB/M01021X/1) and FvE was funded by BBSRC (BB/M02332X/1). The Sheffield zebrafish aquarium and small molecule screening facilities are supported by grants from the MRC (G0700091, G0802527).

References

1. Davis EE, Frangakis S, Katsanis N (2014) Interpreting human genetic variation with in vivo zebrafish assays. Biochim Biophys Acta 1842:1960–1970. doi:10.1016/j.bbadis.2014.05.024
2. Howe K et al (2013) The zebrafish reference genome sequence and its relationship to the human genome. Nature 496:498–503. doi:10.1038/nature12111
3. Cox DB, Platt RJ, Zhang F (2015) Therapeutic genome editing: prospects and challenges. Nat Med 21:121–131. doi:10.1038/nm.3793
4. Reardon S (2015) Leukaemia success heralds wave of gene-editing therapies. Nature 527:146–147. doi:10.1038/nature.2015.18737
5. Doyon Y et al (2008) Heritable targeted gene disruption in zebrafish using designed zinc-finger nucleases. Nat Biotechnol 26:702–708. doi:10.1038/nbt1409
6. Meng X, Noyes MB, Zhu LJ, Lawson ND, Wolfe SA (2008) Targeted gene inactivation in zebrafish using engineered zinc-finger nucleases. Nat Biotechnol 26:695–701. doi:10.1038/nbt1398
7. Sander JD et al (2011) Selection-free zinc-finger-nuclease engineering by context-dependent assembly (CoDA). Nat Methods 8:67–69. doi:10.1038/nmeth.1542
8. Cade L et al (2012) Highly efficient generation of heritable zebrafish gene mutations using homo- and heterodimeric TALENs. Nucleic Acids Res 40:8001–8010. doi:10.1093/nar/gks518
9. Sander JD et al (2011) Targeted gene disruption in somatic zebrafish cells using engineered TALENs. Nat Biotechnol 29:697–698. doi:10.1038/nbt.1934
10. Hwang WY et al (2013) Efficient genome editing in zebrafish using a CRISPR-Cas system. Nat Biotechnol 31:227–229. doi:10.1038/nbt.2501
11. Hruscha A et al (2013) Efficient CRISPR/Cas9 genome editing with low off-target effects in zebrafish. Development 140:4982–4987. doi:10.1242/dev.099085
12. Sertori R, Trengove M, Basheer F, Ward AC, Liongue C (2016) Genome editing in zebrafish: a practical overview. Brief Funct Genomics 15:322–330. doi:10.1093/bfgp/elv051
13. Ear J et al (2016) A zebrafish model of 5q-syndrome using CRISPR/Cas9 targeting RPS14 reveals a p53-independent and p53-dependent mechanism of erythroid failure. J Genet Genomics 43:307–318. doi:10.1016/j.jgg.2016.03.007
14. Zhang Y et al (2014) Defects of protein production in erythroid cells revealed in a zebrafish Diamond-Blackfan anemia model for mutation in RPS19. Cell Death Dis 5:e1352. doi:10.1038/cddis.2014.318
15. Wilkinson RN, Jopling C, van Eeden FJ (2014) Zebrafish as a model of cardiac disease. Prog Mol Biol Transl Sci 124:65–91. doi:10.1016/B978-0-12-386930-2.00004-5
16. Wilkinson RN, van Eeden FJ (2014) The zebrafish as a model of vascular development and disease. Prog Mol Biol Transl Sci 124:93–122. doi:10.1016/B978-0-12-386930-2.00005-7
17. Schmid B, Haass C (2013) Genomic editing opens new avenues for zebrafish as a model for neurodegeneration. J Neurochem 127:461–470. doi:10.1111/jnc.12460
18. Martin-Jimenez R, Campanella M, Russell C (2015) New zebrafish models of neurodegeneration. Curr Neurol Neurosci Rep 15:33. doi:10.1007/s11910-015-0555-z
19. Auer TO, Duroure K, Concordet JP, Del Bene F (2014) CRISPR/Cas9-mediated conversion of eGFP- into Gal4-transgenic lines in zebrafish. Nat Protoc 9:2823–2840. doi:10.1038/nprot.2014.187
20. Auer TO, Duroure K, De Cian A, Concordet JP, Del Bene F (2014) Highly efficient CRISPR/Cas9-mediated knock-in in zebrafish by homology-independent DNA repair. Genome Res 24:142–153. doi:10.1101/gr.161638.113
21. Shin J, Chen J, Solnica-Krezel L (2014) Efficient homologous recombination-mediated genome engineering in zebrafish using TALE nucleases. Development 141:3807–3818. doi:10.1242/dev.108019
22. Zu Y et al (2013) TALEN-mediated precise genome modification by homologous recombination in zebrafish. Nat Methods 10:329–331. doi:10.1038/nmeth.2374
23. Armstrong GA et al (2016) Homology directed knockin of point mutations in the zebrafish tardbp and fus genes in ALS using the CRISPR/Cas9 system. PLoS One 11:–e0150188. doi:10.1371/journal.pone.0150188

24. Bedell VM et al (2012) In vivo genome editing using a high-efficiency TALEN system. Nature 491:114–118. doi:10.1038/nature11537
25. Gagnon JA et al (2014) Efficient mutagenesis by Cas9 protein-mediated oligonucleotide insertion and large-scale assessment of single-guide RNAs. PLoS One 9:e98186. doi:10.1371/journal.pone.0098186
26. Hoshijima K, Jurynec MJ, Grunwald DJ (2016) Precise Editing of the Zebrafish Genome Made Simple and Efficient. Dev Cell 36:654–667. doi:10.1016/j.devcel.2016.02.015
27. Komor AC, Kim YB, Packer MS, Zuris JA, Liu DR (2016) Programmable editing of a target base in genomic DNA without double-stranded DNA cleavage. Nature 533:420–424. doi:10.1038/nature17946
28. Amsterdam A et al (2004) Identification of 315 genes essential for early zebrafish development. Proc Natl Acad Sci U S A 101:12792–12797. doi:10.1073/pnas.0403929101
29. Driever W et al (1996) A genetic screen for mutations affecting embryogenesis in zebrafish. Development 123:37–46
30. Haffter P et al (1996) The identification of genes with unique and essential functions in the development of the zebrafish, *Danio rerio*. Development 123:1–36
31. Kettleborough RN et al (2013) A systematic genome-wide analysis of zebrafish protein-coding gene function. Nature 496:494–497. doi:10.1038/nature11992
32. Shah AN, Davey CF, Whitebirch AC, Miller AC, Moens CB (2015) Rapid reverse genetic screening using CRISPR in zebrafish. Nat Methods 12:535–540. doi:10.1038/nmeth.3360
33. Kim IS et al (2017) Microenvironment-derived factors driving metastatic plasticity in melanoma. Nat Commun 8:14343. doi:10.1038/ncomms14343
34. Sanjana NE (2016) Genome-scale CRISPR pooled screens. Anal Biochem. doi:10.1016/j.ab.2016.05.014
35. Tsai SQ, Joung JK (2016) Defining and improving the genome-wide specificities of CRISPR-Cas9 nucleases. Nat Rev Genet 17:300–312. doi:10.1038/nrg.2016.28
36. Kleinstiver BP et al (2016) High-fidelity CRISPR-Cas9 nucleases with no detectable genome-wide off-target effects. Nature 529:490–495. doi:10.1038/nature16526
37. Feng Y et al (2016) Expanding CRISPR/Cas9 genome editing capacity in zebrafish using SaCas9. G3 (Bethesda) 6:2517–2521. doi:10.1534/g3.116.031914
38. Kleinstiver BP et al (2016) Genome-wide specificities of CRISPR-Cas Cpf1 nucleases in human cells. Nat Biotechnol 34:869–874. doi:10.1038/nbt.3620
39. Kok FO et al (2015) Reverse genetic screening reveals poor correlation between morpholino-induced and mutant phenotypes in zebrafish. Dev Cell 32:97–108. doi:10.1016/j.devcel.2014.11.018
40. Novodvorsky P et al (2015) klf2ash317 mutant zebrafish do not recapitulate morpholino-induced vascular and haematopoietic phenotypes. PLoS One 10:e0141611. doi:10.1371/journal.pone.0141611
41. Shmukler BE et al (2015) Homozygous knockout of the piezo1 gene in the zebrafish is not associated with anemia. Haematologica 100:e483–e485. doi:10.3324/haematol.2015.132449
42. Rossi A et al (2015) Genetic compensation induced by deleterious mutations but not gene knockdowns. Nature 524:230–233. doi:10.1038/nature14580
43. Diss G et al (2017) Gene duplication can impart fragility, not robustness, in the yeast protein interaction network. Science 355:630–634. doi:10.1126/science.aai7685
44. Runtuwene V et al (2011) Noonan syndrome gain-of-function mutations in NRAS cause zebrafish gastrulation defects. Dis Model Mech 4:393–399. doi:10.1242/dmm.007112
45. Sousa SB et al (2014) Gain-of-function mutations in the phosphatidylserine synthase 1 (PTDSS1) gene cause Lenz-Majewski syndrome. Nat Genet 46:70–76. doi:10.1038/ng.2829
46. Thermes V et al (2002) I-SceI meganuclease mediates highly efficient transgenesis in fish. Mech Dev 118:91–98
47. Kawakami K et al (2004) A transposon-mediated gene trap approach identifies developmentally regulated genes in zebrafish. Dev Cell 7:133–144. doi:10.1016/j.devcel.2004.06.005
48. Mosimann C et al (2013) Site-directed zebrafish transgenesis into single landing sites with the phiC31 integrase system. Dev Dyn 242:949–963. doi:10.1002/dvdy.23989
49. Roberts JA et al (2014) Targeted transgene integration overcomes variability of position effects in zebrafish. Development 141:715–724. doi:10.1242/dev.100347
50. Langenau DM et al (2003) Myc-induced T cell leukemia in transgenic zebrafish. Science 299:887–890. doi:10.1126/science.1080280
51. Feng H et al (2007) Heat-shock induction of T-cell lymphoma/leukaemia in conditional Cre/lox-regulated transgenic zebrafish. Br J Haematol 138:169–175. doi:10.1111/j.1365-2141.2007.06625.x
52. Chen J et al (2007) NOTCH1-induced T-cell leukemia in transgenic zebrafish. Leukemia 21:462–471. doi:10.1038/sj.leu.2404546
53. Feng H et al (2010) T-lymphoblastic lymphoma cells express high levels of BCL2, S1P1, and ICAM1, leading to a blockade of tumor cell intravasation. Cancer Cell 18:353–366. doi:10.1016/j.ccr.2010.09.009
54. Patton EE et al (2005) BRAF mutations are sufficient to promote nevi formation and cooperate with p53 in the genesis of melanoma. Curr Biol 15:249–254. doi:10.1016/j.cub.2005.01.031

55. Davies H et al (2002) Mutations of the BRAF gene in human cancer. Nature 417:949–954. doi:10.1038/nature00766
56. O'Donnell KC et al (2014) Axon degeneration and PGC-1alpha-mediated protection in a zebrafish model of alpha-synuclein toxicity. Dis Model Mech 7:571–582. doi:10.1242/dmm.013185
57. Ohki Y et al (2017) Glycine-alanine dipeptide repeat protein contributes to toxicity in a zebrafish model of C9orf72 associated neurodegeneration. Mol Neurodegener 12:6. doi:10.1186/s13024-016-0146-8
58. Jindal GA et al (2017) In vivo severity ranking of Ras pathway mutations associated with developmental disorders. Proc Natl Acad Sci U S A 114:510–515. doi:10.1073/pnas.1615651114
59. Tsetskhladze ZR et al (2012) Functional assessment of human coding mutations affecting skin pigmentation using zebrafish. PLoS One 7:e47398. doi:10.1371/journal.pone.0047398
60. Waters MF et al (2006) Mutations in voltage-gated potassium channel KCNC3 cause degenerative and developmental central nervous system phenotypes. Nat Genet 38:447–451. doi:10.1038/ng1758
61. Issa FA, Mazzochi C, Mock AF, Papazian DM (2011) Spinocerebellar ataxia type 13 mutant potassium channel alters neuronal excitability and causes locomotor deficits in zebrafish. J Neurosci 31:6831–6841. doi:10.1523/JNEUROSCI.6572-10.2011
62. Gonzaga-Jauregui C et al (2015) Exome sequence analysis suggests that genetic burden contributes to phenotypic variability and complex neuropathy. Cell Rep 12:1169–1183. doi:10.1016/j.celrep.2015.07.023
63. Bedell VM, Westcot SE, Ekker SC (2011) Lessons from morpholino-based screening in zebrafish. Brief Funct Genomics 10:181–188. doi:10.1093/bfgp/elr021
64. Sia D, Moeini A, Labgaa I, Villanueva A (2015) The future of patient-derived tumor xenografts in cancer treatment. Pharmacogenomics 16:1671–1683. doi:10.2217/pgs.15.102
65. Malaney P, Nicosia SV, Dave V (2014) One mouse, one patient paradigm: new avatars of personalized cancer therapy. Cancer Lett 344:1–12. doi:10.1016/j.canlet.2013.10.010
66. Garralda E et al (2014) Integrated next-generation sequencing and avatar mouse models for personalized cancer treatment. Clin Cancer Res 20:2476–2484. doi:10.1158/1078-0432.CCR-13-3047
67. Lam SH, Chua HL, Gong Z, Lam TJ, Sin YM (2004) Development and maturation of the immune system in zebrafish, *Danio rerio*: a gene expression profiling, in situ hybridization and immunological study. Dev Comp Immunol 28:9–28
68. Pelster B, Burggren WW (1996) Disruption of hemoglobin oxygen transport does not impact oxygen-dependent physiological processes in developing embryos of zebra fish (*Danio rerio*). Circ Res 79:358–362
69. Rouhi P et al (2010) Hypoxia-induced metastasis model in embryonic zebrafish. Nat Protoc 5:1911–1918. doi:10.1038/nprot.2010.150
70. Schnurr ME, Yin Y, Scott GR (2014) Temperature during embryonic development has persistent effects on metabolic enzymes in the muscle of zebrafish. J Exp Biol 217:1370–1380. doi:10.1242/jeb.094037
71. Haldi M, Ton C, Seng WL, McGrath P (2006) Human melanoma cells transplanted into zebrafish proliferate, migrate, produce melanin, form masses and stimulate angiogenesis in zebrafish. Angiogenesis 9:139–151. doi:10.1007/s10456-006-9040-2
72. Spence R, Gerlach G, Lawrence C, Smith C (2008) The behaviour and ecology of the zebrafish, *Danio rerio*. Biol Rev Camb Philos Soc 83:13–34. doi:10.1111/j.1469-185X.2007.00030.x
73. Tulotta C et al (2016) Imaging of human cancer cell proliferation, invasion, and micrometastasis in a zebrafish xenogeneic engraftment model. Methods Mol Biol 1451:155–169. doi:10.1007/978-1-4939-3771-4_11
74. Drabsch Y, He S, Zhang L, Snaar-Jagalska BE, ten Dijke P (2013) Transforming growth factor-beta signalling controls human breast cancer metastasis in a zebrafish xenograft model. Breast Cancer Res 15:R106. doi:10.1186/bcr3573
75. Pruvot B et al (2011) Leukemic cell xenograft in zebrafish embryo for investigating drug efficacy. Haematologica 96:612–616. doi:10.3324/haematol.2010.031401
76. Nicoli S, Ribatti D, Cotelli F, Presta M (2007) Mammalian tumor xenografts induce neovascularization in zebrafish embryos. Cancer Res 67:2927–2931. doi:10.1158/0008-5472.CAN-06-4268
77. He S et al (2012) Neutrophil-mediated experimental metastasis is enhanced by VEGFR inhibition in a zebrafish xenograft model. J Pathol 227:431–445. doi:10.1002/path.4013
78. Jung DW et al (2012) A novel zebrafish human tumor xenograft model validated for anti-cancer drug screening. Mol BioSyst 8:1930–1939. doi:10.1039/c2mb05501e
79. White RM et al (2008) Transparent adult zebrafish as a tool for in vivo transplantation analysis. Cell Stem Cell 2:183–189. doi:10.1016/j.stem.2007.11.002
80. Stoletov K, Montel V, Lester RD, Gonias SL, Klemke R (2007) High-resolution imaging of the dynamic tumor cell vascular interface in transparent zebrafish. Proc Natl Acad Sci U S A 104:17406–17411. doi:10.1073/pnas.0703446104
81. Tang Q et al (2014) Optimized cell transplantation using adult rag2 mutant zebrafish. Nat Methods 11:821–824. doi:10.1038/nmeth.3031
82. Jung IH et al (2016) Impaired lymphocytes development and xenotransplantation of gastrointestinal tumor cells in Prkdc-Null SCID zebrafish model. Neoplasia 18:468–479. doi:10.1016/j.neo.2016.06.007
83. Zhang B et al (2016) Novel immunologic tolerance of human cancer cell xenotransplants in zebraf-

ish. Transl Res 170:89–98 e81–83. doi:10.1016/j.trsl.2015.12.007
84. Bentley VL et al (2015) Focused chemical genomics using zebrafish xenotransplantation as a pre-clinical therapeutic platform for T-cell acute lymphoblastic leukemia. Haematologica 100:70–76. doi:10.3324/haematol.2014.110742
85. Rampazzo E et al (2013) Wnt activation promotes neuronal differentiation of glioblastoma. Cell Death Dis 4:e500. doi:10.1038/cddis.2013.32
86. Marques IJ et al (2009) Metastatic behaviour of primary human tumours in a zebrafish xenotransplantation model. BMC Cancer 9:128. doi:10.1186/1471-2407-9-128
87. Mercatali, L. et al (2016) Development of a patient-derived xenograft (PDX) of breast cancer bone metastasis in a zebrafish model. Int J Mol Sci 17, doi:10.3390/ijms17081375
88. Gaudenzi G et al (2016) Patient-derived xenograft in zebrafish embryos: a new platform for translational research in neuroendocrine tumors. Endocrine. doi:10.1007/s12020-016-1048-9
89. Lin J et al (2016) A clinically relevant in vivo zebrafish model of human multiple myeloma to study preclinical therapeutic efficacy. Blood 128:249–252. doi:10.1182/blood-2016-03-704460
90. Bansal N et al (2014) Enrichment of human prostate cancer cells with tumor initiating properties in mouse and zebrafish xenografts by differential adhesion. Prostate 74:187–200. doi:10.1002/pros.22740
91. Staal FJ, Spaink HP, Fibbe WE (2016) Visualizing human hematopoietic stem cell trafficking in vivo using a zebrafish xenograft model. Stem Cells Dev 25:360–365. doi:10.1089/scd.2015.0195
92. Li J et al (2015) Xenotransplantation of human adipose-derived stem cells in zebrafish embryos. PLoS One 10:e0123264. doi:10.1371/journal.pone.0123264
93. Patel N et al (2012) Developmental regulation of TAC1 in peptidergic-induced human mesenchymal stem cells: implication for spinal cord injury in zebrafish. Stem Cells Dev 21:308–320. doi:10.1089/scd.2011.0179
94. Xia H et al (2014) Identification of a cell-of-origin for fibroblasts comprising the fibrotic reticulum in idiopathic pulmonary fibrosis. Am J Pathol 184:1369–1383. doi:10.1016/j.ajpath.2014.01.012
95. Lee LM, Seftor EA, Bonde G, Cornell RA, Hendrix MJ (2005) The fate of human malignant melanoma cells transplanted into zebrafish embryos: assessment of migration and cell division in the absence of tumor formation. Dev Dyn 233:1560–1570. doi:10.1002/dvdy.20471
96. Benyumov AO et al (2012) A novel zebrafish embryo xenotransplantation model to study primary human fibroblast motility in health and disease. Zebrafish 9:38–43. doi:10.1089/zeb.2011.0705
97. Chan XY et al (2015) Three- dimensional vascular network assembly from diabetic patient-derived induced pluripotent stem cells. Arterioscler Thromb Vasc Biol 35:2677–2685. doi:10.1161/ATVBAHA.115.306362
98. Orlova VV et al (2014) Functionality of endothelial cells and pericytes from human pluripotent stem cells demonstrated in cultured vascular plexus and zebrafish xenografts. Arterioscler Thromb Vasc Biol 34:177–186. doi:10.1161/ATVBAHA.113.302598
99. Orlova VV et al (2014) Generation, expansion and functional analysis of endothelial cells and pericytes derived from human pluripotent stem cells. Nat Protoc 9:1514–1531. doi:10.1038/nprot.2014.102
100. MacRae CA, Peterson RT (2015) Zebrafish as tools for drug discovery. Nat Rev Drug Discov 14:721–731. doi:10.1038/nrd4627
101. Strange K (2016) Drug discovery in fish, flies, and worms. ILAR J 57:133–143. doi:10.1093/ilar/ilw034
102. Swinney DC (2013) Phenotypic vs. target-based drug discovery for first-in-class medicines. Clin Pharmacol Ther 93:299–301. doi:10.1038/clpt.2012.236
103. Peterson RT, Link BA, Dowling JE, Schreiber SL (2000) Small molecule developmental screens reveal the logic and timing of vertebrate development. Proc Natl Acad Sci U S A 97:12965–12969. doi:10.1073/pnas.97.24.12965
104. Rennekamp AJ, Peterson RT (2015) 15 years of zebrafish chemical screening. Curr Opin Chem Biol 24:58–70. doi:10.1016/j.cbpa.2014.10.025
105. Baxendale S et al (2012) Identification of compounds with anti-convulsant properties in a zebrafish model of epileptic seizures. Dis Model Mech 5:773–784. doi:10.1242/dmm.010090
106. North TE et al (2007) Prostaglandin E2 regulates vertebrate haematopoietic stem cell homeostasis. Nature 447:1007–1011. doi:10.1038/nature05883
107. Robertson AL et al (2014) A zebrafish compound screen reveals modulation of neutrophil reverse migration as an anti-inflammatory mechanism. Sci Transl Med 6:225ra229. doi:10.1126/scitranslmed.3007672
108. Gallardo VE et al (2015) Phenotype-driven chemical screening in zebrafish for compounds that inhibit collective cell migration identifies multiple pathways potentially involved in metastatic invasion. Dis Model Mech 8:565–576. doi:10.1242/dmm.018689
109. Kokel D et al (2010) Rapid behavior-based identification of neuroactive small molecules in the zebrafish. Nat Chem Biol 6:231–237. doi:10.1038/nchembio.307
110. Rihel J et al (2010) Zebrafish behavioral profiling links drugs to biological targets and rest/wake regulation. Science 327:348–351. doi:10.1126/science.1183090
111. Asimaki A et al (2014) Identification of a new modulator of the intercalated disc in a zebrafish model of arrhythmogenic cardiomyopathy. Sci Transl Med 6:240ra274. doi:10.1126/scitranslmed.3008008

112. Peal DS et al (2011) Novel chemical suppressors of long QT syndrome identified by an in vivo functional screen. Circulation 123:23–30. doi:10.1161/CIRCULATIONAHA.110.003731
113. Yeh JR et al (2008) AML1-ETO reprograms hematopoietic cell fate by downregulating scl expression. Development 135:401–410. doi:10.1242/dev.008904
114. Owens KN et al (2008) Identification of genetic and chemical modulators of zebrafish mechanosensory hair cell death. PLoS Genet 4:e1000020. doi:10.1371/journal.pgen.1000020
115. White RM et al (2011) DHODH modulates transcriptional elongation in the neural crest and melanoma. Nature 471:518–522. doi:10.1038/nature09882
116. Kaufman CK et al (2016) A zebrafish melanoma model reveals emergence of neural crest identity during melanoma initiation. Science 351:aad2197. doi:10.1126/science.aad2197
117. Kalueff AV et al (2013) Towards a comprehensive catalog of zebrafish behavior 1.0 and beyond. Zebrafish 10:70–86. doi:10.1089/zeb.2012.0861
118. Kalueff AV et al (2016) Zebrafish neurobehavioral phenomics for aquatic neuropharmacology and toxicology research. Aquat Toxicol 170:297–309. doi:10.1016/j.aquatox.2015.08.007
119. Stewart AM et al (2015) A novel 3D method of locomotor analysis in adult zebrafish: implications for automated detection of CNS drug-evoked phenotypes. J Neurosci Methods 255:66–74. doi:10.1016/j.jneumeth.2015.07.023
120. Rennekamp AJ et al (2016) sigma1 receptor ligands control a switch between passive and active threat responses. Nat Chem Biol 12:552–558. doi:10.1038/nchembio.2089
121. Bruni G et al (2016) Zebrafish behavioral profiling identifies multitarget antipsychotic-like compounds. Nat Chem Biol 12:559–566. doi:10.1038/nchembio.2097
122. Cunliffe VT (2016) Building a zebrafish toolkit for investigating the pathobiology of epilepsy and identifying new treatments for epileptic seizures. J Neurosci Methods 260:91–95. doi:10.1016/j.jneumeth.2015.07.015
123. Winter MJ et al (2008) Validation of a larval zebrafish locomotor assay for assessing the seizure liability of early-stage development drugs. J Pharmacol Toxicol Methods 57:176–187. doi:10.1016/j.vascn.2008.01.004
124. Baraban SC, Taylor MR, Castro PA, Baier H (2005) Pentylenetetrazole induced changes in zebrafish behavior, neural activity and c-fos expression. Neuroscience 131:759–768. doi:10.1016/j.neuroscience.2004.11.031
125. Dravet C, Bureau M, Oguni H, Fukuyama Y, Cokar O (2005) Severe myoclonic epilepsy in infancy: Dravet syndrome. Adv Neurol 95:71–102
126. Baraban SC, Dinday MT, Hortopan GA (2013) Drug screening in Scn1a zebrafish mutant identifies clemizole as a potential Dravet syndrome treatment. Nat Commun 4:2410. doi:10.1038/ncomms3410
127. Griffin A et al (2017) Clemizole and modulators of serotonin signalling suppress seizures in Dravet syndrome. Brain. doi:10.1093/brain/aww342
128. Bracken MB (2009) Why animal studies are often poor predictors of human reactions to exposure. J R Soc Med 102:120–122. doi:10.1258/jrsm.2008.08k033
129. Seok J et al (2013) Genomic responses in mouse models poorly mimic human inflammatory diseases. Proc Natl Acad Sci U S A 110:3507–3512. doi:10.1073/pnas.1222878110
130. Rice J (2012) Animal models: not close enough. Nature 484:S9
131. Eliceiri BP, Gonzalez AM, Baird A (2011) Zebrafish model of the blood-brain barrier: morphological and permeability studies. Methods Mol Biol 686:371–378. doi:10.1007/978-1-60761-938-3_18
132. Fleming A, Diekmann H, Goldsmith P (2013) Functional characterisation of the maturation of the blood-brain barrier in larval zebrafish. PLoS One 8:e77548. doi:10.1371/journal.pone.0077548
133. Tam SJ et al (2012) Death receptors DR6 and TROY regulate brain vascular development. Dev Cell 22:403–417. doi:10.1016/j.devcel.2011.11.018
134. Goldstone JV et al (2010) Identification and developmental expression of the full complement of Cytochrome P450 genes in Zebrafish. BMC Genomics 11:643. doi:10.1186/1471-2164-11-643
135. Verbueken E et al (2017) In vitro biotransformation of two human CYP3A probe substrates and their inhibition during early zebrafish development. Int J Mol Sci 18. doi:10.3390/ijms18010217
136. Martignoni M, Groothuis G, de Kanter R (2006) Comparison of mouse and rat cytochrome P450-mediated metabolism in liver and intestine. Drug Metab Dispos 34:1047–1054. doi:10.1124/dmd.105.009035
137. Poon KL et al (2016) Humanizing the zebrafish liver shifts drug metabolic profiles and improves pharmacokinetics of CYP3A4 substrates. Arch Toxicol. doi:10.1007/s00204-016-1789-5
138. Gootenberg DB, Turnbaugh PJ (2011) Companion animals symposium: humanized animal models of the microbiome. J Anim Sci 89:1531–1537. doi:10.2527/jas.2010-3371
139. Rawls JF, Mahowald MA, Goodman AL, Trent CM, Gordon JI (2007) In vivo imaging and genetic analysis link bacterial motility and symbiosis in the zebrafish gut. Proc Natl Acad Sci U S A 104:7622–7627. doi:10.1073/pnas.0702386104
140. Wittbrodt JN, Liebel U, Gehrig J (2014) Generation of orientation tools for automated zebrafish screening assays using desktop 3D printing. BMC Biotechnol 14:36. doi:10.1186/1472-6750-14-36
141. Yanik MF, Rohde CB, Pardo-Martin C (2011) Technologies for micromanipulating, imaging, and phenotyping small invertebrates and vertebrates.

Annu Rev Biomed Eng 13:185–217. doi:10.1146/annurev-bioeng-071910-124703
142. Pulak R (2016) Tools for automating the imaging of zebrafish larvae. Methods 96:118–126. doi:10.1016/j.ymeth.2015.11.021
143. White DT et al (2016) ARQiv-HTS, a versatile whole-organism screening platform enabling in vivo drug discovery at high-throughput rates. Nat Protoc 11:2432–2453. doi:10.1038/nprot.2016.142
144. Collins FS, Varmus H (2015) A new initiative on precision medicine. N Engl J Med 372:793–795. doi:10.1056/NEJMp1500523
145. Gahl WA et al (2016) The NIH undiagnosed diseases program and network: applications to modern medicine. Mol Genet Metab 117:393–400. doi:10.1016/j.ymgme.2016.01.007
146. Wienholds E, Schulte-Merker S, Walderich B, Plasterk RH (2002) Target-selected inactivation of the zebrafish rag1 gene. Science 297:99–102. doi:10.1126/science.1071762
147. Varshney GK et al (2013) The Zebrafish Insertion Collection (ZInC): a web based, searchable collection of zebrafish mutations generated by DNA insertion. Nucleic Acids Res 41:D861–D864. doi:10.1093/nar/gks946
148. Nasevicius A, Ekker SC (2000) Effective targeted gene 'knockdown' in zebrafish. Nat Genet 26:216–220. doi:10.1038/79951
149. Schulte-Merker S, Stainier DY (2014) Out with the old, in with the new: reassessing morpholino knockdowns in light of genome editing technology. Development 141:3103–3104. doi:10.1242/dev.112003
150. Larson MH et al (2013) CRISPR interference (CRISPRi) for sequence-specific control of gene expression. Nat Protoc 8:2180–2196. doi:10.1038/nprot.2013.132
151. Liu SJ et al (2017) CRISPRi-based genome-scale identification of functional long noncoding RNA loci in human cells. Science 355. doi:10.1126/science.aah7111
152. Weber T, Koster R (2013) Genetic tools for multicolor imaging in zebrafish larvae. Methods 62:279–291. doi:10.1016/j.ymeth.2013.07.028
153. Halpern ME et al (2008) Gal4/UAS transgenic tools and their application to zebrafish. Zebrafish 5:97–110. doi:10.1089/zeb.2008.0530
154. Mosimann C, Zon LI (2011) Advanced zebrafish transgenesis with Tol2 and application for Cre/lox recombination experiments. Methods Cell Biol 104:173–194. doi:10.1016/B978-0-12-374814-0.00010-0
155. Pan YA et al (2013) Zebrabow: multispectral cell labeling for cell tracing and lineage analysis in zebrafish. Development 140:2835–2846. doi:10.1242/dev.094631
156. Henninger J et al (2017) Clonal fate mapping quantifies the number of haematopoietic stem cells that arise during development. Nat Cell Biol 19:17–27. doi:10.1038/ncb3444
157. Moro E et al (2013) Generation and application of signaling pathway reporter lines in zebrafish. Mol Gen Genomics 288:231–242. doi:10.1007/s00438-013-0750-z
158. Shimozono S, Iimura T, Kitaguchi T, Higashijima S, Miyawaki A (2013) Visualization of an endogenous retinoic acid gradient across embryonic development. Nature 496:363–366. doi:10.1038/nature12037
159. Thisse B, Thisse C (2014) In situ hybridization on whole-mount zebrafish embryos and young larvae. Methods Mol Biol 1211:53–67. doi:10.1007/978-1-4939-1459-3_5
160. Choi HM et al (2016) Mapping a multiplexed zoo of mRNA expression. Development 143:3632–3637. doi:10.1242/dev.140137
161. Dang M, Henderson RE, Garraway LA, Zon LI (2016) Long-term drug administration in the adult zebrafish using oral gavage for cancer preclinical studies. Dis Model Mech 9:811–820. doi:10.1242/dmm.024166
162. Olt J, Allen CE, Marcotti W (2016) In vivo physiological recording from the lateral line of juvenile zebrafish. J Physiol 594:5427–5438. doi:10.1113/JP271794
163. Keller PJ (2013) In vivo imaging of zebrafish embryogenesis. Methods 62:268–278. doi:10.1016/j.ymeth.2013.03.015
164. Burgess HA, Granato M (2007) Sensorimotor gating in larval zebrafish. J Neurosci 27:4984–4994. doi:10.1523/JNEUROSCI.0615-07.2007
165. Weber M, Huisken J (2015) In vivo imaging of cardiac development and function in zebrafish using light sheet microscopy. Swiss Med Wkly 145:w14227. doi:10.4414/smw.2015.14227
166. Muto A, Kawakami K (2011) Imaging functional neural circuits in zebrafish with a new GCaMP and the Gal4FF-UAS system. Commun Integr Biol 4:566–568. doi:10.4161/cib.4.5.15848
167. Prajsnar TK, Cunliffe VT, Foster SJ, Renshaw SA (2008) A novel vertebrate model of *Staphylococcus aureus* infection reveals phagocyte-dependent resistance of zebrafish to non-host specialized pathogens. Cell Microbiol 10:2312–2325. doi:10.1111/j.1462-5822.2008.01213.x
168. Bojarczuk A et al (2016) *Cryptococcus neoformans* intracellular proliferation and capsule size determines early macrophage control of infection. Sci Report 6:21489. doi:10.1038/srep21489
169. Harvey SA et al (2013) Identification of the zebrafish maternal and paternal transcriptomes. Development 140:2703–2710. doi:10.1242/dev.095091
170. Wardle FC, Muller F (2014) Fish genomics: casting the net wide. Brief Funct Genomics 13:79–81. doi:10.1093/bfgp/elt055

11 Personalized Medicine and Resurrected Hopes for the Management of Alzheimer's Disease: A Modular Approach Based on GSK-3β Inhibitors

Reem K. Arafa and Nehal H. Elghazawy

Abstract

Alzheimer's disease (AD) is one of the most common neurological disorders with vast reaching worldwide prevalence. Research attempts to decipher what's happening to the human mind have shown that pathogenesis of AD is associated with misfolded protein intermediates displaying tertiary structure conformational changes eventually leading to forming large polymers of unwanted aggregates. The two hallmarks of AD pathological protein aggregates are extraneuronal β-amyloid (Aβ) based senile plaques and intraneuronal neurofibrillary tangles (NFTs). As such, AD is categorized as a protein misfolding neurodegenerative disease (PMND). Therapeutic interventions interfering with the formation of these protein aggregates have been widely explored as potential pathways for thwarting AD progression. One such tactic is modulating the function of enzymes involved in the metabolic pathways leading to formation of these misfolded protein aggregates. Much evidence has shown that glycogen synthase kinase-3β (GSK-3β) plays a key role in hyperphosphorylation of tau protein leading eventually to its aggregation to form NFTs. Data presented hereby will display a plethora of information as to how to interfere with progression of AD through the route of GSK-3β activity control.

Keywords

Alzheimer's disease • GSK-3β inhibitors • Extraneuronal senile plaques • Intraneuronal neurofibrillary tangles • Protein misfolding neurodegenerative disease • Tau-hyperphosphorylation

R.K. Arafa (✉) • N.H. Elghazawy
Zewail City of Science and Technology,
Cairo 12588, Egypt
e-mail: rkhidr@zewailcity.edu.eg

S. El-Khamisy (ed.), *Personalised Medicine*, Advances in Experimental Medicine and Biology 1007,
DOI 10.1007/978-3-319-60733-7_11

11.1 Introduction

Alzheimer's disease (AD) is the most common form of dementia. It is a neurodegenerative disorder defined by progressive memory loss and cognitive impairment. It was discovered in 1906 by Alois Alzheimer, the German neuropathologist and clinician, after the clinicopathological study of a 51-year-old woman who presented a dementia syndrome [1].

AD is a severely debilitating disease which affects more than 35 million patients worldwide [2, 3]. An estimated 5.3 million Americans of all ages have Alzheimer's disease in 2015, where almost 5.1 million people are age 65 and older, and approximately 200,000 individuals are under age 65 (younger-onset Alzheimer's [4]. A review of many studies concluded that older African-Americans are about twice as likely to have Alzheimer's and other dementias as older whites [5, 6] and Hispanics are about one and one-half times as likely to have Alzheimer's and other dementias as older whites [6, 7]. Moreover, the WHO 2012 Report "Dementia: a public health priority" estimates that the encounter of dementia worldwide is around 35.6 million people (Fig. 11.1) [8]. As the world population ages, the frequency is expected to double by 2030 and triple by 2050 [9, 10].

Earlier approaches towards the therapeutic management of AD were based on the "one-size-fits-all-concept" regardless of the fact that some patients are less likely than others to respond to a particular therapeutic agent by virtue of their individual's specific genetic, biomarker, phenotypic and psychosocial makeup. In contrast, with the introduction of the concept of precision medicine, also named "personalized or individualized medicine", as a rapidly advancing field in medical clinical and research settings, new horizons for optimizing accuracy of disease diagnosis and precision of prevention and/or treatment together with minimizing side effects are being explored. The measurement of molecular, environmental, and behavioral factors contributing to a specific disease improves the understanding of disease onset and progression as well as response to treatment. In addition, it allows a more accurate

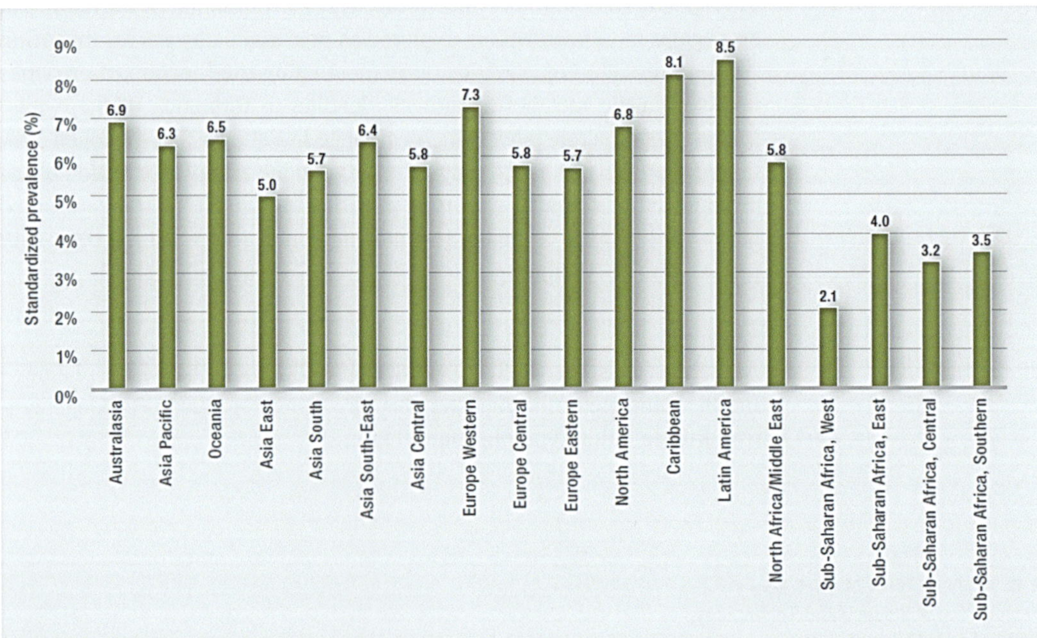

Fig. 11.1 Estimated prevalence of dementia for persons aged 60 and over, standardized to Western Europe population, by Global Burden of Disease region [8]

diagnosis and more effective disease prevention and treatment strategies specifically personalized to the individual.

11.2 Genetic and Molecular Considerations in AD

Many scientific hypotheses have been explored in an attempt to decrypt the different histopathological lesions found in the brain of AD patients. The first one is the cholinergic hypothesis that considers the disease as a consequence of a deficit in the neurotransmitter acetylcholine [11] making the acetylcholinesterase inhibitors drugs of choice in AD patients [12].

The two other hypotheses are based on the biochemical notion of AD being a protein misfolding neurodegenerative disease (PMND) [13] where accumulation of two hallmark pathological protein aggregates, extraneuronal senile plaques and intraneuronal neurofibrillary tangles (NFTs), is associated with the progression thereof (Fig. 11.2) [14].

The extraneuronal senile plaques are composed of the poorly-soluble β-amyloid (Aβ) peptide polymers that arise from the cleavage of transmembrane amyloid precursor protein (APP) by two proteases known as β and ɣ secretases [16, 17]. On the other hand, the intraneuronal NFTs are polymers generated by the aggregation of hyperphosphorylated tau proteins [18, 19].

As per the plaques, three heritable mutations of the APP, presenilin-1 (PS-1) and presenilin-2 (PS-2) genes were found to affect APP processing and result in the increased Aβ protein formation [3]. These three mutations were linked to early-onset AD and are said to account for almost 5% of observed AD cases. On the molecular level, Aβ monomers are soluble with structural short regions of beta sheets and polyproline II helices. Yet, they undergo a dramatic conformational alteration to form a beta sheet-rich tertiary structure that aggregates to form amyloid fibrils at high concentration. These fibrils aggregate and deposit densely outside neurons giving rise to what is called senile plaques [20–22]. With their deposition into plaques, these aggregated forms of Aβ peptide have been shown to be neurotoxic contributing to cellular death and neuronal loss through the apoptosis seen in AD [23–25].

Regarding the second hallmark, the tau protein which was found to be associated with late-onset AD, it is a multifunctional microtubule-associated protein that stabilizes the neuronal cytoskeleton. In a normal brain, the equilibrium between phosphorylations and dephosphorylations of tau pro-

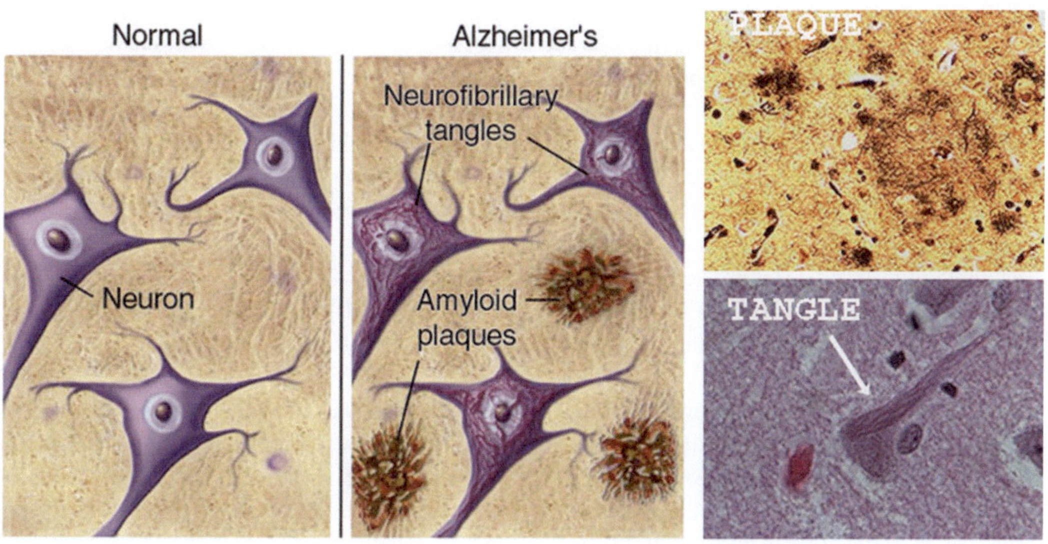

Fig. 11.2 Hallmarks of Alzheimer's disease: neurofibrillary tangles and amyloid plaques [15]

tein modulates the stability of the cytoskeleton. Owing to the importance of phosphorylation in cellular and physiological processes, it is not surprising that abnormal phosphorylation turns out to be a cause or consequence of numerous human diseases such as cancers, diabetes, and AD [26]. Tau hyperphosphorylation is considered one of the earliest modifications found in Alzheimer's brains and is believed to first develop in a key staging area for memory coordination in the brain called the entorhinal cortex. Hyperphosphorylated tau accumulates as paired helical filaments [27] that in turn aggregate into masses inside nerve cell bodies known as neurofibrillary tangles thus displaying the second form of protein misfolding abnormalities associated with AD. Tau hyperphosphorylation is affected by the action of different protein kinase and phosphatase systems including proline-directed kinases such as mitogen-activated protein kinase 1 (MAPK1), glycogen synthase kinase 3 (GSK-3) and cyclin dependent kinase 5 (Cdk5), as well as non-proline-directed enzymes such as casein kinase1, protein kinase A, and MAP/microtubule affinity-regulating kinase 1 (MARK1) [28–30]. Intensive research on the physiology and pathology of tau protein led to the discovery that the two kinases; cyclin dependent kinase 5 (Cdk-5) and glycogen synthase kinase-3*β* (GSK-3*β*) are responsible for the tau posttranslational aberrant modifications [12, 31].

First, Cdk5 is activated by factors like p35 and p39, and is involved in tau phosphorylations as related to normal neurogenesis. Pathological change in Cdk5 regulatory patterns were found to be associated with neuronal death of hippocampal neurons and tau hyperphosphorylation. However, pretreatment of cells with Cdk5 specific inhibitors such as butyrolactone I or by using anti-sense probes for Cdk5 was shown to protect cells against neuronal death and tau phosphorylation [31].

On the other hand, GSK-3 is a proline-directed serine-threonine kinase first identified in the late 1970s as an enzyme that phosphorylates glycogen synthase in the glycogen synthesis pathway. It plays an important role in many vital processes such as cellular signaling pathways, metabolic control, embryogenesis, cell death and oncogenesis [32]. Unlike other protein kinases, GSK-3 is normally constitutively active in all cells, and can be regulated through inhibition [33]. GSK-3 has two distinctive isoforms GSK-3*α* and GSK-3*β*, however it has been suggested that GSK-3*β* plays various functions in neurogenesis, differentiation during nervous system development [34–37] and axon development [38]. Thus, GSK-3*β* is a potential target in several neurological diseases in which its activity is increased such as in AD [39–41]. Moreover, evidence showed that progression of AD is mainly due to accumulation of a complexes of various molecules and gene products, including APP, A*β* peptide, presenilins, apo E4, tau, Wnt and Notch [42, 43] and products of oxidative stress [44, 45], as well as mediators of apoptosis (Fig. 11.3) [46].

Furthermore, a direct relation has been obtained between the GSK-3*β* and tau phosphorylation, since overexpression of GSK-3*β* in transgenic mice has been reported to increase tau hyperphosphorylation and to cause some behavioral deficits [47, 48]. GSK-3*β*, has also been shown to be associated with NFTs as co-expression of p25 and mutant human tau in mice led to the formation of NFTs with resulting neurodegeneration. Interestingly, GSK-3*β* has been implicated in facilitating (APP) processing resulting in upregulation of the synthesis and aggregation of Aβ, with inhibition of GSK-3*β* reported to decrease Aβ level [28, 49–51].

Involvement of GSk-3*β* in many of the interactions with AD related factors made this biomolecule a promising therapeutic target for AD management, which is the main focus of this review [25].

11.3 Insights into the Structure of GSK-3*β*

Structural analysis demonstrated that GSK-3*β* is a 47 kD cytosolic protein. The enzyme adopts the typical two-domain kinase fold with a β-strand domain (residues 25–138) at the N-terminal end and an α-helical domain at the C-terminal end

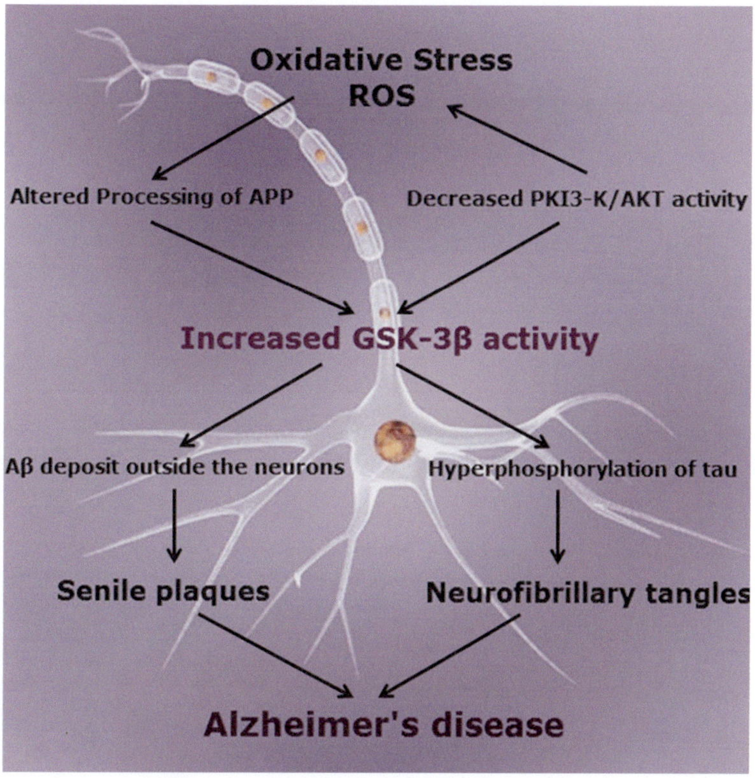

Fig. 11.3 Role of GSK-3*β* in the pathogenesis of AD

(residues 139–343) (Fig. 11.4). For optimal positioning of the catalytic groups involved in the ɣ-phosphate transfer, these two domains must exhibit certain alignment to ensure optimal configuration of the substrate-binding site and catalytic site of the kinase [52, 53]. The ATP-binding site is at the interface of the α-helical and β-strand domains and is bordered by the glycine-rich loop and the hinge. At the ATP binding site lie two conserved lysine residues, Lys85/86, that are important for binding ATP and stabilizing the ɣ-phosphate during transfer to the substrate [52, 54–57]. The activation loop (residues 200–226) runs along the surface of the substrate binding groove [52]. It contains a conserved tyrosine residue, Tyr216, which, when phosphorylated, is believed to increase GSK-3*β* activity approximately 200-fold [58]. However, in case of absence of Tyr216 phosphorylation, the activation loop is still able to achieve a conformation that strongly resembles the phosphorylated activation loop structure [52, 53, 55, 59, 60]. The most distal N- and C-terminal regions of GSK-3*β* are structurally disordered and are believed to be very flexible [52, 53, 56].

Moreover, outside the catalytic core, distinct amino acids in the C-terminal (approximate amino acids 344–388) are known for having a unique structure consisting of short helices and loops that pack against the large core helical domain [52, 53, 55, 61]. The β-strand domain consists of seven, antiparallel β-strands: strands 2–6 form a β-barrel that is interrupted between strand 4 and 5 by a short helix (residue 96–102) that packs against the β-barrel. This helix is conserved in all kinases, and two of its residues play key roles in the catalytic activity of the enzyme [52].

GSK-3*β* has a particular and unique requirement for two divalent magnesium ions allowing magnesium to bind to ATP for coordinating ɣ-phosphate transfer (Fig. 11.4) [62].

The key amino acids involved in functioning of GSK-3*β* are Arg96 that is involved in the alignment of the two domains and Glu97 which is positioned in the active site and forms a salt

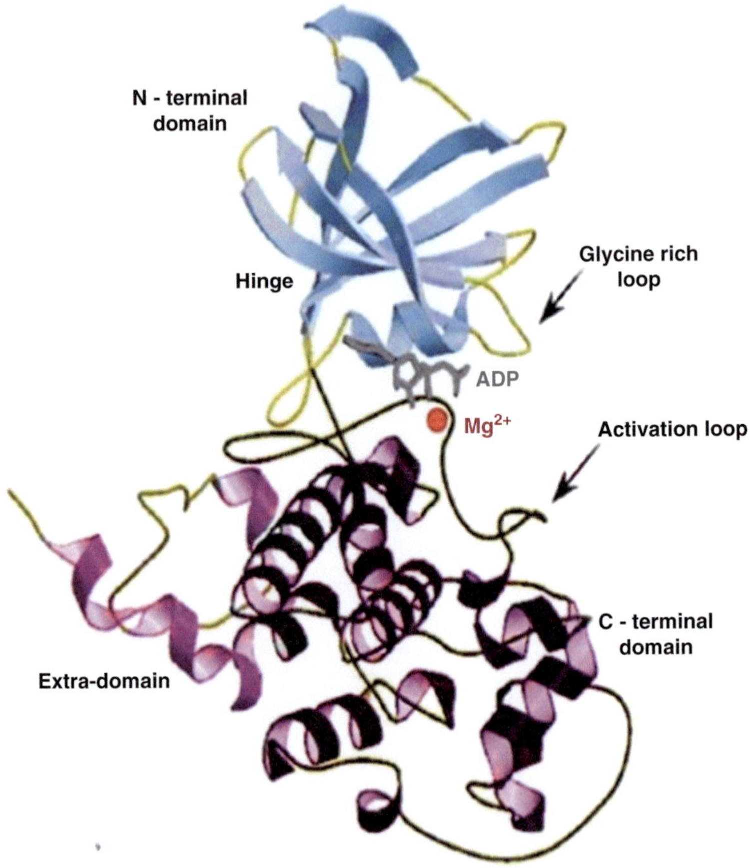

Fig. 11.4 Structure of GSK-3*β* complexed with an ADP molecule [55]

bridge with Lys85, being considered a key residue in catalysis. Finally, GSK-3*β* has two phosphorylation sites that influence the catalytic activity of the protein, Ser9 which is the phosphorylation site for AKT, and whose phosphorylation inactivates GSK-3*β* and Tyr216, located in the activation loop, where phosphorylation of which increases the catalytic activity of the enzyme [52].

11.4 GSK-3*β* Regulation and Inhibition

For GSK-3*β* to be inhibited, phosphorylation at the specific serine residue Ser9 occurs, allowing the N-terminus of the GSK molecule to bind within its own active-site-binding pocket [63].

GSK-3*β* can also be regulated by the Wnt signaling pathway. In the absence of Wnt, GSK-3*β* activity is enhanced due to the formation of a complex with adenomatosis polyposis coli (APC) protein, Axin and β-catenin (Fig. 11.5). This complex in turn phosphorylates the β-catenin to be recognized by the ubiquitin ligase βTrCP, where it gets ubiquinated leading to its degradation [64, 65]. However, in case of Wnt incorporation, it binds both Frizzled and LRP5/6 receptors to initiate GRK5/6-mediated LRP phosphorylation as well as dishevelled/β-arrestin-mediated Frizzled incorporation. Consequently, dishevelled protein (DVL) is recruited, where its membrane translocation and phosphorylation leads to dissociation of β-catenin from the axin/APC/GSK3β complex, which in turn inhibits GSK-3*β* through formation of a complex with GSK-3*β*-binding proteins (GBPs) [66] or through activation of protein kinase C (PKC) [67] and stabilization of β-catenin [25]. Hence, β-catenin phosphorylation is inhibited and it accumulates in the cytosol. The

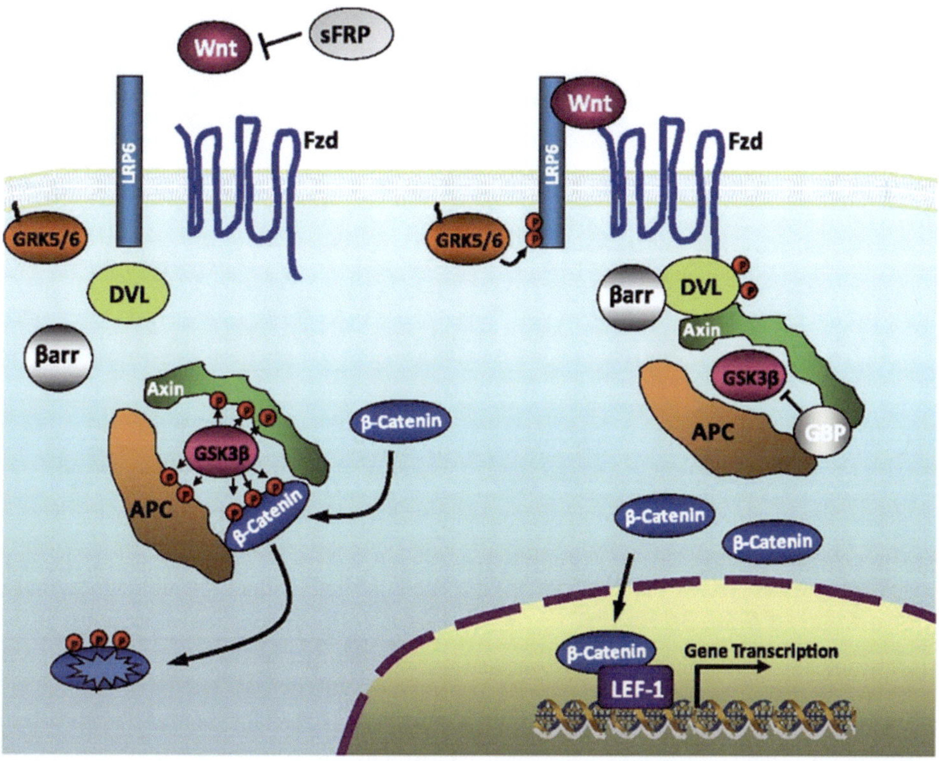

Fig. 11.5 Wnt signaling regulation of GSK-3*β*. Abbreviations: *Fzd* Frizzled, *GBP* GSK3*β* binding proteins, *DVL* Dishevelled, *βarr* β-arrestin, *GRK* G protein-coupled receptor kinase [68]

accumulated cytosolic β-catenin translocates into the nucleus to bind to LEF/TCFs co-transcription factors, which results in the Wnt-responsive gene transcription (Fig. 11.5) [68].

The phosphatidylinositol 3-kinase (PI3K)/Akt (also called protein kinase B) signaling pathway was also identified as an important mechanism supporting cellular proliferation and survival. Activated Akt is able to phosphorylate and modulate the activity of multiple proteins, which influences several cellular functions such as glycogen synthesis, protein synthesis, gene expression, and the proliferation and survival of cells [69–71]. One of the targets of Akt is GSK-3*β*, where it phosphorylates Ser9 of the GSK-3*β* [63]. This regulatory action of Akt has been further targeted by certain compounds that act as GSK-3*β* inhibitors [72]. Potent selective small molecule GSK-3*β* inhibitors have been shown to protect primary neurons from death induced by reduced PI-3k activity [73].

However, for designing GSK-3*β* inhibitors, the binding sites present were extensively explored. Examining almost 25 different GSK-3 structures showed that GSK-3 has seven different pockets. The first three cavities were found to be the known binding sites of GSK-3, where the ATP, the substrate, and the peptides axin/fratide bind to this protein. Also, four new druggable cavities on GSK-3 in which different ligands could interact have also been discovered. One of them is located on the C-terminal lobe of the kinase and it is very exposed to solvent, another is located in the hinge region between the C- and N-terminal lobes, and finally, two of them are situated on the N-lobe of GSK-3 (Fig. 11.6) [74].

Most kinase inhibitors act by competition with either ATP or the metal-binding sites that are involved directly in the catalytic process. However, small molecular weight compounds might regulate GSK-3*β* activity by inhibiting the protein-protein interactions that are necessary for substrate binding by modulating the Tyr216 activation sites and the Ser9 inhibition sites, and by interfering with the intracellular targeting domain of GSK-3*β* [75].

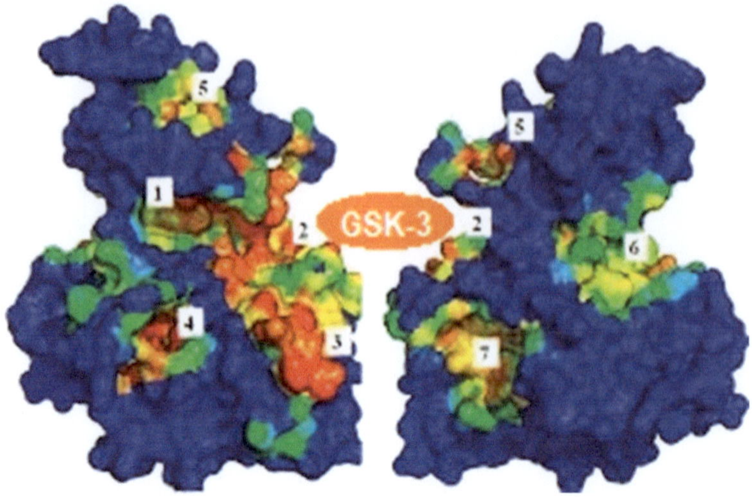

Fig. 11.6 Potential sites for inhibition of GSK-3. Legend of the binding sites: *1* ATP, *2* substrate, *3* axin/fratide, *4–7* new druggable cavities [74]

11.5 Therapeutic Interventions Related to GSK-3*β* Based on Small-Molecule Inhibitors

Since GSK-3*β* is embedded in multi-protein complexes, various small molecules are designed to target the interaction sites between GSK-3*β* and other proteins. Although this process is a major challenge in drug discovery, it has attracted more attention following recent successes and thereby three main classes of GSK-3*β* inhibitors have been introduced; metal cations, ATP competitive and non-ATP competitive. Structure-based approaches are used to provide the insights into the key interactions shown by selective and nonselective ATP-competitive GSK-3*β* inhibitors. Several other computational approaches have also been employed for the design and development of the GSK-3*β* inhibitors like Quantitative Structure Activity Relationship (QSAR) studies, pharmacophore map generation and molecular field approaches [73, 76, 77].

11.5.1 Metal Cations

Lithium was the first drug to be used as GSK-3*β* inhibitor even before evolution of the GSK3 hypothesis. It has been used for more than 50 years in treatment of neurological diseases. It acts via the GSK-3*β* by two distinct and interrelated mechanisms. First, the direct inhibition, where lithium competes with magnesium (essential for GSK-3*β* constitutive activity) at the cationic binding site, dislocating Mg^{2+} from the enzyme catalytic core and inhibiting the enzyme activity. This mechanism is attributed to the similarities in properties between lithium and magnesium, allowing lithium to bind to and inhibit magnesium dependent substrates [78–81].

The Second is the indirect inhibition which involves the lithium induced activation of protein kinase C *via* Akt. This takes place usually in response to insulin or insulin growth factors, leading to phosphorylation of the Ser9 residue of the regulatory N terminal domain leading to conformational changes and inactivation of GSK-3*β* (Fig. 11.7) [82–84].

Another putative mechanism of action of lithium is its ability to inhibit IMP and inositol polyphosphate 1-phosphatase activity by noncompetitive dislocation of Mg^{2+} from enzyme's catalytic sites. Consequently, significant reduction of inositol triphosphate formation is noticed, which leads to modulation of many intracellular pathways relevant to neuropsychiatric disorders.

Finally, lithium can stimulate gene expression as well as the release of neurotrophic factors e.g.: brain-derived neurotrophic factor (BDNF) and vascular endothelial growth factor [85, 86] reducing the neurotrophic factors that play an important role in the physiopathology of AD [87].

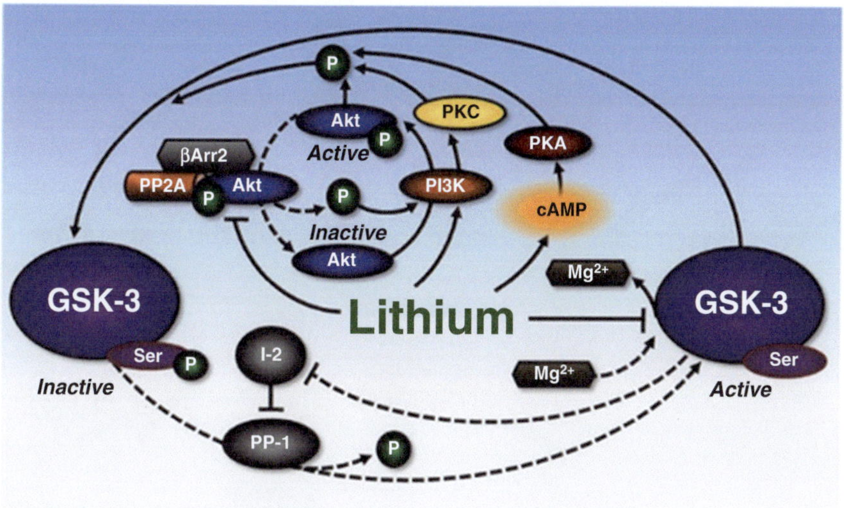

Fig. 11.7 Inhibitory regulation of GSK-3*β* by lithium. *Lines* with *solid arrows* represent stimulatory connections; *lines* with flattened ends represent inhibitory connections. *Dashed lines* represent pathways with reduced activity as a result of lithium treatment. *I-2* inhibitor-2, *PP-1* protein phosphatase-l [76]

The therapeutic range of lithium is 0.5–1.5 mM, and its IC_{50} toward GSK-3*β* is 1–2 mM [88]. Upon testing lithium's effect against Alzheimer's and related neurodegenerative models, studies demonstrated that lithium blocks amyloid APP deposits and reduces A*β* secretion in cells and transgenic mice overexpressing APP [49, 51, 89]. Treatment with lithium also prevented A*β* neurotoxicity in rat brain [90] and reduced tauopathy in transgenic mice overexpressing human mutant tau [91–93].

11.5.2 ATP-Competitive GSK-3*β* Inhibitors

For inhibitors to act by ATP-competitive inhibition, specific interactions with the key amino acids in the ATP-binding site must be formed. These interactions include hydrogen bonds with the backbone atoms of Asp133 and Val135. Pro136 seems to strengthen the interaction of the inhibitor with the backbone. For enhanced activity and selectivity, the amino acids Lys85, Glu97, and Asp200 are essential. Lys85 was observed to form two simultaneous salt bridges with Glu97 and Asp200 (Fig. 11.8) [94].

11.5.2.1 Thiazoles

N-(4-methoxybenzyl)-N-(5-nitro-1,3-thiazol-2-yl)urea also known as AR-A014418 (Compound **1**, Table 11.1) is considered the most important thiazole derivative. Uniqueness of this compound arises from the fact that, unlike other most reported GSK-3*β* inhibitors, it is not a powerful Cdk inhibitor. Moreover, its specificity against GSK-3*β* was demonstrated when tested and compared to 26 different kinases. Co-crystals of AR-A014418 and GSK-3*β* revealed that it resides at the ATP pocket with interactions along the hinge/linker region of the GSK-3*β* through three hydrogen bond interactions to the main chain atoms of the protein. The nitro, group of the inhibitor occupies the inner part of the ATP pocket; the closest distance between the nitro O to the selectivity residue Leu-132 is only 3.03 Å. The other end group from the inhibitor, the phenyl ring, takes an orientation that is ~108° out of the plane of the core inhibitor, such that it fits in π-cationic stacking interaction to the guanidine group of Arg-141 (3.8 Å) (Fig. 11.9). Based on its capacity as a GSK-3*β* inhibitor, AR-A014418 showed inhibition of tau phosphorylation in cells overexpressing tau protein. The importance of AR-A014418 as a specific GSK-3*β* inhibitor

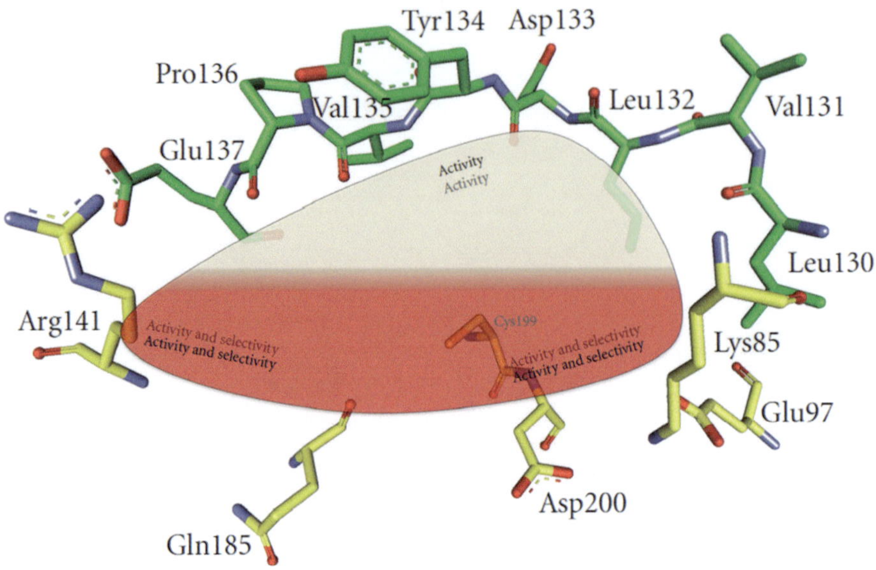

Fig. 11.8 Schematic view of the ATP binding pocket of GSK-3β; important areas for activity and selectivity are denoted by PDB 1I09 code [52]

arises from its ability to interfere with both tau phosphorylation and β-amyloid-induced toxicity. AR-A014418 inhibits recombinant human GSK-3β with an IC_{50} value of 104 ± 27 nM. Moreover, it inhibits tau phosphorylation in the transfected cells in a dose-dependent fashion exhibiting an IC_{50} of 2.7 μM, and it showed to be a more potent inhibitor when compared with lithium chloride (IC_{50} = 1.5 mM). Finally, AR-A014418 protects neuroblastoma N2A cells (a neuronal-like phenotype) in culture from death induced by reduced PI3K pathway activity in a dose-dependent manner where its half-maximal effect of protection against N2A cell death is at a concentration of 0.5 μM, and the maximal effect at 50 μM [95].

11.5.2.2 Indirubins

This is a family of bis-indoles extracted from various natural sources such as indigo-producing plants, several species of Gastropod mollusks and various wild-type or recombinant bacteria. Indirubins (Compound **2**, Table 11.1) have been known for clear antiproliferative effects due to their ability to inhibit Cdk's and GSK-3 [26]. Structure-activity relationship (SAR) studies suggested that indirubins bind to GSK-3β's ATP binding pocket *via* hydrogen bonds with amino acids, Arg, Asn, Lys, Asp, Cys present in its binding pocket. These interactions assure the strong binding of indirubins and thus their effectiveness to revert the GSK-3β's function and stop the hyperphosphorylation of the microtubule and prevent NFT formation in manifestations of AD [96].

A variety of indirubins were identified as powerful inhibitors of GSK-3β while others were inactive [97]. Indirubins' analogues such as indiribin-3′-oxime (Compound **3**, Table 11.1) is known to possess better pharmacological effect and less toxicity than other indirubins. The crystal structure of indirubin-3′-oxime with GSK-3β shows that the binding pocket is divided into three parts [56]. The pocket which encloses the inhibitor between Ile62, Val70, and Ala83 on the top and Leu188 on the bottom and the hinge segment which is formed using the chain of Leu132-Asp133-Tyr134-Val135-Pro136. Interactions with this segment encompass three hydrogen bonds between the amino acids Asp133 and Val135 of the protein and indirubin-3′-oxime are formed as follows: The N1 atom of the inhibitor forms a hydrogen bond with the carbonyl oxygen of Asp133. The backbone nitrogen and carbonyl oxygen of Val135 are involved to form

Table 11.1 ATP competitive *GSK-3β* inhibitors

Compound number, name	Chemical structure
1. AR-A014418	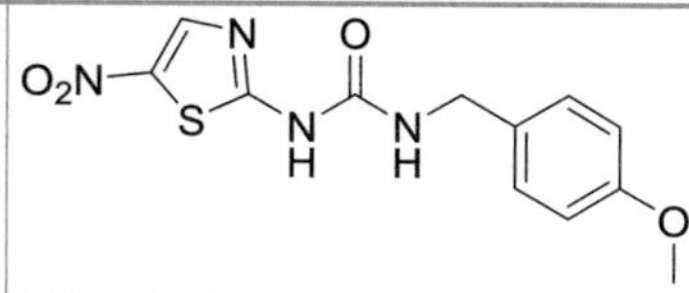
2. Indirubins general structure	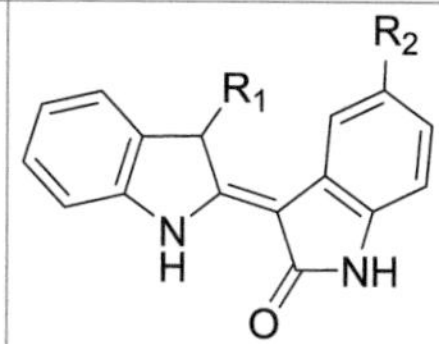
3. Indirubin-3-monoxime	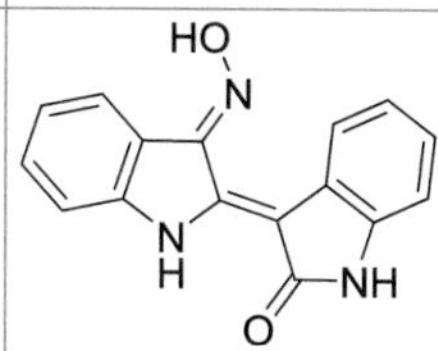
4. 6-Bromoindirubin-3′-oxime	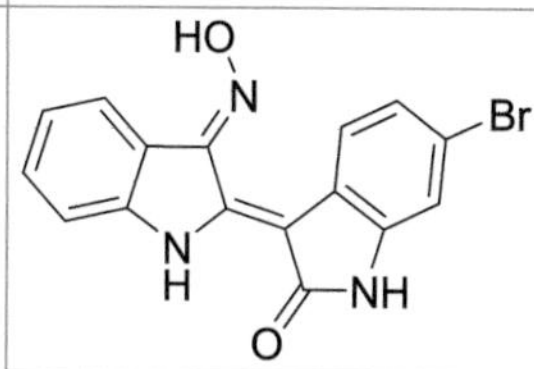
5. 6-BIDECO	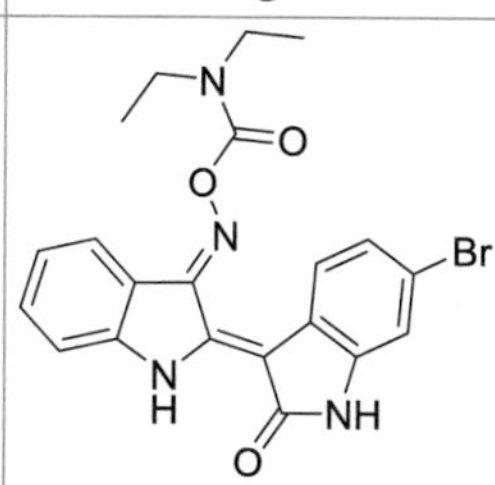
6. 6-BIMYEO	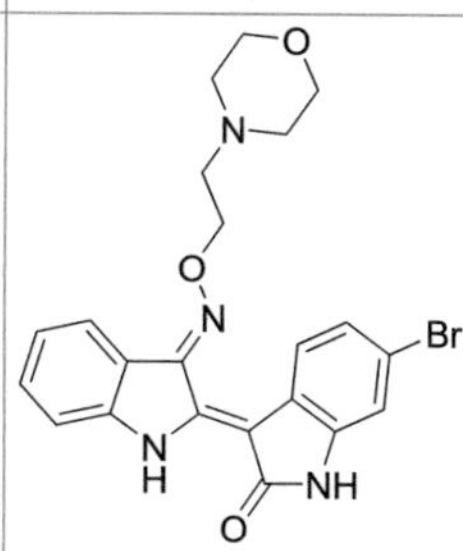
7. Ruboxistaurin	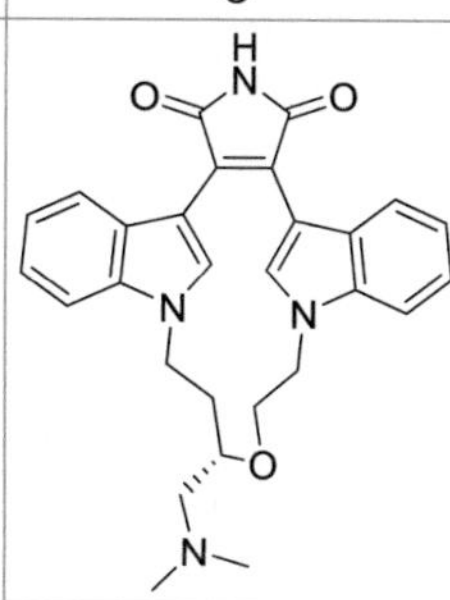

(continued)

Table 11.1 (continued)

Compound number, name	Chemical structure
8. GF 109203X	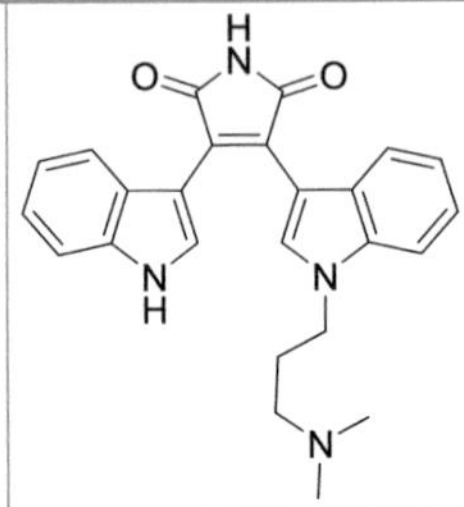
9. Ro 31-8820	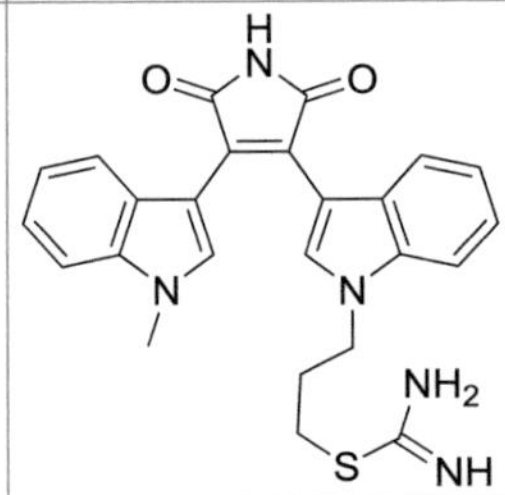
10. Staurosporine	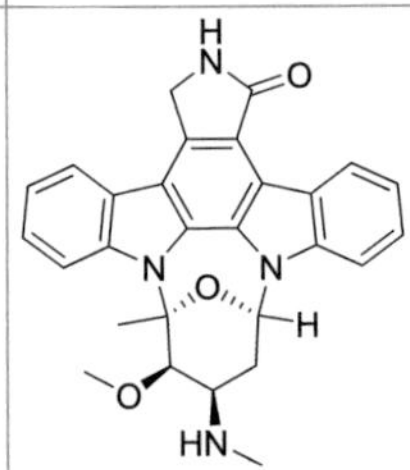
11. Synthesized maleimide structure	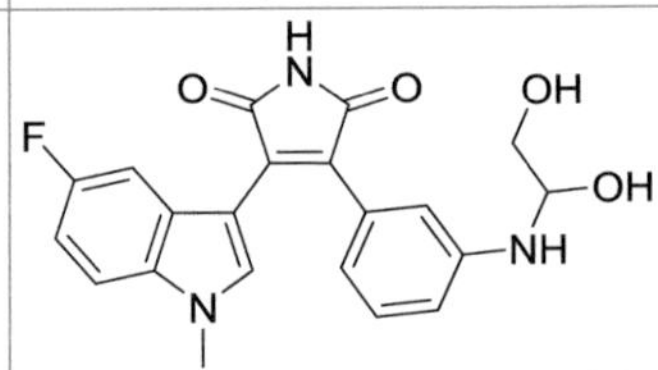
12. SB-216763	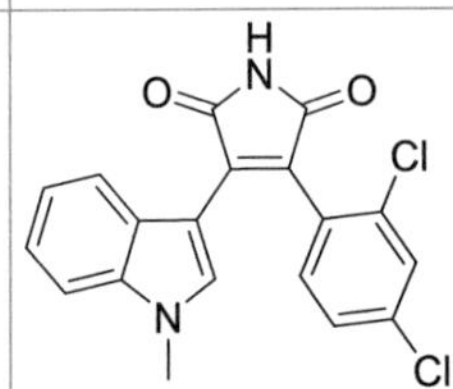
13. SB- 415286	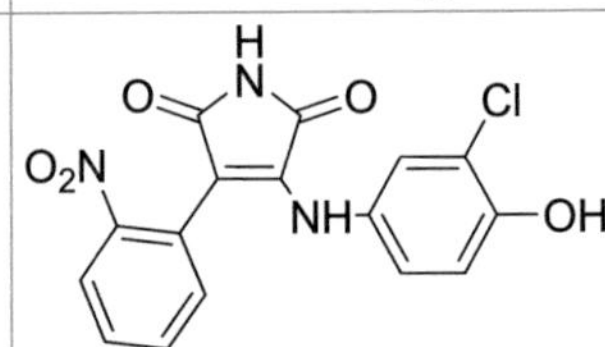
14. Paullone	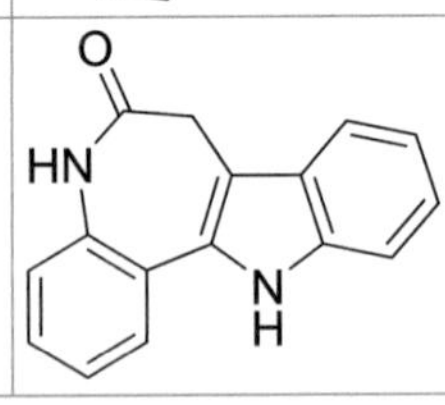

(continued)

Table 11.1 (continued)

Compound number, name	Chemical structure
15. Alsterpaullone	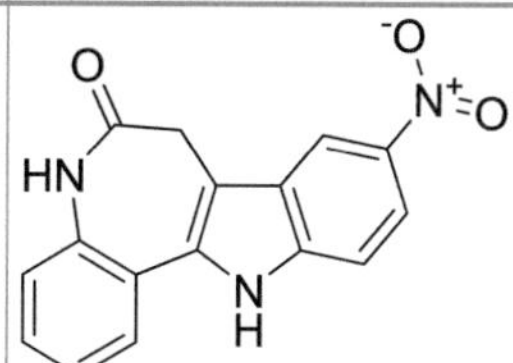
16. Kenpaullone	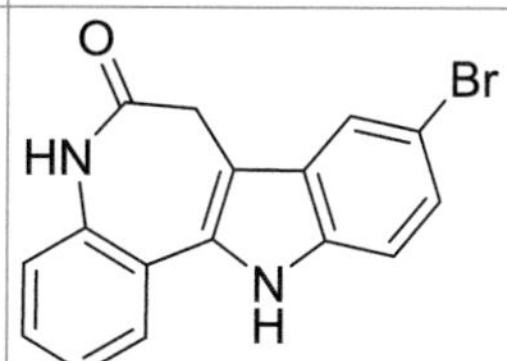
17. Aloisines prototype structure	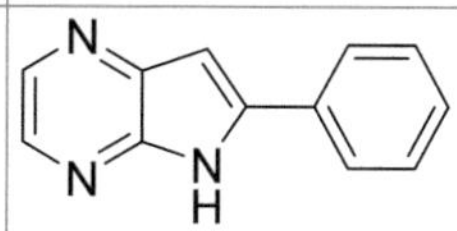
18. Aloisine A	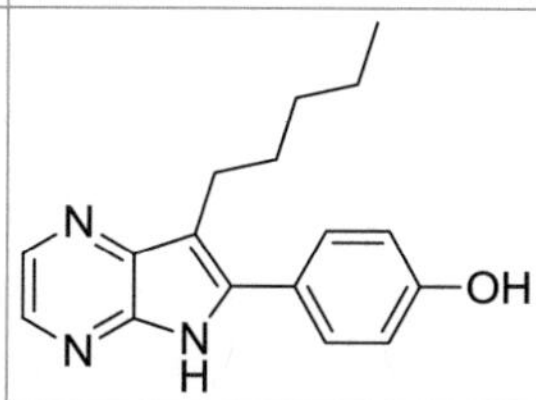
19. Aloisine B	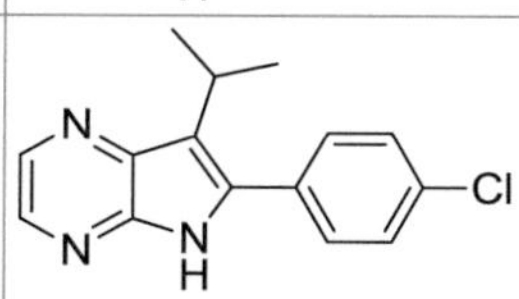
20. Oxadiazole derivative	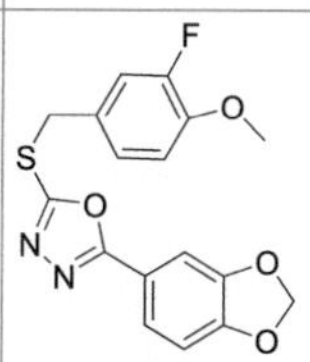
21. Oxadiazole derivative	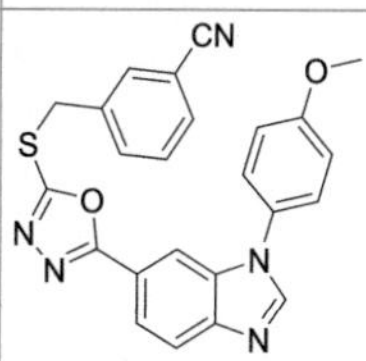
22. Hymenialdisine	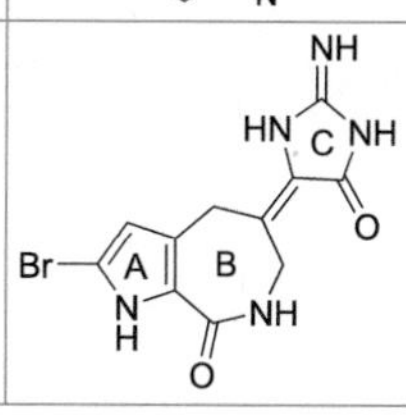

(continued)

Table 11.1 (continued)

Compound number, name	Chemical structure
23. Dibromocantharelline	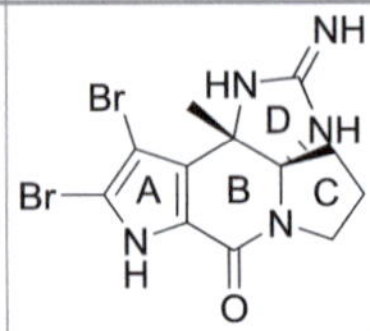
24. AZD 1080	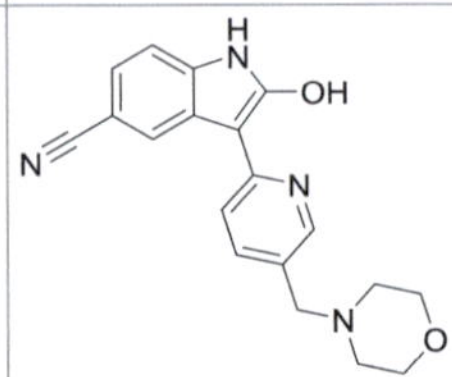
25. Meridianin derivative	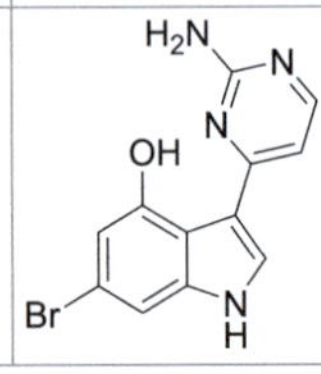

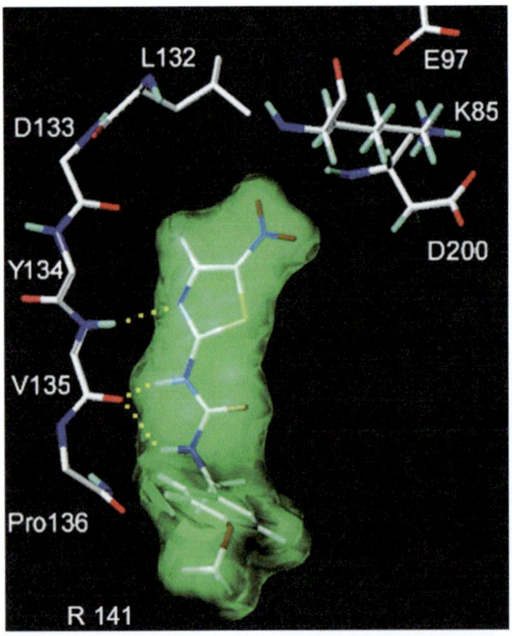

Fig. 11.9 Binding of AR-A014418 to GSK-3*β*. Hydrogen bonds between the inhibitor and the protein molecule are shown as *yellow dotted lines* [95]

the other two hydrogen bonds with O2 and N1 of the inhibitor, respectively. Finally, Arg141 shields the edge of the inhibitor's aromatic ring from the bulk solvent by orienting its side-chain (Fig. 11.10) [56].

One indirubin, 6-BIO (6-bromoindirubin-3′-oxime) (Compound **4**, Table 11.1), widely used to investigate the physiological role of GSK-3*β*, has been considered as a lead compound for designing indirubins with better selectivity towards GSK-3*β* and optimum solubility. Consequently, the two recently developed indirubin derivatives 6-BIDECO (6-bromoindirubin-3-[O-(*N,N*-diethylcarbamyl)oxime) (Compound **5**, Table 11.1) and 6-BIMYEO (6-bromoindirubin-3-[O-(2-morpholin-1-ylethyl)oxime) (Compound **6**, Table 11.1), have shown higher selectivity toward GSK-3*β* activities and less cytotoxicity compared with classical GSK-3*β* inhibitors [98]. These compounds retain the pharmacophoric features of indirubins; the lactam nitrogen, the carbonyl and the heterocyclic nitrogen, which form key hydrogen bonds with the active site, and the 6-bromo group, which is a selectivity determinant for GSK-3*β* [99, 100].

11.5.2.3 Maleimides

Bisindolylmaleimides represent a class of potent GSK-3*β* inhibitors such as Ruboxistaurin

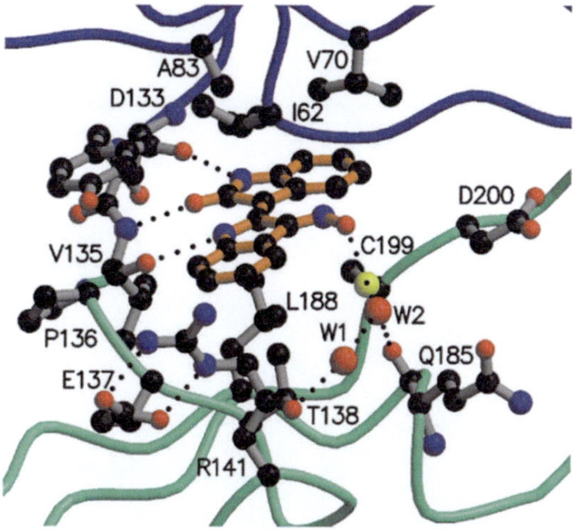

Fig. 11.10 Diagram showing the binding of indirubin-3-monoxime to GSK-3*β*. Inhibitor molecule is shown in tan; water molecules and Mg^{2+} are shown in *red* and *yellow*, respectively. The N- and C-terminal domains are in *blue* and *green*, respectively [56]

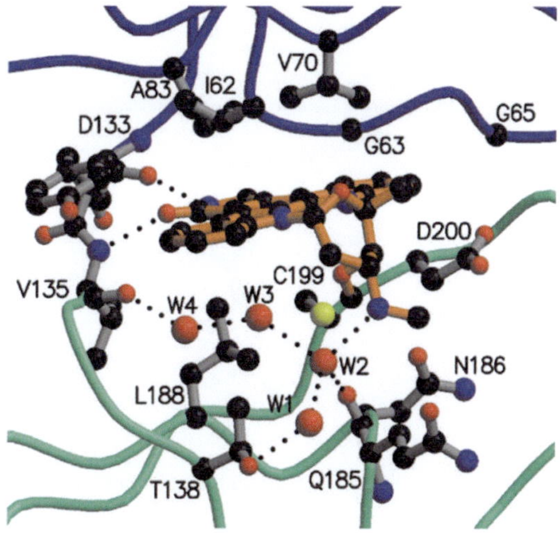

Fig. 11.11 Binding of staurosporine to GSK-3*β* [56]

(Compound **7**, Table 11.1), GF 109203X (Compound **8**, Table 11.1) and Ro 31–8820 (Compound **9**, Table 11.1). They have been developed based on staurosporine (Compound **10**, Table 11.1), a microbial alkaloid that was identified as an early potent GSK-3*β* inhibitor (IC_{50} = 15.18 nM) [101]. Co-crystal structure of staurosporine with GSK-3*β* reveals its binding in the ATP-binding site. The hinge interactions include two hydrogen bonds, one from N1 of staurosporine to the Asp133 carbonyl oxygen and another from O5 of staurosporine to the backbone nitrogen of Val135. Another polar interaction is a water-mediated interaction from the methylamino nitrogen (N4) of the glycosidic ring to the carbonyl oxygen, of Gln185 [102–106]. In the staurosporine complex, a water molecule is part of a hydrogen-bonding network that starts with O^{γ} of Thr138, passes through four water molecules and ends with the carbonyl oxygen of Val135 (Fig. 11.11). Finally, residues that contribute to the GSK-3*β*/staurosporine complex include Ile62, Gly63, Gly65, Val70, Ala83, Asp133, Tyr134, Gln185, Asn186, Leu188, Cys199 and Asp200 [56, 102–106].

Unfortunately, most of the bisindolylmaleimides have suffered issues of toxicity, bad solubility and poor selectivity, making them unsuitable for treatment of diseases such as AD [107, 108]. Hence, recent efforts in replacing one indole with other heteroaryl substituents led to the emergence of some monoindolylmaleimides such as imidazo[1,2-a]pyridinylindolylmaleimides, 7-azaindazolylindolylmaleimides, benzofuranylindolylmaleimides, 4-azaindolylindolylmaleimides and3-([1,2,4]triazolo[4,3-a]pyridin-3-yl)-4-(indol-3-yl)maleimides that have been identified as potent GSK-3*β* inhibitors. Among these maleimides, studies revealed that the introduction of a nitrogen atom at the 4-position of the indole ring could remarkably increase the selectivity towards GSK-3*β* [101, 109–112].

By having a closer look on an X-ray structure of a synthesized maleimide inhibitor (Compound **11**, Table 11.1) (K_d 0.05 nM on GSK-3*β*), it is clear that it occupies the ATP binding pocket of GSK-3*β*. Moreover, the structure revealed several key interactions between the compound and GSK-3*β*. The maleimide NH acts as H bond donor interacting with Asp133 carbonyl group and one of the carbonyl groups from the maleimide acts as a H-bond acceptor to interact with Val135 NH. Together, they form the hinge interaction as seen in most kinase inhibitors. The other carbonyl group from the maleimide interacts with Asp200 through water. The side chain shows additional polar interactions: the NH with

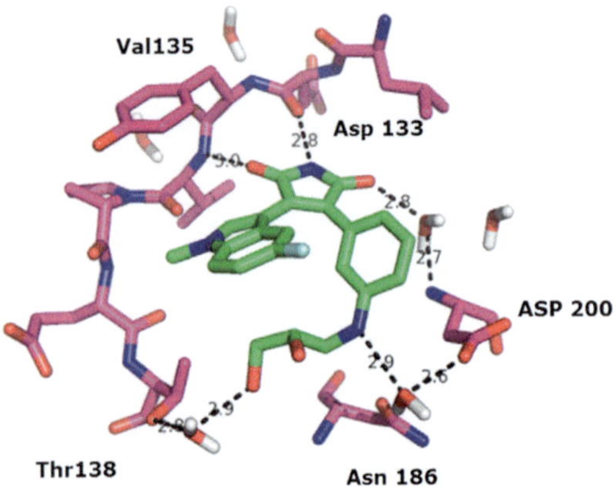

Fig. 11.12 X-ray of maleimide inhibitor bound to GSK-3β [113]

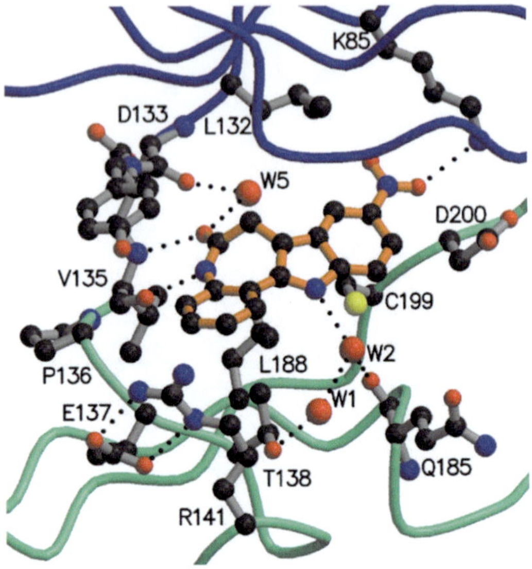

Fig. 11.13 Alsterpaullone interactions with GSK-3β [56]

Asn186 via water and the terminal OH with Thr138 via water (Fig. 11.12) [113, 114].

Among the maleimides that have been developed as highly selective GSK-3β inhibitors are arylindolemaleimide SB-216763 (Compound **12**, Table 11.1) and the anilinomaleimide SB-415286 (Compound **13**, Table 11.1) that are developed by GlaxoSmithKline as potent GSK-3β inhibitors with IC_{50} values within the low nanomolar range [100, 115].

11.5.2.4 Paullones

Paullone (7,12-dihydroindolo[3,2-*d*][1] benzazepine-6(5H)-ones) (Compound **14**, Table 11.1), and its derivatives were identified as novel antiproliferative compounds during the high-throughput screening campaign performed at the National Cancer Institute, USA (NCI) in 1999 [116].

Alsterpaullone (9-nitropaullone) (Compound **15**, Table 11.1), is considered the most potent GSK-3β inhibitor of the series (IC_{50} value of 4 nM). The co-crystal structure of alsterpaullone bound in the GSK-3β ATP-active site showed that Alsterpaullone's hinge interactions include two direct hydrogen bonds with Val135 and one water mediated interaction with Asp133. The N5 and carbonyl oxygen atoms of alsterpaullone make a pair of hydrogen bonds with the backbone nitrogen, and carbonyl oxygen of Val135, respectively, and a water molecule bridges between the carbonyl oxygen atoms of alsterpaullone and Asp133. Moreover, alsterpaullone makes polar interactions between the nitro group in position 9 and the side-chain amino group of Lys85. The final polar interaction between alsterpaullone and GSK-3β occurs through a bridging water molecule; the water hydrogen bonds with N12 of alsterpaullone and the carbonyl oxygen of Gln185. A water molecule in this position is oriented by a hydrogen bond network with Thr138 O^{γ} (Fig. 11.13) [56].

On the other hand, kenpaullone (Compound **16,** Table 11.1) displays neuroprotective effects against GSK-3β mediated mitochondrial dysfunction and stress-induced cell death [117]. The introduction of a 9-halogen in the indolobenzazepinone scaffold favors improved inhibitory activity toward GSK-3β due to extensive interaction with the Val135 residue justifying the enhanced selectivity for GSK-3β [100, 118].

11.5.2.5 Aloisines

Aloisines represent a family of compounds that is called following the first name of Dr. Alois Alzheimer. They are represented by the unsubstituted prototype 6-phenyl[5H]pyrrolo[2,3-b]pyrazines (Compound **17**, Table 11.1). Two aloisines, aloisine A and aloisine B, are considered among the most well-known as well as potent aloisine analogues. Aloisine A (IC_{50} = 0.65 μM) (Compound **18**, Table 11.1) is the most potent of those analogs tested and showed anti-proliferative effects in differentiated post mitotic neurons [119]. Complex structure of aloisine B (IC_{50} = 0.75 μM) (Compound **19**, Table 11.1) with GSK-3*β*, showed that aloisine B is located in the cleft between two domains of GSK-3*β* which are the beta-sheet and alpha-helix. It reveals that substituent on position 3 of the pyrrole ring is confined by the kinase residues near it, making too large substituent at this position detrimental for the inhibitory activity. As for the substituent on position 4 of the benzene ring, it points to the opening of the cleft, allowing bulky and hydrophilic substituents to contribute positively to the inhibition activity. Near that position, there is an apolar residue, Leu188, which interacts with the substituent *via* hydrophobic interaction. The positive charged residue Arg141 near position 4 of the benzene ring makes negative-rich substituent favored at this position, and the O atom in residue Val135, which is pointing to the position 5, makes a positive-rich substituent helpful (Fig. 11.14) [120].

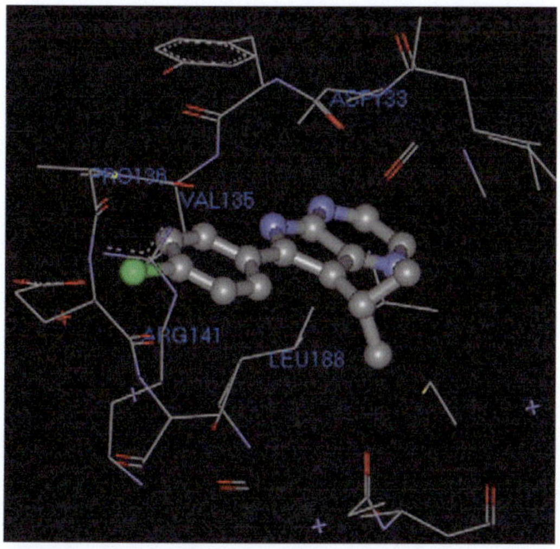

Fig. 11.14 Binding of Aloisine B with GSK-3*β* [120]

11.5.2.6 Oxadiazoles

1,3,4-Oxadiazole-moiety is considered a new backbone scaffold of great potential for small molecules acting as ATP-competitive GSK-3*β* inhibitors. Various size aryls/heteroaryls have been introduced to position 2 and 5 of the 1,3,4-oxadiazole ring to construct new molecules as potential enzyme inhibitors. Co-crystal structure of GSK-3*β* and the oxadiazole derivative **20** (Table 11.1) (IC_{50} value of 65 nM in *in vitro* assay) showed multiple sets of interactions where the O1 oxygen and the hydrogen on the C2-carbon of the benzodioxole made hydrogen bonds with the amide NH hydrogen and carbonyl oxygen of Val135 in the hinge region, respectively. The 4-methoxy-3-fluorobenzyl group fills the hydrophobic site and both the N3 and N4-nitrogen atoms of the oxadiazole are incorporated into the unique hydrogen bond network between Lys85-Glu97-Asp200 through two water molecules (Fig. 11.15). In addition, hydrophobic amino acids were observed near the benzodioxole ring

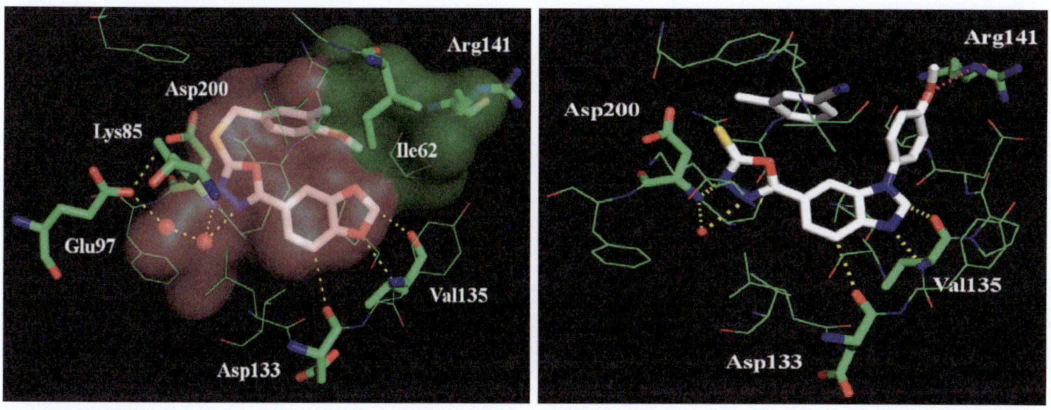

Fig. 11.15 Interactions of oxadiazole derivatives with GSK-3*β* [121]

and Arg141 was found adjacent to the gatekeeper. Based on the previous interactions, designing and synthesizing new compounds bearing similar groups to maintain the essential interactions was performed. As a result, a new compound (Compound **21,** Table 11.1) having 4-methoxyphenyl group on the core heterocycles and 3-cyano groups on the S-benzyl group to act as electron withdrawing group showed single-digit nanomolar potent inhibitory activity (IC_{50} = 2.3 nM) as well as 1000-fold selectivity towards GSK-3*β* when compared to other protein kinases. The major interactions of this compound with GSK-3*β* were hydrogen bonding of the benzimidazole core with the hinge region and the oxadiazole with Asp200. Finally, interaction of the 4-methoxyphenyl group with Arg141 was observed [121].

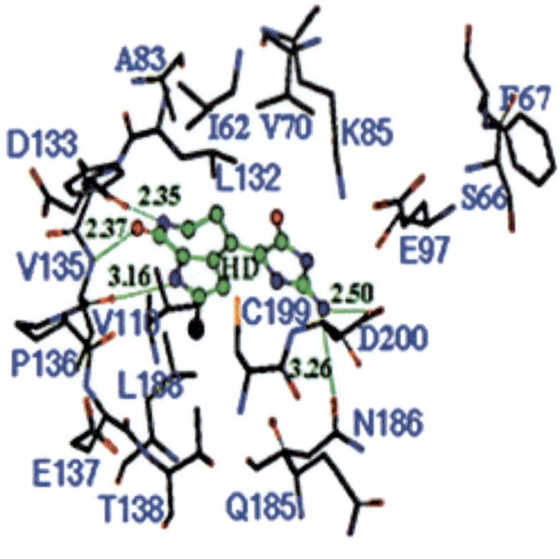

Fig. 11.16 Binding mode of hymenialdisine with GSK-3*β* [123]

11.5.2.7 Miscellaneous

Hymenialdisine

The marine sponge constituent hymenialdisine (Compound **22**, Table 11.1) is a potent inhibitor of GSK-3*β*. It competes at the ATP binding site where the hydrophobic residues lining the ATP binding cleft such as Ile62, Val110, Leu188, and Leu132 surround it. The two residues Asp133 and Val135 are part of the kinase hinge region that forms 1–3 H-bonds with the hymenialdisine [75, 122]. In addition, electrostatic interactions exist between the O atom of the C ring and Lys85, as well as the nitrogen atoms of the cyclic guanidine and Asn186 and Asp200 in the GSK-3*β* (Fig. 11.16) [123].

Hymenialdisine also blocks the *in vivo* phosphorylation of the microtubule-binding protein tau at sites that are hyper-phosphorylated by GSK-3*β* in Alzheimer's disease [124].

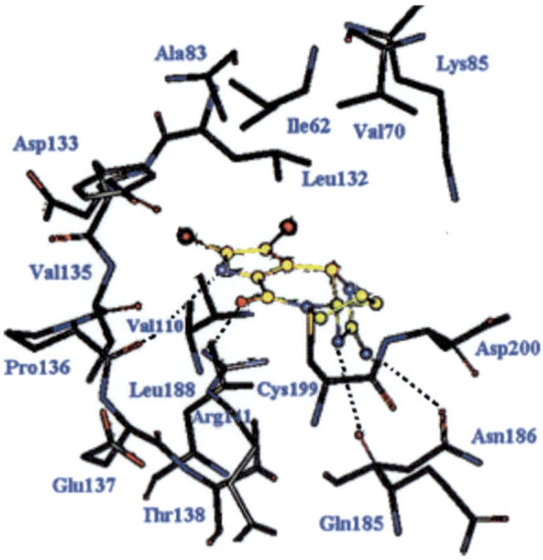

Fig. 11.17 Binding mode of dibromocantharelline with GSK-3*β* [123]

Dibromocantharelline

Dibromocantharelline is another marine sponge extracted compound. The initial docking results of dibromocantharelline (Compound **23**, Table 11.1) presents some unique behaviors including the H-bond between the N1 atom and carbonyl oxygen of Val135, and the salt bridge involving the O atom of the B ring and the side chain of Arg141, as well as the electrostatic interactions between the cyclic guanidine moiety and Gln185 and Asn186 (Fig. 11.17) [123].

AZD1080

AZD1080, 2-hydroxy-3-[5-[(morpholin-4-yl) methyl]pyridin-2-yl]-1H-indole-5-carbonitrile (Compound **24,** Table 11.1), is a potent and selective small molecule inhibitor of GSK-3*β* with a pKi of 7.5 (IC_{50} = 31 nM) that was discovered using structure-based drug design methods. High resolution X-ray crystal structure showed that AZD1080 binds in the ATP pocket of GSK-3β where the oxindole ring system forms hydrogen bonds to the back-bone of the ATP pocket. The cyano group is directed toward the conserved salt bridge and the solubilizing morpholine ring is pointed out toward the solvent area [125].

Meridianins

It is a family of brominated 3-(2-amino-pyrimidine)-indoles (Compound **25,** Table 11.1) that are isolated from the tunicate Aplidium-meridianum, an ascidian collected near the South Georgia Islands. The very limited available SAR suggests that the primary amine of the pyrimidine and the hydroxyl of the indole act as H-bond donors while the nitrogen of the pyrimidine could act as a H-bond acceptor [93, 126]. Although attempts have been performed to prepare more selective Meridianins GSK-3β inhibitors [127]. However, in all cases, they were most potent toward CDKs, and inhibition of GSK-3β was marginal [93, 128].

11.5.3 Non-ATP Competitive GSK-3β Inhibitors

11.5.3.1 The Thiadiazolidindione Family (TDZDs)

In 2002, the family of 1,2,4-thiadiazole-3,5-dione (TDZD) was reported as the first non-ATP competitive GSK-3β inhibitors [129]. A wide range of TDZDs inhibits GSK-3β with IC_{50} values in the micromolar range. Regarding the SAR of this class, the size of the substituent attached to the *N*2 of the thiadiazolidinone ring seems to be crucial for GSK-3β inhibition with the methyl moiety being the best substitution obtained. On the other hand, the nature of the substituent of *N*4 is also important for inhibition since potency is enhanced with the introduction of an aromatic moiety, such as phenyl, methylphenyl, or naphthyl groups, suggesting favorable hydrophobic interactions with the enzyme. Regarding the alkyl substituents in

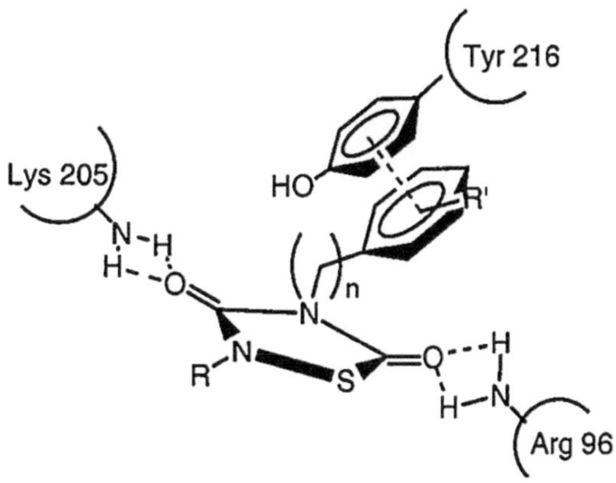

Fig. 11.18 Proposed binding mode of TDZD to GSK-3β [129]

this *N*4 position, only the smallest ones, such as ethyl moiety, result in a GSK-3β inhibitor. Carbonyl 3 of the framework is indispensable for activity as its substitution led to derivatives that mainly retain the inhibitory potency but decreased compound solubility and stability. Regarding the *C*5 carbonyl group, when it is replaced by bioisosteric imino moiety, a dramatic decrease in the inhibition is observed. This fact might suggest that the C5-carbonyl group is critical for binding however some alkyl/aryl or amino fragments can be tolerated at this position. Based on the 3D crystalline structure of GSK-3β a hypothetical binding mode is proposed where the negative charge on the TDZD heterocycle may be the driving force to recognize the oxyanion binding site of the enzyme. Moreover, interactions between the side chain of residues Arg96 and Lys205 and the crucial carbonyl groups of TDZD might be possible. An additional disposition of the inhibitor with the *N*4 pointing out to the inside of the activation loop toward Tyr216 might be explain the potency of the *N*4-aryl TDZD by potential π-π stacking interactions (Fig. 11.18) [129, 130].

Among the drugs that fall in this class are TDZD-8 (Compound **1,** Table 11.2), NP00111, NP031115 and Tideglusib (Compound **2,** Table 11.2). They have been identified as neuroprotective drugs that decrease the tau phosphorylation [93, 131–134]. Only Tideglusib has reached phase II safety studies which showed

Table 11.2 Non-ATP competitive GSK-3β inhibitors

Compound number, name	Chemical structure
1. TDZD-8	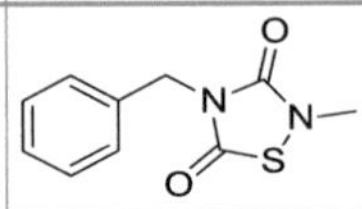
2. Tideglusib	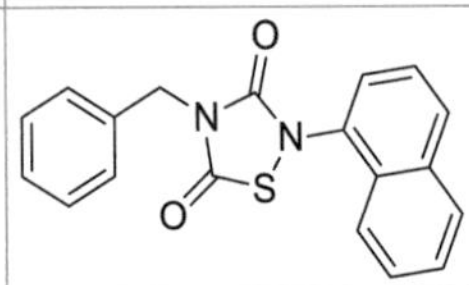
3. Manzamine A	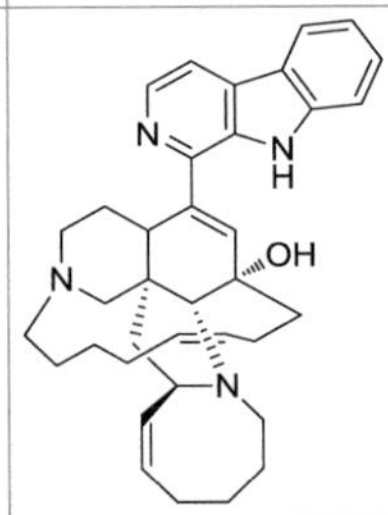
4. Palinurin	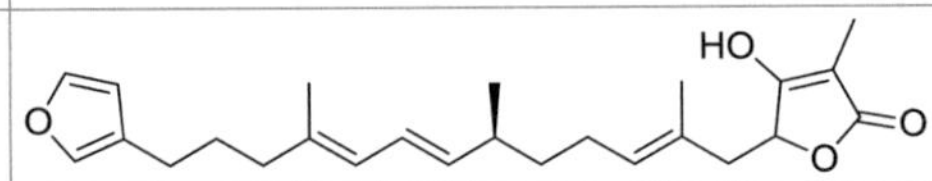
5. Halomethylketone general structure	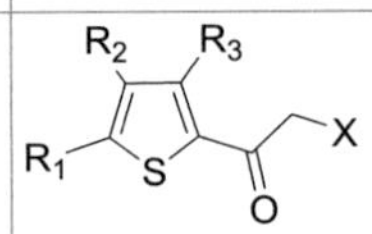 X = Cl or Br
6. 6-(4-Pyridyl)pyrimidin-4(3H)-one derivative	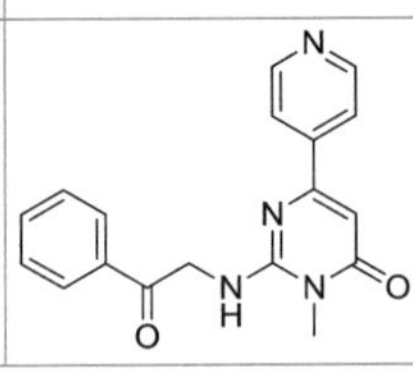

that it is generally well tolerated and have a potential therapeutic efficacy in cases of mild to moderate AD patients that are already on cholinesterase inhibitor treatment for several months [135, 136]. As per the mode of inhibition of the tideglusib to GSK-3β, it was demonstrated that, tideglusib is an irreversible inhibitor of GSK-3β, thus explaining the non-competitive inhibition pattern with respect to ATP that was previously reported for other TDZDs. By comparing it to hypothemycin (molecule reported to inhibit GSK-3β *via* Cys-199 in the ATP-binding site) the role of Cys-199 on the inhibition caused by tideglusib is less clear. Although replacing Cys-199 impaired notably the inhibitory effect of tideglusib, such an effect was not fully abolished [137].

11.5.3.2 Marine Organism Extracted GSK-3β Inhibitors

Several GSK-3β inhibitors are isolated from marine organisms and have the potential to provide new scaffolds comparable to the already established inhibitors. From these natural inhibitors are the two marine compounds, the alkaloid manzamine A and the sesquiterpene palinurin (Compound **3** and **4**, Table 11.2, respectively). First, Manzamines are complex β-carboline alkaloids isolated from Indo-Pacific sponges and characterized as having an intricate and novel polycyclic system [138]. The binding site of manzamine A has been postulated by molecular modeling studies as an allosteric site at the back of the ATP site, just in the junction of C-terminal and N-terminal globes of GSK-3β, being the first GSK-3β allosteric modulator described [139]. As per the binding, the hydroxyl group of Tyr288 can form hydrogen bonds with the pyrrole hydrogen atom or with the hydroxyl group of the ligand (Fig. 11.19). Moreover, the ligand binding indirectly affects the conformation of the activation loop owing to the interaction with Phe229. As a consequence, a strong salt bridge is formed between the residues Arg96 and Glu211 and the loop C moves toward the activation loop [140]. Manzamine A was able to inhibit GSK-3β with an IC_{50} of 10 μM. Moreover, treatment of the SH-SY5Y cells (often used as *in vitro* models of neuronal function and differentiation) with manzamine A at different concentrations (5, 15, and 50 μM) resulting in a decrease of tau phosphorylation [138].

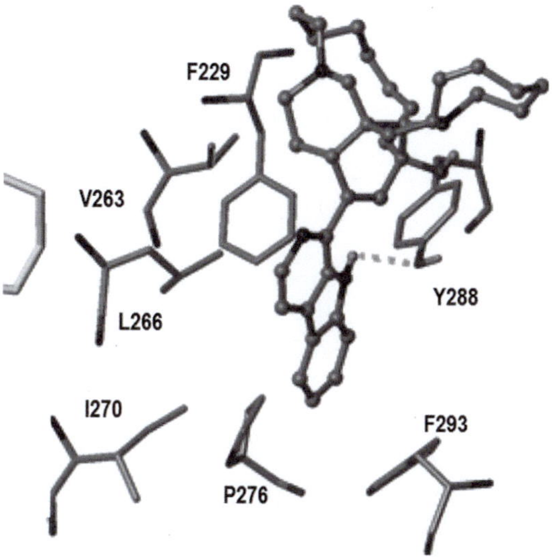

Fig. 11.19 Binding of Manzamine A with GSK-3β [140]

Second, the sesquiterpene palinurin has been announced as cell permeable non-ATP competitive GSK-3β inhibitor able to reduce tau phosphorylation in cell cultures [141]. Its molecule can be differentiated into two parts: the hydrophilic, negatively charged tetronic ring, and the hydrophobic sesquiterpene fragment [142]. Docking of the molecule with GSK-3β showed

Fig. 11.20 Binding of Pallinurin, with GSK-3β [143]

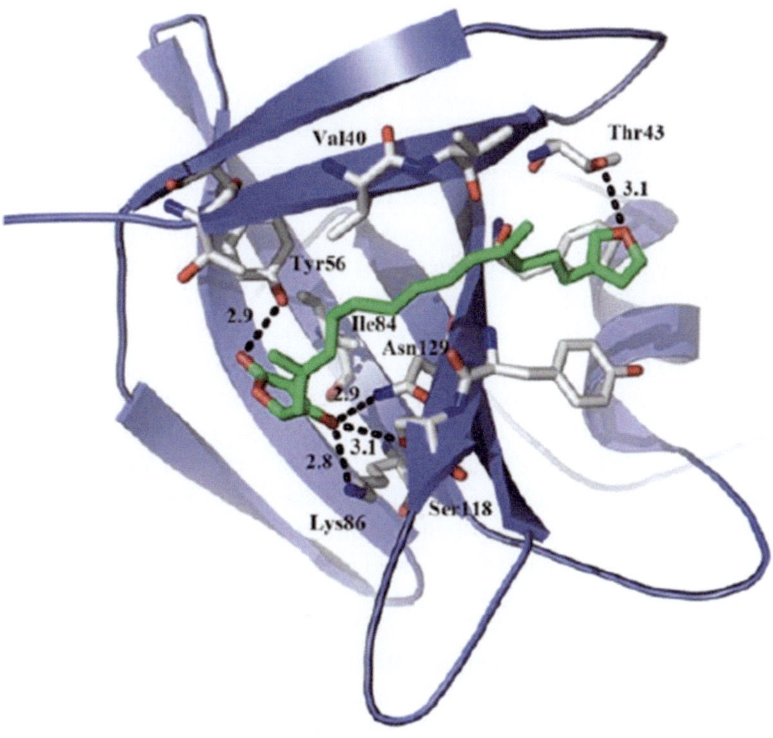

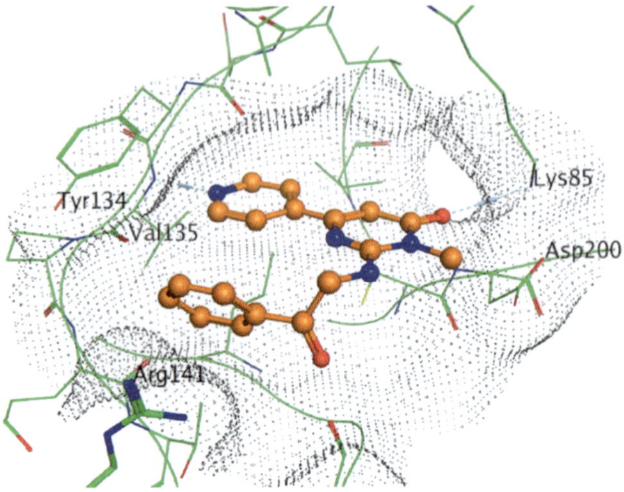

Fig. 11.21 Binding of HMK derivative with GSK-3β [149]

possible binding in more than one site. The first pocket is located at the bottom of the C-terminal lobe, the ring was captured in a small cavity formed by the side chains of residues Thr152, Val155, Arg306 and Pro278. The ring shape fitted very well inside the cavity, but only one interaction was formed with the positively charged side chain of Arg306 [143].

The second most populated pocket, seeming to be a better binding site for palinurin, is located at the N-terminal lobe. In this pocket, Lys86 formed a salt-bridge and a hydrogen bond with the deprotonated hydroxyl of the tetronic ring, and Tyr56 was hydrogen bonded to the carbonyl group of the ring [143]. These compounds are valuable candidates, with privileged scaffolds provided by nature, to be considered for further optimization of synthetic, biological, and ADME properties in a drug development process (Fig. 11.20) [12].

To confirm the inhibitory effect of pallinurin on GSK-3β activity, the isolated natural compound was tested showing IC_{50} values of 2.6 mM. Finally, treatment of human neuroblastoma SH-SY5Y cells with palinurin at different concentrations resulted in a decrease of tau phosphorylation starting at 35–50 mM [143].

11.5.3.3 Halomethylketones (HMKs)

Synthesized derivatives of halomethylketone (Compound **5**, Table 11.2) share the same structural features: a substituted thiophene ring and a ketone group. They represent the first known irreversible inhibitors of GSK-3β with IC_{50} values in the low micromolar range. They are reported to decrease tau phosphorylation in cell cultures, good kinase and neurotransmitter selectivity, and ability to cross the blood-brain barrier. Their inhibitory activity is mediated by covalent modification of Cys199 residue [12, 144–146].

11.5.3.4 Pyrimidinones

Those are class members that have been recently studied as potential GSK-3β inhibitors [147–149]. Docking study of a 6-(4-pyridyl)pyrimidin-4(3H)-one derivative (Compound **6**, Table 11.2) with GSK-3β showed that the nitrogen atom on the pyridine ring made a hydrogen bond with the amide of Val135 and the oxygen atom of the carbonyl moiety in the pyrimidone ring made a hydrogen bonding network with Lys85. An additional interaction was observed between the phenyl group and the guanidinyl moiety of Arg141 through a cation–π interaction. A further hydrogen bonding was observed between the hydrogen donor moiety on the 3-position of pyrimidone with amino acid residues of the external region in the ATP-binding site (Fig. 11.21). This compound has shown subnanomolar inhibitory activity (IC_{50} = 8.9 nM) and good brain permeability, and reduced tau phosphorylation by 24% in mouse brain [149].

11.5.3.5 Others

Some drugs are thought to bind through other binding sites rather than that of ATP or substrate. The GSK-3β surface has been mapped and four potential allosteric sites were discovered. These sites should be used for future rational drug design and discovery of small selective inhibitors that may reach clinical development as future therapies for severe diseases where GSK-3β is up-regulated [74]. One of the recently discovered inhibitors that bind allosterically to GSK-3β is the quinolone derivative VP0.7, that is neither considered a non-ATP nor substrate competitive GSK-3β inhibitor, where it binds to an allosteric pocket in the C-terminal lobe of the enzyme. Docking studies proposed a change in the activation loop of the enzyme that may be responsible for this allosteric modulation [74, 143].

11.6 Conclusion

Playing a key role in the hyperphosphorylation of tau protein, one of the two major hallmarks of AD, glycogen synthase kinase-3β (GSK-3β) signified to the research community a thriving target for the management of AD. Consequently, many GSK-3β inhibitors have been developed over the past years in an attempt to find biologically active molecules for the management of AD. These inhibitors have been classified into metal cations, ATP-competitive, and non-ATP competitive. Most of these discovered classes include potent compounds showing high inhibitory activity, good brain permeability, as well as remarked tau phosphorylation reduction in animal models which led to the progression of some of them to, the clinical trials stage. Data presented hereby beacons the various classes of GSK-3β inhibitors shedding light on their pharmacophoric structural features, SAR and modes of molecular interactions with their biological target. It is believed that information displayed herein pave the way for future design and discovery of more GSK-3β inhibitors based on a combined understanding of the various presented chemical backbone scaffolds and personalizing the interventions to an individual's molecular risk and disease pathology profile.

References

1. Ramirez-Bermudez J (2012) Arch Med Res 43:595
2. Querfurth HW, LaFerla FM (2010) N Engl J Med 362:329
3. Hooper C, Killick R, Lovestone S (2008) J Neurochem 104:1433
4. Alzheimer's Association (2015) Alzheimers Dement. 11:332
5. Potter GG, Plassman BL, Burke JR, Kabeto MU, Langa KM, Llewellyn DJ, Rogers MA, Steffens DC (2009) Alzheimers Dement 5:445
6. Gurland BJ, Wilder DE, Lantigua R, Stern Y, Chen J, Killeffer EH, Mayeux R (1999) Int J Geriatr Psychiatry 14:481
7. Haan MN, Mungas DM, Gonzalez HM, Ortiz TA, Acharya A, Jagust WJ (2003) J Am Geriatr Soc 51:169
8. http://www.who.int/mental_health/publications/dementia_report_2012/en/. Last accessed 5 Jan 2017
9. Blennow K, de Leon MJ, Zetterberg H (2006) Lancet 368:387
10. Waring SC, Rosenberg RN (2008) Arch Neurol 65:329
11. Micheau J, Marighetto A (2011) Behav Brain Res 221:424
12. Martinez A, Gil C, Perez DI (2011) Int J Alzheimers Dis 2011:280502
13. Ashraf GM, Greig NH, Khan TA, Hassan I, Tabrez S, Shakil S, Sheikh IA, Zaidi SK, Akram M, Jabir NR, Firoz CK, Naeem A, Alhazza IM, Damanhouri GA, Kamal MA (2014) CNS Neurol Disord Drug Targets 13:1280
14. Lewis AJ, Tierney MC, Fisher RH, Zorzitto ML, Snow WG, Reid DW, Nieuwstraten P (1988) Neurology 38:1660
15. http://mmcneuro.wordpress.com/2012/12/23/diagnostic-testing-for-alzheimers/. Last accessed 23 Jan 2017
16. Joachim CL, Selkoe DJ (1989) J Gerontol 44:B77
17. Marotta CA, Majocha RE, Tate B (1992) J Mol Neurosci 3:111
18. Crowther RA, Olesen OF, Jakes R, Goedert M (1992) FEBS Lett 309:199
19. Lloret A, Fuchsberger T, Giraldo E, Vina J (2015) Free Radic Biol Med 83:186
20. Danielsson J, Andersson A, Jarvet J, Graslund A (2006) Magn Reson Chem 44. Spec No:S114
21. Tomaselli S, Esposito V, Vangone P, van Nuland NA, Bonvin AM, Guerrini R, Tancredi T, Temussi PA, Picone D (2006) Chembiochem 7:257
22. Ohnishi S, Takano K (2004) Cell Mol Life Sci 61:511
23. Yaar M, Zhai S, Pilch PF, Doyle SM, Eisenhauer PB, Fine RE, Gilchrest BA (1997) J Clin Invest 100:2333
24. Estus S, Tucker HM, van Rooyen C, Wright S, Brigham EF, Wogulis M, Rydel RE (1997) J Neurosci 17:7736
25. Balaraman Y, Limaye AR, Levey AI, Srinivasan S (2006) Cell Mol Life Sci 63:1226

26. Polychronopoulos P, Magiatis P, Skaltsounis AL, Myrianthopoulos V, Mikros E, Tarricone A, Musacchio A, Roe SM, Pearl L, Leost M, Greengard P, Meijer L (2004) J Med Chem 47:935
27. Goedert M, Klug A, Crowther RA (2006) J Alzheimers Dis 9:195
28. Brunden KR, Trojanowski JQ, Lee VM (2009) Nat Rev Drug Discov 8:783
29. Maccioni RB, Cambiazo V (1995) Physiol Rev 75:835
30. Schweers O, Mandelkow EM, Biernat J, Mandelkow E (1995) Proc Natl Acad Sci U S A 92:8463
31. Maccioni RB, Munoz JP, Barbeito L (2001) Arch Med Res 32:367
32. Grimes CA, Jope RS (2001) Prog Neurobiol 65:391
33. Doble BW, Woodgett JR (2003) J Cell Sci 116:1175
34. Hur EM, Zhou FQ (2010) Nat Rev Neurosci 11:539
35. Chen L, Zhou W, Chen PC, Gaisina I, Yang S, Li X (2011) Mol Pharmacol 79:974
36. Kim WY, Wang X, Wu Y, Doble BW, Patel S, Woodgett JR, Snider WD (2009) Nat Neurosci 12:1390
37. Sirerol-Piquer M, Gomez-Ramos P, Hernandez F, Perez M, Moran MA, Fuster-Matanzo A, Lucas JJ, Avila J, Garcia-Verdugo JM (2011) Hippocampus 21:910
38. Garrido JJ, Simon D, Varea O, Wandosell F (2007) FEBS Lett 581:1579
39. Hernandez F, de Barreda EG, Fuster-Matanzo A, Goni-Oliver P, Lucas JJ, Avila J (2009) Brain Res Bull 80:248
40. Chico LK, Van Eldik LJ, Watterson DM (2009) Nat Rev Drug Discov 8:892
41. Sayas C, Jurado J, Avila J, Villanueva N (2012) Curr Biotechnol 1:80
42. De Strooper B, Annaert W (2001) J Cell Biol 152:F17
43. Anderton BH, Dayanandan R, Killick R, Lovestone S (2000) Mol Med Today 6:54
44. Retz W, Gsell W, Munch G, Rosler M, Riederer P (1998) J Neural Transm Suppl 54:221
45. Behl C (1999) Prog Neurobiol 57:301
46. Li WP, Chan WY, Lai HW, Yew DT (1997) J Mol Neurosci 8:75
47. Lucas JJ, Hernandez F, Gomez-Ramos P, Moran MA, Hen R, Avila J (2001) EMBO J 20:27
48. Hernandez F, Borrell J, Guaza C, Avila J, Lucas JJ (2002) J Neurochem 83:1529
49. Phiel CJ, Wilson CA, Lee VM, Klein PS (2003) Nature 423:435
50. Aplin AE, Jacobsen JS, Anderton BH, Gallo JM (1997) Neuroreport 8:639
51. Rockenstein E, Torrance M, Adame A, Mante M, Bar-on P, Rose JB, Crews L, Masliah E (2007) J Neurosci 27:1981
52. ter Haar E, Coll JT, Austen DA, Hsiao HM, Swenson L, Jain J (2001) Nat Struct Biol 8:593
53. Dajani R, Fraser E, Roe SM, Young N, Good V, Dale TC, Pearl LH (2001) Cell 105:721
54. Hanks SK, Quinn AM, Hunter T (1988) Science 241:42
55. Aoki M, Yokota T, Sugiura I, Sasaki C, Hasegawa T, Okumura C, Ishiguro K, Kohno T, Sugio S, Matsuzaki T (2004) Acta Crystallogr D Biol Crystallogr 60:439
56. Bertrand JA, Thieffine S, Vulpetti A, Cristiani C, Valsasina B, Knapp S, Kalisz HM, Flocco M (2003) J Mol Biol 333:393
57. Carrera AC, Alexandrov K, Roberts TM (1993) Proc Natl Acad Sci U S A 90:442
58. Hughes K, Nikolakaki E, Plyte SE, Totty NF, Woodgett JR (1993) EMBO J 12:803
59. Bax B, Carter PS, Lewis C, Guy AR, Bridges A, Tanner R, Pettman G, Mannix C, Culbert AA, Brown MJ, Smith DG, Reith AD (2001) Structure 9:1143
60. Dajani R, Fraser E, Roe SM, Yeo M, Good VM, Thompson V, Dale TC, Pearl LH (2003) EMBO J 22:494
61. Buescher J (2010) Integrated Biomedical Science Graduate. Doctor of Philosophy
62. Ryves WJ, Dajani R, Pearl L, Harwood AJ (2002) Biochem Biophys Res Commun 290:967
63. Cross DA, Alessi DR, Cohen P, Andjelkovich M, Hemmings BA (1995) Nature 378:785
64. Hart MJ, de los Santos R, Albert IN, Rubinfeld B, Polakis P (1998) Curr Biol 8:573
65. van Noort M, Meeldijk J, van der Zee R, Destree O, Clevers H (2002) J Biol Chem 277:17901
66. Yost C, Farr GH 3rd, Pierce SB, Ferkey DM, Chen MM, Kimelman D (1998) Cell 93:1031
67. Cook D, Fry MJ, Hughes K, Sumathipala R, Woodgett JR, Dale TC (1996) EMBO J 15:4526
68. Chen W, Chen M, Barak LS (2010) Am J Physiol Gastrointest Liver Physiol 299:G293
69. Datta SR, Brunet A, Greenberg ME (1999) Genes Dev 13:2905
70. Brazil DP, Hemmings BA (2001) Trends Biochem Sci 26:657
71. Brunet A, Datta SR, Greenberg ME (2001) Curr Opin Neurobiol 11:297
72. De Sarno P, Li X, Jope RS (2002) Neuropharmacology 43:1158
73. Dessalew N, Patel DS, Bharatam PV (2007) J Mol Graph Model 25:885
74. Palomo V, Soteras I, Perez DI, Perez C, Gil C, Campillo NE, Martinez A (2011) J Med Chem 54:8461
75. Meijer L, Flajolet M, Greengard P (2004) Trends Pharmacol Sci 25:471
76. Gadakar PK, Phukan S, Dattatreya P, Balaji VN (2007) J Chem Inf Model 47:1446
77. Lather V, Kristam R, Saini J, Kristam R, Karthikeyan N, Balaji V (2008) QSAR Comb Sci 27:718
78. Pasquali L, Busceti CL, Fulceri F, Paparelli A, Fornai F (2010) Behav Pharmacol 21:473
79. Frausto da Silva JJ, Williams RJ (1976) Nature 263:237

80. Amari L, Layden B, Rong Q, Geraldes CF, Mota de Freitas D (1999) Anal Biochem 272:1
81. Wallace J (2014) Cell Calcium 55:175
82. Chalecka-Franaszek E, Chuang DM (1999) Proc Natl Acad Sci U S A 96:8745
83. Ryves WJ, Harwood AJ (2001) Biochem Biophys Res Commun 280:720
84. Zhang F, Phiel CJ, Spece L, Gurvich N, Klein PS (2003) J Biol Chem 278:33067
85. Sugawara H, Iwamoto K, Bundo M, Ishiwata M, Ueda J, Kakiuchi C, Ishigooka J, Kato T (2010) J Neural Transm 117:155
86. Yasuda S, Liang MH, Marinova Z, Yahyavi A, Chuang DM (2009) Mol Psychiatry 14:51
87. Diniz BS, Machado-Vieira R, Forlenza OV (2013) Neuropsychiatr Dis Treat 9:493
88. Klein PS, Melton DA (1996) Proc Natl Acad Sci U S A 93:8455
89. Sun X, Sato S, Murayama O, Murayama M, Park JM, Yamaguchi H, Takashima A (2002) Neurosci Lett 321:61
90. De Ferrari GV, Chacon MA, Barria MI, Garrido JL, Godoy JA, Olivares G, Reyes AE, Alvarez A, Bronfman M, Inestrosa NC (2003) Mol Psychiatry 8:195
91. Noble W, Planel E, Zehr C, Olm V, Meyerson J, Suleman F, Gaynor K, Wang L, LaFrancois J, Feinstein B, Burns M, Krishnamurthy P, Wen Y, Bhat R, Lewis J, Dickson D, Duff K (2005) Proc Natl Acad Sci U S A 102:6990
92. Caccamo A, Oddo S, Tran LX, LaFerla FM (2007) Am J Pathol 170:1669
93. Eldar-Finkelman H, Martinez A (2011) Front Mol Neurosci 4:32
94. Lloyd DG, Smith HM, O'Sullivan T, Zisterer DM, Meegan MJ (2005) Med Chem 1:335
95. Bhat R, Xue Y, Berg S, Hellberg S, Ormo M, Nilsson Y, Radesater AC, Jerning E, Markgren PO, Borgegard T, Nylof M, Gimenez-Cassina A, Hernandez F, Lucas JJ, Diaz-Nido J, Avila J (2003) J Biol Chem 278:45937
96. Yellamma K, Praveen K, Peera K (2014) Int J Pharm Biol Sci 5:94
97. Leclerc S, Garnier M, Hoessel R, Marko D, Bibb JA, Snyder GL, Greengard P, Biernat J, Wu YZ, Mandelkow EM, Eisenbrand G, Meijer L (2001) J Biol Chem 276:251
98. Martin L, Magnaudeix A, Wilson CM, Yardin C, Terro F (2011) J Neurosci Res 89:1802
99. Vougogiannopoulou K, Ferandin Y, Bettayeb K, Myrianthopoulos V, Lozach O, Fan Y, Johnson CH, Magiatis P, Skaltsounis AL, Mikros E, Meijer L (2008) J Med Chem 51:6421
100. Silva T, Reis J, Teixeira J, Borges F (2014) Ageing Res Rev 15:116
101. Ye Q, Shen Y, Zhou Y, Lv D, Gao J, Li J, Hu Y (2013) Eur J Med Chem 68:361
102. Lawrie AM, Noble ME, Tunnah P, Brown NR, Johnson LN, Endicott JA (1997) Nat Struct Biol 4:796
103. Lamers MB, Antson AA, Hubbard RE, Scott RK, Williams DH (1999) J Mol Biol 285:713
104. Prade L, Engh RA, Girod A, Kinzel V, Huber R, Bossemeyer D (1997) Structure 5:1627
105. Zhao B, Bower MJ, McDevitt PJ, Zhao H, Davis ST, Johanson KO, Green SM, Concha NO, Zhou BB (2002) J Biol Chem 277:46609
106. Zhu X, Kim JL, Newcomb JR, Rose PE, Stover DR, Toledo LM, Zhao H, Morgenstern KA (1999) Structure 7:651
107. Gani OA, Engh RA (2010) Nat Prod Rep 27:489
108. Pajak B, Orzechowska S, Gajkowska B, Orzechowski A (2008) Adv Med Sci 53:21
109. Engler TA, Henry JR, Malhotra S, Cunningham B, Furness K, Brozinick J, Burkholder TP, Clay MP, Clayton J, Diefenbacher C, Hawkins E, Iversen PW, Li Y, Lindstrom TD, Marquart AL, McLean J, Mendel D, Misener E, Briere D, O'Toole JC, Porter WJ, Queener S, Reel JK, Owens RA, Brier RA, Eessalu TE, Wagner JR, Campbell RM, Vaughn R (2004) J Med Chem 47:3934
110. Gaisina IN, Gallier F, Ougolkov AV, Kim KH, Kurome T, Guo S, Holzle D, Luchini DN, Blond SY, Billadeau DD, Kozikowski AP (2009) J Med Chem 52:1853
111. Ye Q, Xu G, Lv D, Cheng Z, Li J, Hu Y (2009) Bioorg Med Chem 17:4302
112. Ye Q, Mao W, Zhou Y, Xu L, Li Q, Gao Y, Wang J, Li C, Xu Y, Xu Y, Liao H, Zhang L, Gao J, Li J, Pang T (2015) Bioorg Med Chem 23:1179
113. Gong L, Hirschfeld D, Tan YC, Heather Hogg J, Peltz G, Avnur Z, Dunten P (2010) Bioorg Med Chem Lett 20:1693
114. Ye Q, Li M, Zhou YB, Cao JY, Xu L, Li YJ, Han L, Gao JR, Hu YZ, Li J (2013) Arch Pharm (Weinheim) 346:349
115. Coghlan MP, Culbert AA, Cross DA, Corcoran SL, Yates JW, Pearce NJ, Rausch OL, Murphy GJ, Carter PS, Roxbee Cox L, Mills D, Brown MJ, Haigh D, Ward RW, Smith DG, Murray KJ, Reith AD, Holder JC (2000) Chem Biol 7:793
116. Zaharevitz DW, Gussio R, Leost M, Senderowicz AM, Lahusen T, Kunick C, Meijer L, Sausville EA (1999) Cancer Res 59:2566
117. Petit-Paitel A, Brau F, Cazareth J, Chabry J (2009) PLoS One 4:e5491
118. Chen Q, Cui W, Cheng Y, Zhang F, Ji M (2011) J Mol Model 17:795
119. Mettey Y, Gompel M, Thomas V, Garnier M, Leost M, Ceballos-Picot I, Noble M, Endicott J, Vierfond JM, Meijer L (2003) J Med Chem 46:222
120. Zeng M, Jiang Y, Zhang B, Zheng K, Zhang N, Yu Q (2005) Bioorg Med Chem Lett 15:395
121. Saitoh M, Kunitomo J, Kimura E, Hayase Y, Kobayashi H, Uchiyama N, Kawamoto T, Tanaka T, Mol CD, Dougan DR, Textor GS, Snell GP, Itoh F (2009) Bioorg Med Chem 17:2017
122. Noble ME, Endicott JA, Johnson LN (2004) Science 303:1800
123. Zhang N, Zhong R, Yan H, Jiang Y (2011) Chem Biol Drug Des 77:199
124. Meijer L, Thunnissen AM, White AW, Garnier M, Nikolic M, Tsai LH, Walter J, Cleverley KE, Salinas

PC, Wu YZ, Biernat J, Mandelkow EM, Kim SH, Pettit GR (2000) Chem Biol 7:51
125. Georgievska B, Sandin J, Doherty J, Mortberg A, Neelissen J, Andersson A, Gruber S, Nilsson Y, Schott P, Arvidsson PI, Hellberg S, Osswald G, Berg S, Falting J, Bhat RV (2013) J Neurochem 125:446
126. Gompel M, Leost M, De Kier Joffe EB, Puricelli L, Franco LH, Palermo J, Meijer L (2004) Bioorg Med Chem Lett 14:1703
127. Akue-Gedu R, Debiton E, Ferandin Y, Meijer L, Prudhomme M, Anizon F, Moreau P (2009) Bioorg Med Chem 17:4420
128. Echalier A, Bettayeb K, Ferandin Y, Lozach O, Clement M, Valette A, Liger F, Marquet B, Morris JC, Endicott JA, Joseph B, Meijer L (2008) J Med Chem 51:737
129. Martinez A, Alonso M, Castro A, Perez C, Moreno FJ (2002) J Med Chem 45:1292
130. Castro A, Encinas A, Gil C, Brase S, Porcal W, Perez C, Moreno FJ, Martinez A (2008) Bioorg Med Chem 16:495
131. Sereno L, Coma M, Rodriguez M, Sanchez-Ferrer P, Sanchez MB, Gich I, Agullo JM, Perez M, Avila J, Guardia-Laguarta C, Clarimon J, Lleo A, Gomez-Isla T (2009) Neurobiol Dis 35:359
132. Ribe EM, Perez M, Puig B, Gich I, Lim F, Cuadrado M, Sesma T, Catena S, Sanchez B, Nieto M, Gomez-Ramos P, Moran MA, Cabodevilla F, Samaranch L, Ortiz L, Perez A, Ferrer I, Avila J, Gomez-Isla T (2005) Neurobiol Dis 20:814
133. Beaulieu JM, Sotnikova TD, Yao WD, Kockeritz L, Woodgett JR, Gainetdinov RR, Caron MG (2004) Proc Natl Acad Sci USA 101:5099
134. Lipina TV, Kaidanovich-Beilin O, Patel S, Wang M, Clapcote SJ, Liu F, Woodgett JR, Roder JC (2011) Synapse 65:234
135. del Ser T, Steinwachs KC, Gertz HJ, Andres MV, Gomez-Carrillo B, Medina M, Vericat JA, Redondo P, Fleet D, Leon T (2013) J Alzheimers Dis 33:205
136. Lovestone S, Boada M, Dubois B, Hull M, Rinne JO, Huppertz HJ, Calero M, Andres MV, Gomez-Carrillo B, Leon T, del Ser T, A. investigators (2015) J Alzheimers Dis 45:75
137. Dominguez JM, Fuertes A, Orozco L, del Monte-Millan M, Delgado E, Medina M (2012) J Biol Chem 287:893
138. Hamann M, Alonso D, Martin-Aparicio E, Fuertes A, Perez-Puerto MJ, Castro A, Morales S, Navarro ML, Del Monte-Millan M, Medina M, Pennaka H, Balaiah A, Peng J, Cook J, Wahyuono S, Martinez A (2007) J Nat Prod 70:1397
139. Peng J, Kudrimoti S, Prasanna S, Odde S, Doerksen RJ, Pennaka HK, Choo YM, Rao KV, Tekwani BL, Madgula V, Khan SI, Wang B, Mayer AM, Jacob MR, Tu LC, Gertsch J, Hamann MT (2010) J Med Chem 53:61
140. Osolodkin DI, Shulga DA, Palyulin VA, Zefirov NS (2010) Russ Chem Bull, Int Ed 59:1983
141. Martinez A, Castro A, Medina M (2006) Marine compounds as a new source for glycogen synthase kinase 3 inhibitors. In: Glycogen synthase kinase 3 (GSK-3) and its inhibitors. Wiley, Hoboken, p 307
142. Klumber WD (1938) J Am Chem Soc 60:859
143. Bidon-Chanal A, Fuertes A, Alonso D, Perez DI, Martinez A, Luque FJ, Medina M (2013) Eur J Med Chem 60:479
144. Conde S, Perez DI, Martinez A, Perez C, Moreno FJ (2003) J Med Chem 46:4631
145. Perez DI, Conde S, Perez C, Gil C, Simon D, Wandosell F, Moreno FJ, Gelpi JL, Luque FJ, Martinez A (2009) Bioorg Med Chem 17:6914
146. Perez DI, Palomo V, Perez C, Gil C, Dans PD, Luque FJ, Conde S, Martinez A (2011) J Med Chem 54:4042
147. Fukunaga K, Sakai D, Watanabe K, Nakayama K, Kohara T, Tanaka H, Sunada S, Nabeno M, Okamoto M, Saito K, Eguchi J, Mori A, Tanaka S, Inazawa K, Horikawa T (2015) Bioorg Med Chem Lett 25:1086
148. Fukunaga K, Uehara F, Aritomo K, Shoda A, Hiki S, Okuyama M, Usui Y, Watanabe K, Yamakoshi K, Kohara T, Hanano T, Tanaka H, Tsuchiya S, Sunada S, Saito K, Eguchi J, Yuki S, Asano S, Tanaka S, Mori A, Yamagami K, Baba H, Horikawa T, Fujimura M (2013) Bioorg Med Chem Lett 23:6933
149. Uehara F, Shoda A, Aritomo K, Fukunaga K, Watanabe K, Ando R, Shinoda M, Ueno H, Kubodera H, Sunada S, Saito K, Kaji T, Asano S, Eguchi J, Yuki S, Tanaka S, Yoneyama Y, Niwa T (2013) Bioorg Med Chem Lett 23:6928

Regenerative Medicine: Advances from Developmental to Degenerative Diseases

12

Nicholas F. Blair, Thomas J.R. Frith, and Ivana Barbaric

Abstract

Chronic tissue and organ failure caused by an injury, disease, ageing or congenital defects represents some of the most complex therapeutic challenges and poses a significant financial healthcare burden. Regenerative medicine strategies aim to fulfil the unmet clinical need by restoring the normal tissue function either through stimulating the endogenous tissue repair or by using transplantation strategies to replace the missing or defective cells. Stem cells represent an essential pillar of regenerative medicine efforts as they provide a source of progenitors or differentiated cells for use in cell replacement therapies. Whilst significant leaps have been made in controlling the stem cell fates and differentiating them to cell types of interest, transitioning bespoke cellular products from an academic environment to off-the-shelf clinical treatments brings about a whole new set of challenges which encompass manufacturing, regulatory and funding issues. Notwithstanding the need to resolve such issues before cell replacement therapies can benefit global healthcare, mounting progress in the field has highlighted regenerative medicine as a realistic prospect for treating some of the previously incurable conditions.

Keywords

Regenerative medicine • Stem cells • Spinal cord injury • Parkinson's • Hirschprung's

Nicholas F. Blair and Thomas J.R. Frith contributed equally to this work.

N.F. Blair
Wellcome Trust – MRC Cambridge Stem Cell Institute, University of Cambridge, Cambridge, UK

T.J.R. Frith • I. Barbaric (✉)
Centre for Stem Cell Biology, Department of Biomedical Science, The University of Sheffield, Sheffield, UK
e-mail: i.barbaric@sheffield.ac.uk

12.1 Introduction

The ultimate goal of regenerative medicine is to heal diseased or injured tissues and organs either by replacing them or enhancing their regeneration potential *in situ* [1]. Curing the disease using innovative regenerative medicine therapies prom-

S. El-Khamisy (ed.), *Personalised Medicine*, Advances in Experimental Medicine and Biology 1007,
DOI 10.1007/978-3-319-60733-7_12

ises to revolutionise the healthcare of the future. The need for effective regenerative medicine therapies has been intensified by the projections for an increasingly ageing world population and the consequent predicted rise in age-associated degenerative diseases [2]. Against this daunting background, the historical precedent of allogeneic transplantation highlights cell replacement as a conceivable approach to treating degenerative diseases [3]. Nonetheless, the large-scale deployment of such an approach has been limited by the lack of an adequate supply of cells, as the demand for donated tissues and organs by far outweighs the current and future clinical need. The advent of stem cell technologies has had a profound impact on the field of regenerative medicine, providing exciting new perspectives promising to overcome the existing limitations. Indeed, recent years have witnessed tremendous progress towards this goal, with several ongoing clinical trials involving stem cell-derived cells for treatment of degenerative diseases. Here, we start by providing a brief overview of the main types and characteristics of stem cells as the main sources of cells for regenerative medicine therapies. Furthermore, we discuss several examples of the development of stem cell-based therapies for currently incurable diseases caused either by injury (spinal cord injury), degeneration (Parkinson's disease) or developmental anomalies (Hirschprung's disease). Finally, based on the current data and lessons learnt from the past and current stem cell-based clinical studies, we highlight the main outstanding hurdles hampering the translation of stem cell-based cellular therapies into standard clinical practice.

12.2 Stem Cells as a Source of Cells for Regenerative Medicine

Stem cells are broadly defined as cells that have the ability to replenish their own population (the feature known as self-renewal) and the ability to produce more specialised cell types (differentiation) [4]. These unique features make stem cells an ideal source of cells for regenerative medicine, as they allow production of an unlimited number of cells of a particular type that could be used to replace the missing or diseased cells in the body. Although by definition all stem cells possess the ability to self-renew whilst retaining the ability to differentiate, different types of stem cells can be distinguished based on various criteria. For example, according to their developmental origin, stem cells can be categorised as either adult or embryonic. The adult stem cells are typically found in adult somatic tissues where they maintain tissue homeostasis and are hence also termed tissue-specific stem cells. On the other hand, embryonic stem cells originate from the early embryos [5–7]. The adult and embryonic stem cells also differ in their ability to give rise to differentiated cell types. Adult stem cell differentiation is typically limited to the cell types of the tissue where they reside, a feature known as multipotency. In contrast to this, embryonic stem cells have the ability to produce all of the cell types in the body, and this broad developmental potential of embryonic stem cells is termed pluripotency [5, 6].

12.2.1 Multipotent Stem Cells

Multipotent stem cells support the life-long tissue regeneration and homeostasis due to their ability to produce all of the cell types of their residential tissue or organ. Through seminal work of two Canadian scientists, Till and McCulloch, the hematopoietic stem cell was the first multipotent stem cell identified, and it remains the best characterised stem cell to date [8, 9]. Capable of multilineage differentiation to all of the blood lineages, hematopoietic stem cells have to daily replenish billions of cells lost from the hematopoietic system due to the limited life-span of specialised blood cells. Hematopoietic stem cells have also provided a paradigm for cell replacement therapies. Indeed, the transplantation of hematopoietic stem cells has been clinically used since the 1950s as a treatment for blood and bone marrow cancers [10]. The treatments are based on the ability of transplanted hematopoietic stem cell from a tissue-matched donor to reconstitute all of the blood cells in a patient whose bone marrow has been ablated using irradiation or chemotherapy [11, 12].

Another example of a tissue in which a rapid turn-over of specialised cells is underpinned by a self-renewing stem cell population is the intestinal system. The intestine is one of the fastest renewing tissues in the body, with an entire intestinal epithelium being replaced every 4–5 days, hence warranting a constant production of the differentiated cells [13]. Unlike the hematopoietic stem cells, which are relatively easily accessible and whose functional identity can be shown by a transplantation of a single cell, the identification of stem cells in the gut relied on the lineage tracing analyses [14]. Such analyses revealed the intestinal stem cell at the apex of the intestinal tissue hierarchy, giving rise to differentiated cell types of the gut which carry out their specialised functions [15, 16].

In contrast to the rapidly renewing tissues such as blood, gut, and skin, the regenerative capacity of some other tissues, such as the central nervous system is less apparent. Nonetheless, neural stem cells have been identified in the adult central nervous system, albeit mainly limited to restricted regions of the hippocampal dentate gyrus [17] and the subventricular zone of the lateral ventricular wall [18]. Harnessing the therapeutic potential of the neural stem cells could be possible either through stimulating their regenerative capacity *in vivo*, or purifying them and expanding *in vitro* prior to the therapeutic applications [19]. However, given the difficulties in isolating neural stem cells from *in vivo* sources, a promising alternative supply of neural stem cells are human pluripotent stem cells, which appear to have the ability to generate large numbers of neural stem cells that can be patterned to various sub-types useful for regenerative medicine [20].

12.2.2 Pluripotent Stem Cells

Defined by the ability to self-renew and give rise to cells from all three embryonic germ layers (ectoderm, mesoderm, and endoderm), the two types of pluripotent stem cells with likely clinical applications are human embryonic stem cells (hESCs) and human induced pluripotent stem cells (hiPSCs). HESCs were first derived in 1998, almost 20 years after the establishment of mouse embryonic stem cell lines [7]. The publication of the seminal paper describing the process of derivation of hESCs from donated surplus IVF blastocysts spurred a flurry of interest into stem cell research. The ability of hESCs to differentiate into somatic cell types *in vitro* was quickly recognised as an enormous opportunity for basic research, disease modelling and, most importantly, as a long-awaited source of cells for regenerative medicine. In another remarkable breakthrough in the field, Yamanaka and colleagues generated human induced pluripotent stem cells (hiPSCs) by reprogramming somatic cells using only four transcription factors [21]. In addition to alleviating some of the ethical issues associated with the derivation of hESCs, reprogramming of somatic cells allows derivation of patient-specific pluripotent cells. This, in turn, provides a platform for personalised approach to medicine, be it for disease modelling and drug discovery or for the production of patient-specific (and hence immuno-compatible) cells for cell replacement therapy (Fig. 12.1).

A number of intracellular and cell-surface markers are associated with the undifferentiated state of hPSCs and hence used to identify undifferentiated cells in culture. These include core pluripotency transcription factors POU5F1 (OCT4) and NANOG, and cell surface antigens such as TRA-1-60, TRA-1-81, SSEA3, and SSEA4 [22]. However, it should be noted that whilst the aforementioned markers can be used to assess hPSC phenotypes, the true definition of hPSCs is based on their functional features of self-renewal and differentiation. Therefore, assessing whether a cell is a true stem cell should ultimately test its functional attributes. This is one of the major difficulties when assessing hPSCs, since their true developmental potency can only be demonstrated by placing cells in an environment where they can differentiate to cells from all three parent lineages that go on to generate the complete embryo. Equivalent experiments are performed with murine PSCs, whereby the

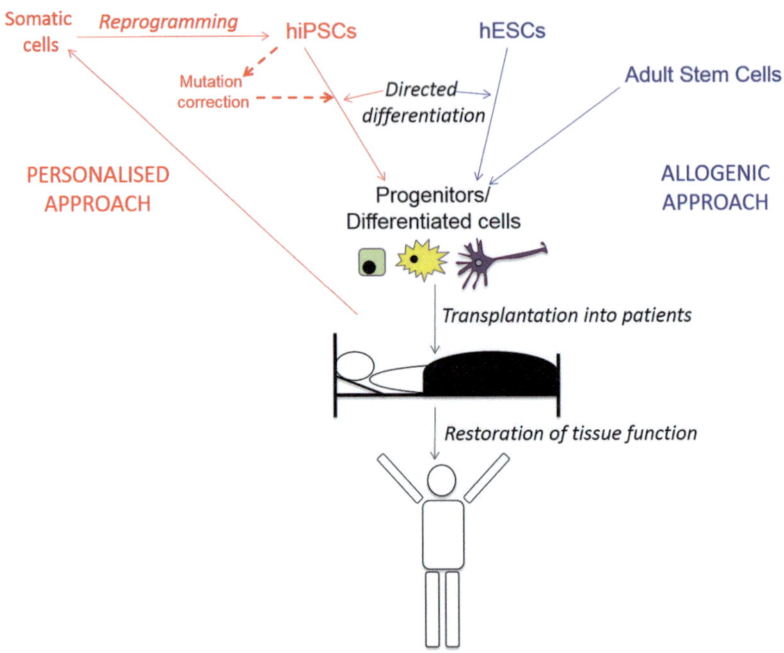

Fig. 12.1 The cell replacement therapy paradigm. Two main approaches include allogeneic approach using adult stem cells or human embryonic stem cells (hESCs) (*right*), and personalised approach, which utilises patient-derived human induced pluripotent stem cells (hiPSCs) (*left*). In either approach, stem cells are directed to differentiate to desired cell types prior to transplantation into patients. In the case of genetic disorders, it may be necessary to correct the disease-causing mutation in hiPSCs by genetic engineering in order to generate functional patient-specific differentiated cells (mutation correction)

cells are injected into a mouse blastocyst, followed by embryo transfer into a pseudopregnant foster female. If the injected PSCs are truly pluripotent, they will contribute to all the cell lineages in the chimeric mouse, including the germ line. Obviously, ethical principles do not allow this type of functional assessment of hPSCs, and alternative *in vitro* and *in vivo* assays are used as surrogate tests for assessing functional aspects of hPSCs. In particular, the teratoma assay has been considered a gold standard test of pluripotency [23]. The assay entails injecting hPSCs into an ectopic site of an immunodeficient mouse. In such an *in vivo* environment, hPSCs tend to form complex tumours (teratomas), containing differentiated cells and haphazardly organized tissues. Importantly, the cells and rudimentary tissues in teratomas are of ectodermal, mesodermal and endodermal origin, and the presence of cells from all three embryonic germ layers has been considered as evidence of pluripotency of injected hPSCs [24].

12.2.3 Differentiation of Human Pluripotent Stem Cells

Differentiation of stem cells to desired specialised cell types is an essential prerequisite to utilising these remarkable cells for therapeutic applications. Nonetheless, although in theory hPSCs can make any cell type in the body, deciphering instructive cues that drive these unspecialised cells to a fully functioning mature cell type of choice has proven an arduous task. Early efforts of finding the appropriate differentiation protocols for hPSCs have been focused on the production of just a handful of cell types out of over two hundred possible differentiated types that build the human body. The cell types in question were deemed to have the greatest therapeutic significance, including pancreatic beta cells, hepatocytes, cardiomyocytes, and neurons [25]. These early efforts of producing specialised cell types from hPSCs were plagued by issues concerning differentiation efficiency, robustness, and reproducibility. It is worth noting that the early methods for culturing hPSCs entailed growing them on a layer of mitotically inactivated mouse embryonic fibroblasts in a media that included fetal bovine serum. Not surprisingly, such a chemically undefined culture system suffered from batch-to-batch variability and a consequent lack of reproducibility. Some of the robustness and reproducibility issues also appeared to be due to seemingly differing propensities of hPSC lines for differentiation to specific lineages [26]. In the years that followed, meticulous studies contributed to vastly improved differentiation protocols, directing hPSC differentiation to a number of cell types of interest. Although arguably each of the differentiation protocols developed had specific intricacies, some of the common denominators started to emerge as key principles that can be applied to instructing hPSC differentiation. In particular, the majority of successful protocols for hPSC differentiation in a monolayer are based on mimicking cues that the cells experience during normal embryonic development [25]. Admittedly, not much is known about the very early stages of human embryonic development *in vivo*, due to the inaccessibility of the early embryo and the ethical concerns with performing human developmental studies. Nonetheless, very informative studies on the development of other mammalian species and the differentiation studies of the mouse embryonic stem cells have provided the crucial insight into the signalling prompts that hPSCs may experience during development. In line with mimicking the developmental processes, the successful differentiation of hPSCs typically requires stepwise protocols, whereby each stage of differentiation is carefully instructed with specific signalling cues before the ensuing progenitor cells are exposed to a new set of signals. A seminal study by Wichterle et al. [27] demonstrated this paradigm by differentiating hPSCs to motor neurons through sequential manipulation of signalling pathways that underpin motor neuron specification during embryo development. This concept was subsequently applied to generate numerous cell types from hPSCs, including various neuronal subtypes (spinal motor, cortical, DA and GABA neurons), cardiomyocytes, hepatocytes and β-cells (summarised in [28]).

12.3 Progress in the Development of hPSC-Based Cell Replacement Therapies

The establishment of protocols for hPSC differentiation to various differentiated cell types has spurred progress of hPSC-based cell replacement therapies towards clinical trials. Here we give a brief overview of the progress in the trials for spinal cord injury and Parkinson's disease. Several other ongoing clinical trials are examining the safety/efficacy of cell replacement therapies for the treatment of chronic conditions such as retinal degeneration, heart failure and diabetes (reviewed in [29]). In addition, driven by immense clinical need and the ability to obtain appropriate cell types, further clinical studies may be on the horizon. We highlight a developmental disorder, Hirschprung's disease, as a condition potentially amenable to treatment by cell replacement therapy.

12.3.1 Regenerative Medicine Approach to Treatment of Spinal Cord Injury

Spinal cord injury is one of the key target injuries for a regenerative medicinal approach. There are more than 10,000 new cases per year in the USA, with long-term repercussions for sufferers requiring constant care resulting with an estimated cost of $4 billion annually (reviewed in [30]). Permanent paralysis and loss of sensation upon traumatic spinal cord injury is caused by the death of neurons and glia cells. In some cases, a key issue arises from demyelination of otherwise intact axons, leading to the loss of function and degeneration of neurons [31]. In such cases, a potential approach for treating spinal cord injury could entail transplanting the patients with cells capable of remyelinating spinal cord neurons in order to prevent their degeneration. Such an approach was tested in animal models of spinal cord injury, whereby animals were transplanted with progenitor cells capable of differentiating into oligodendrocytes *in vivo*. Cell types that have been tested as a source of cells for generating oligodendrocyte progenitors prior to transplantation include hESCs [32, 33], neural stem cells [34] and hiPSCs [35]. Given the ability of hPSCs to give rise to an unlimited number of cells *in vitro*, they were considered a particularly promising source of cells for therapeutic applications [32, 33]. Recovery of motor function in animal models of spinal cord injury provided an impetus for clinical trials to test safety and efficacy of hESC-derived oligodendrocytes for the treatment of spinal cord injury [36]. Clinical trials were commenced by the Geron corporation in 2010, with the Phase I of the trial designed to test the safety of the product through dose escalation. The starting dose was two million cells injected into the spinal cord of each patient. For spinal cord injury, this represents a relatively low dose as calculations based on the equivalent experiments in rat models indicate that 20 million cells would need to be transplanted for any rescue of function. In line with that, no major improvements were noted in the patients' motor function in the safety trial. Minor adverse events were reported when patients were checked 1 week to 1 year post-transplantation, but there was no evidence of serious adverse events, tumours or rejection of the transplanted cells. Although this clinical trial was initially met with optimism, it was terminated after two years for commercial reasons [37]. Recently, Geron's oligodendrocyte differentiation protocol was acquired by Asterias Biotherapeutics, who are in the process of recruiting for a follow-up safety trial (http://www.scistar-study.com/).

12.3.2 Regenerative Medicine Approach to Treatment of Parkinson's Disease

Parkinson's disease (PD) is a neurodegenerative condition with the characteristic clinical features of tremor, rigidity, and slowness of movement, together with a range of non-motor features. It affects 1–2% of the population over the age of 65 [38] and has a significant burden of disease. There is currently no treatment that alters the course of the disease and 60% of patients progress to severe disability or death within 8 years of diagnosis [39]. The pathological hallmark of the disease is the loss of a specific subtype of dopaminergic neurons from the substantia nigra within the midbrain. The focal loss of this relatively rare population of cells makes the disease a prime target for cell replacement therapy.

Efforts to identify a viable source of dopaminergic cells for transplantation to the PD-affected brain began in the 1970s. Grafts derived from fetal ventral mesencephalon (fVM) showed the most promise with evidence of successful engraftment into the host brain, the ability to release dopamine and to ameliorate motor deficits in experimental animals [40]. The outcome of human transplantation of fVM tissue has met with variable results but there it is clear that in some cases it provides an effective and durable therapy with some patients able to remain off pharmacotherapy for over 15 years after transplantation [41]. Whilst this work provides a proof of concept that cell replacement strategies can be a successful treatment for Parkinson's Disease, the ethical and availability issues associated with fetal tissue preclude this from being a viable therapy outside of research studies.

Advances in stem cell and neural differentiation techniques now raise the prospect of being able to replicate the positive clinical outcomes using pluripotent stem-cell derived graft material. A major achievement in the field was the development of protocols, which can generate high yields of the specific A9 dopaminergic neuron subtype that is affected in the disease [42]. These protocols have now been adapted to clinical grade reagents and culture conditions and preclinical work has demonstrated these cells to be safe and have a similar efficacy to fetal-derived cells when transplanted in animal models [43]. It is expected clinical trials will begin over the next few years at a number of centres around the world [44].

For these initial trials, an allogeneic approach using a single hESC or hiPSC source cell line has been favoured. The relatively immunologically privileged status of the brain means that the lifelong immunosuppression may not necessarily be essential in CNS transplantation. In patients who have been transplanted with fetal cells from an allogenic source, it has been demonstrated that a finite period of immunosuppression following transplantation (ranging from 12 months to 5 years) is sufficient for tolerance to the cells to be induced, with evidence that the grafts can then continue to survive for decades in the absence of immunosuppression [41, 45]. Despite this, two groups have been working towards an autologous hiPSC-derived cell therapy for Parkinson's disease [46, 47], although one of these groups appears to have shifted focus to allogeneic haplobanked hiPSCs. One alternative approach that has already reached clinical trial has involved the use of parthenogenic stem cells. This is the first clinical trial to be approved for a stem-cell derived therapy in Parkinson's disease, with the first patient treated in 2016. There are, however, concerns that the differentiated cell type used in this trial may not be optimal and that the supporting pre-clinical data for this approach was limited [48]. It will be several years before it will be known if cell replacement therapies can provide an effective and viable therapy for Parkinson's disease. Not only will this potentially provide a first example of the use of stem cell-based therapy for a neurodegenerative disease, but will also provide information about the relative merits the different source material and differentiation strategies being employed by different groups to produce their cell transplantation product.

12.3.3 Regenerative Medicine Approach to Treatment of Hirschprung's Disease

Hirschsprung's disease is a congenital disorder with an incidence of 1 in 5000 live births (reviewed in [49]). The patients are born with a segment of gut that is not innervated by the enteric nervous system, resulting in the constricted colon and the inability of patients to defecate [50]. Unless there is surgical intervention to remove non-innervated part of the gut within 24 h of birth, Hirschsprung's disease is fatal [51]. Given that the disease is underpinned by an absence of a particular cell type – enteric neurons – cell replacement therapies have been thought to be the ideal treatment for Hirschsprung's disease [52]. The key regenerative medicine approaches for Hirschsprung's disease would involve deriving the correct precursors for the enteric nervous system, transplanting them *en masse* and allowing them to migrate, differentiate and integrate with the gut, thus allowing for the rescue of peristalsis and relaxation of the constricted gut [53]. Due to the sheer length of the gut, it is essential for sufficient numbers of cells to be generated for any regenerative therapy, which has led to significant work into conditions that will allow for expansion of enteric progenitors prior to differentiation into enteric neurons. Considerable promise has been demonstrated with studies from mouse gut stem cells, where both fetal and adult stem cell populations have been isolated, expanded and shown to form neural and glial derivatives after transplantation *in vivo* [54, 55]. The ability to form neurospheres that generate neurons and glia is not limited to gut stem cells. Central nervous system-derived stem cells have also been touted as a source of cells for enteric nervous system transplantation [53]. In addition, there has been significant progress in generating enteric neurons from hPSCs [56]. Transplantation of hPSC-derived enteric neuron precursors into a mouse model of Hirschsprung's disease (Ednrb−/−) led to the migration of cells along the gut and rescued the mutant mice from dying [56]. HPSC-derived enteric neurons can also innervate hPSC-derived gut organoids, which represent the three-dimensional models of the gut tissue comprising various cell types present in the gut epithelia as well as the smooth muscle that surrounds it [57]. Combining the enteric neural progenitors with gut organoids led to the formation of enteric ganglia and innervation of the smooth muscle, thus allowing the control of peristalsis [57].

Whilst such preclinical studies provide proof of concept for cellular replacement approaches for the treatment of Hirschsprung's disease, more work is warranted to specifically assess long-term safety and functionality of any transplanted cells. The presence of immune cells in the gut is an added complication to this therapy that may not present an issue in the treatment of some other diseases, such as Parkinson's. In addition, the number of cells required for treatment of Hirschsprung's disease is a major hurdle to be overcome. Indeed, due to the length of the gut, it is anticipated that transplantation of vast amount of cells will be required to sufficiently reinnervate aganglionic areas. Apart from the issues of producing the large numbers of cells, this will also have implications for the method of transplantation. For example, an injection of cells, which appears a choice delivery of cells for Parkinson's disease, may not be the best method for Hirschsprung's disease. Current preclinical methods are utilising neurospheres or cells encased in extracellular matrix, but these methods have not been optimised as yet to achieve the best functional rescue. Potentially the best method will be a combination of hPSC-derived enteric neural crest cells in a bioengineered device, which can assist in cell grafting and reducing immunogenicity [58].

12.4 Lessons Gleaned from Past and Current (Pre)Clinical Studies

As we await results from current clinical trials on the safety and efficacy of hPSC-derived cellular products in regenerative medicine therapies, it is appropriate that we take stock of key challenges that have plagued clinical translation thus far, with a view of informing future developments in the field.

12.4.1 The Challenge of Producing Specific Mature Cell Types

The ability to control and direct differentiation of hPSCs to desired functional cell types is an essential prerequisite for regenerative medicine efforts. Significant progress has been made towards establishing chemically-defined protocols for hPSC differentiation to a variety of cells types, including cardiomyocytes [59], hindbrain and spinal cord neural stem cells [60], epicardial cells [61], and vascular smooth muscle subtypes [62]. However, many of the protocols yield the differentiated cells that exhibit a relatively immature phenotype. For example, phenotypes of hPSC-derived cardiomyocytes reflect structural, molecular and electrophysiology phenotypes of fetal, rather than fully mature adult cardiomyocytes [63, 64]. Similarly, phenotypic and functional features of hPSC-derived hepatocytes [65] and β cells also appear to align more closely with their fetal rather than the adult counterparts [66]. Although fetal-like cells will undoubtedly prove useful in developmental studies and some aspects of disease modelling, cell replacement therapies necessitate the production of cells capable of generating fully functional adult cell types when transplanted. Several strategies are being explored to promote maturity of the hPSC-derived fetal-like cells, encompassing both *in vitro* and *in vivo* approaches (reviewed in [67]).

A further issue hindering the formulation of robust differentiation protocols is the inter-line variability of hPSCs in the propensity to differentiate into particular cell types. The differentiation bias of hPSCs was revealed in studies that examined the efficiency of the same differentiation protocol on a variety of different hESC or hiPSC lines in parallel [26, 68, 69]. The conclusions drawn from such studies indicated that some lines readily differentiate to cell types of interest, whilst others yield a very low efficiency of desired differentiation. A low efficiency of differentiation may result in the exclusion of a cell line from use, a practical solution that is particularly undesirable when small numbers of patient-specific or haplotype-matched hPSC lines are available. Alternatively, the differences in the differentiation propensity may warrant optimisation of the differentiation protocols for each hPSC line, which can be time consuming and expensive. Hence, future research is needed to unravel the factors that underlie the observed differences in differentiation capacity of hPSC lines. An important step towards this goal was made in a recent study that examined the molecular features of hiPSC lines that exhibited high and low propensity to differentiate to hematopoietic stem cells [69]. Based on this study, the analysis of epigenetic landscape of hPSCs appears to be a promising way forward for predicting the differentiation potential of hPSC lines and selecting the optimal lines for downstream applications.

12.4.2 The Outcome of the Transplantation: The Importance of the Supportive Niche and Absence of Immune Reaction

Obtaining appropriate cell types for transplantation *in vivo* represents only a part of the challenge in restoring normal tissue function, with another major hurdle being the survival and functionality of the transplanted cells. Indeed, it appears that less than 1–3% of total transplanted cells survive initial transplantation *in vivo* [70, 71]. One of the major reasons behind a failure of cells to thrive upon transplantation is thought to be the absence of supportive environment or a niche. Diseased, aged or injured tissues may not provide sufficient levels of oxygen or present the signals necessary for cell survival. On the other hand, the engraftment of cells even in healthy adult tissues is generally limited, possibly due to the lack of available niches for the transplanted cells. In that respect, it is telling that successful bone marrow transplants require ablation of the bone marrow to kill off host cells occupying the niche before repopulation with transplanted cells. Nonetheless, the approach of killing off host cells occupying the niche is clearly not a feasible approach for many diseases, including Parkinson's. For some diseases, it has been speculated that a transplantation of stromal cell types might aid in rescuing tissue function through helping to generate a supportive niche for transplanted cells. For example, oligodendrocyte precursors for spinal cord injury have been demonstrated to release trophic factors after transplantation, which show positive effects on spinal cord neurons *in vitro* [72].

In addition to the lack of a supportive environment, the death of transplanted cells can also be mediated by the immune reaction of the host. Regenerative medicine encompasses a wide range of potential therapeutic strategies, from the transplantation of allogeneic replacement tissue generated *in vitro* to the use reprogrammed cells transplanted autologously, and potentially the *in vivo* transdifferentiation of supportive cells to perform the function of a disease cell type. The ability to avoid the use of immunotherapy is one of the reasons put forward in favour of autologous forms of treatment. However, many of the therapies that are closest to, or currently in, clinical trials are those that involve allogeneic grafts generated from hPSCs of a single cell line. In these circumstances, it is necessary to achieve immune tolerance of the graft, either through the use of immunosuppressive agents or other means. This may not necessarily be at the same high doses required for solid-organ transplantation and may not necessarily be life-long. In circumstances where the cells are transplanted to an immunologically privileged site such as the brain or the anterior chamber of the eye, a finite period of immunosuppression may be sufficient. An alternative to the use of immunosuppression may be the induction of tolerance. Recent work has indicated this may be possible to generate long-term tolerance to stem cell-derived grafts by using CD4/CD8 coreceptor and costimulation (CD40L) blockade with monoclonal antibodies given at the time of transplantation [73]. A further alternative strategy in development is the use of genetic engineering of the HLA locus to create a universal cell that is able to evade the alloimmune response [74]. With these developments, the issue of immunosuppression is not necessarily an overriding consideration and it will be of interest to see whether the advances in technologies supporting the efficient production of clinical-grade, regulator-approved, autologous iPSC lines outpaces the advances in strategies to obviate the need for immunosuppression in the allogeneic setting.

12.4.3 Safety of the hPSC-Derived Cellular Products

Safety of the hPSC-derived cell replacement therapies is at the forefront of concerns in the regenerative medicine field, with a particularly critical issue being the potential tumorigenicity of transplanted cells. This issue stems partly from the fact that the undifferentiated hPSCs have the ability to form teratomas when placed into ectopic sites in immunocompromised mice [24]. In this context, it is important to note that cell replacement therapies are based on using derivatives of hPSCs and not the undifferentiated cells *per se*. Thus, strategies for minimising the risk of remnant undifferentiated hPSCs following the differentiation, for example by sorting the cell populations or by eliminating undifferentiated cells through chemical treatment, should be effective in minimising the risk of teratomas. A similar strategy could be used for eliminating other unwanted cell types that may be present in a cellular preparation at the end of the differentiation protocol. It has been speculated that 'contaminating' cell types could also present a safety issue in some situations, particularly if they are transplanted to a tissue or a niche in which they do not typically reside [75]. Whilst efficient purifying and monitoring methods should alleviate the tumorigenic risk of undifferentiated hPSCs or contaminating cell types, more challenging to tackle is the potential tumorigenicity of hPSC-derived differentiated derivatives. The observation that hPSCs acquire genetic aberrations during culture [76] has raised concerns that some of the genetic changes may go undetected at both genotype and phenotype levels in hPSCs [77], but may confer malignant properties to differentiated derivatives when placed in an *in vivo* environment. Such a concern precipitated a halt of a clinical trial for age-related macular degeneration in Japan when patient-derived hiPSCs were found to contain several genetic changes that were not present in the somatic cells used for reprogramming [78]. In light of these findings, the scientists involved in the trial decided to err on the side of caution, thus suspending the trial and changing their strategy to using haplotype-matched donor cells [78]. The use of partially matched donor cells will allow extensive genetic characterisation of a large batch of cells which should be time- and cost-efficient compared to characterising individual patient-specific hiPSC lines. Nonetheless, the challenge remains to determine which genetic changes represent a potential safety issue for cellular replacement and which are merely innocuous genetic events. In addition to potential tumorigenicity, another risk factor for cellular therapies is the presence of adventitious agents and disease transmission from transplanted cells. Traditional sterilization is not applicable in case of cellular products, hence mitigating the risk of viral and bacterial transmission includes both testing for adventitious agents and manufacturing in compliance with Good Manufacturing Practice (GMP).

12.4.4 Regulatory Landscape

The challenges faced by developers of regenerative therapies do not end with the successful generation of a target cell type and the demonstration of efficacy in preclinical studies. To proceed to a Phase I clinical trial, approval for use of the therapy in humans is required from the relevant national or international regulatory bodies such as the US FDA or European EMA. In general terms, to satisfy regulatory requirements a cell therapy must have a production process that is well-controlled, reproducible and capable of generating a cell product within well-defined specifications. All reagents and processes must comply with clinical-grade Good Manufacturing Practices (GMP). In addition, the safety of the cell product must be demonstrated using data combined from animal studies, cell karyotyping or other genetic analyses, as well as testing using standard assays for sterility and adventitious agents. For cell products that have been derived from hPSCs, it is critical that the cell product is evaluated for tumorigenicity through the use of animal transplantation and biodistribution studies as well as flow cytometry or other single cell analyses to exclude the possibility of contamination of the final cell product with potentially oncogenic pluripotent cells.

Demonstrating safety and meeting regulatory requirements for a therapy in which the therapeutic agent is a population of living cells is, unsurprisingly, more difficult than a conventional pharmacological drug. The inherent heterogeneity of hPSC cultures and variability of differentiation procedures is a fundamental issue. Even in well-established clinical grade protocols, it remains difficult to completely eliminate all run-to-run variation. For allogeneic stem cell therapies, another challenge is the identification of a suitable source stem cell line. There are many requirements that need to be considered including whether the cell line was generated in clinical GMP conditions, whether the donor consented to use of the donated material for use in commercial product, the country of origin in relation to prion disease and other infectious risks, and whether the cell line carries any potentially harmful mutations. For example, it has recently been shown that some of the global hESC lines carry mutations in *TP53* (Merkle and Eggan, webinar https://www.stemcell.com/pluripotent-lounge). Whilst the final safety testing, cell production and quality control assays are performed in certified GMP and GLP laboratories, the development of these methods is performed in a standard research environment, usually in an iterative process until the necessary parameters are met to justify moving to the next phase with much higher associated costs (Fig. 12.2).

12.4.5 Regenerative Medicine: The Feasibility of Personalised Cell Products

The advent of techniques for generating induced pluripotent stem cells has given rise to much hope about the prospects for personalized cell therapies that are generated specifically for each individual patient and transplanted autologously, circumventing the need for immunosuppression. It is now technically possible to achieve this, but stem cell lines need to be generated for each individual patient, and these each need to individually pass through extensive safety testing and regulatory requirements before proceeding to transplantation. It is estimated that safety testing alone cost US$500,000 [79], with the total cost per patient estimated to be US$1,000,000. This was the approach attempted by a clinical trial based at the RIKEN Institute in Japan for the treatment of age-related macular degeneration, which was halted due to mutations detected in hiPSCs of one of the patients [80]. The suspension of the trial brought sharply into focus the fact that, at the present time, the logistical and financial challenges of developing an autologous hPSC-based therapy are very significant. This does not necessarily mean that the barriers will remain as high. With technical advances and improving understanding, personalised cell therapies may become a more feasible option in the future, with many research groups focussed on this as an objective.

12.5 Concluding Remarks

Regenerative medicine is on the cusp of transforming healthcare by delivering curative treatments for many life-threatening or debilitating diseases. The major driving force behind the dynamic evolution of regenerative medicine has been the remarkable progress in the field of stem

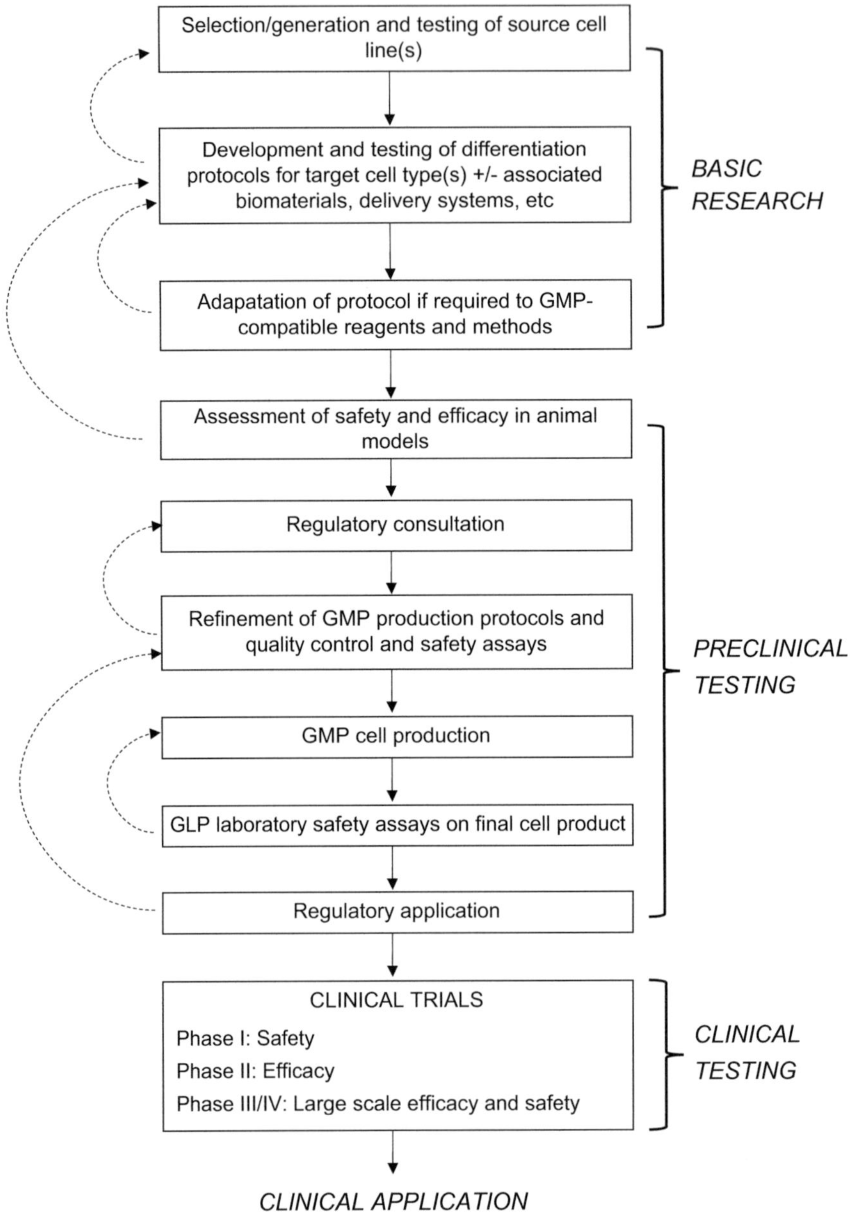

Fig. 12.2 Flow chart of typical steps in development of cell therapy products. Starting with basic biology experiments, which encompass development of differentiation protocols and *in vitro* characterisation of differentiated cells, the process is continued by testing the safety and functionality of derived cells in animal models *in vivo*. Positive outcome of pre-clinical testing provides a base for clinical trials in humans. The *dashed lines* represent iterative loops that may be necessary to optimize the final product

cells and related technologies. If we look forward, it seems that the rate-limiting step for the development of cell replacement therapies will not be the production of desired cell types, but rather, translation of the developments from an academic into the clinical setting. Unlike drug discovery, which has a well-established manufacturing and regulatory trajectory, when it comes to hPSC-derived cell replacement therapies, we are navigating unchartered waters, full of unforeseen scientific, manufacturing, regulatory and funding complexities. Nonetheless, the preliminary results of the safety studies are encouraging and the prospects for the hPSC-derived cellular therapies appear positive. As highlighted in this review, several hurdles are still hampering the translation but they are surmountable. The continuation of efforts to develop a sound translational framework will undoubtedly help regenerative medicine to deliver its full potential and become an important part of modern healthcare.

Acknowledgements We would like to thank Dr Paul J. Gokhale for critical reading of the manuscript. NFB and IB are supported by the UK Regenerative Medicine Platform (grant number MR/L012537/1). IB is also funded by the Medical Research Council (grant number MR/N009371/1) and the European Union's Horizon 2020 research and innovation programme under grant agreement No 668724.

References

1. Mason C, Dunnill P (2008) A brief definition of regenerative medicine. Regen Med 3:1–5. doi:10.2217/17460751.3.1.1
2. Nikolich-Zugich J et al (2016) Preparing for an aging world: engaging biogerontologists, geriatricians, and the society. J Gerontol A Biol Sci Med Sci 71:435–444. doi:10.1093/gerona/glv164
3. Burt RK et al (2008) Clinical applications of blood-derived and marrow-derived stem cells for nonmalignant diseases. JAMA 299:925–936. doi:10.1001/jama.299.8.925
4. Moore KA, Lemischka IR (2006) Stem cells and their niches. Science 311:1880–1885. doi:10.1126/science.1110542
5. Evans MJ, Kaufman MH (1981) Establishment in culture of pluripotential cells from mouse embryos. Nature 292:154–156
6. Martin GR (1981) Isolation of a pluripotent cell line from early mouse embryos cultured in medium conditioned by teratocarcinoma stem cells. Proc Natl Acad Sci U S A 78:7634–7638
7. Thomson JA et al (1998) Embryonic stem cell lines derived from human blastocysts. Science 282:1145–1147
8. Till JE, Mc CE (1961) A direct measurement of the radiation sensitivity of normal mouse bone marrow cells. Radiat Res 14:213–222
9. Becker AJ, Mc CE, Till JE (1963) Cytological demonstration of the clonal nature of spleen colonies derived from transplanted mouse marrow cells. Nature 197:452–454
10. Thomas ED (1999) A history of haemopoietic cell transplantation. Br J Haematol 105:330–339
11. Osawa M, Hanada K, Hamada H, Nakauchi H (1996) Long-term lymphohematopoietic reconstitution by a single CD34-low/negative hematopoietic stem cell. Science 273:242–245
12. Majeti R, Park CY, Weissman IL (2007) Identification of a hierarchy of multipotent hematopoietic progenitors in human cord blood. Cell Stem Cell 1:635–645. doi:10.1016/j.stem.2007.10.001
13. Barker N, van de Wetering M, Clevers H (2008) The intestinal stem cell. Genes Dev 22:1856–1864. doi:10.1101/gad.1674008
14. Potten CS, Kovacs L, Hamilton E (1974) Continuous labelling studies on mouse skin and intestine. Cell Tissue Kinet 7:271–283
15. Barker N, Clevers H (2007) Tracking down the stem cells of the intestine: strategies to identify adult stem cells. Gastroenterology 133:1755–1760. doi:10.1053/j.gastro.2007.10.029
16. Sato T et al (2009) Single Lgr5 stem cells build crypt-villus structures in vitro without a mesenchymal niche. Nature 459:262–265. doi:10.1038/nature07935
17. Eriksson PS et al (1998) Neurogenesis in the adult human hippocampus. Nat Med 4:1313–1317. doi:10.1038/3305
18. Lois C, Alvarez-Buylla A (1993) Proliferating subventricular zone cells in the adult mammalian forebrain can differentiate into neurons and glia. Proc Natl Acad Sci U S A 90:2074–2077
19. Casarosa S, Bozzi Y, Conti L (2014) Neural stem cells: ready for therapeutic applications? Mol Cell Ther 2:31. doi:10.1186/2052-8426-2-31
20. Tabar V, Studer L (2014) Pluripotent stem cells in regenerative medicine: challenges and recent progress. Nat Rev Genet 15:82–92. doi:10.1038/nrg3563
21. Takahashi K et al (2007) Induction of pluripotent stem cells from adult human fibroblasts by defined factors. Cell 131:861–872. doi:10.1016/j.cell.2007.11.019
22. International Stem Cell, I et al (2007) Characterization of human embryonic stem cell lines by the International Stem Cell Initiative. Nat Biotechnol 25:803–816. doi:10.1038/nbt1318
23. Hentze H et al (2009) Teratoma formation by human embryonic stem cells: evaluation of essential parameters for future safety studies. Stem Cell Res 2:198–210. doi:10.1016/j.scr.2009.02.002
24. Damjanov I, Andrews PW (2016) Teratomas produced from human pluripotent stem cells xenografted into immunodeficient mice – a histopathology atlas. Int J Dev Biol 60:337–419. doi:10.1387/ijdb.160274id
25. Murry CE, Keller G (2008) Differentiation of embryonic stem cells to clinically relevant populations: lessons from embryonic development. Cell 132:661–680. doi:10.1016/j.cell.2008.02.008
26. Osafune K et al (2008) Marked differences in differentiation propensity among human embryonic stem cell lines. Nat Biotechnol 26:313–315. doi:10.1038/nbt1383

27. Wichterle H, Lieberam I, Porter JA, Jessell TM (2002) Directed differentiation of embryonic stem cells into motor neurons. Cell 110:385–397
28. Williams LA, Davis-Dusenbery BN, Eggan KC (2012) SnapShot: directed differentiation of pluripotent stem cells. Cell 149:1174–1174 e1171. doi:10.1016/j.cell.2012.05.015
29. Trounson A, DeWitt ND (2016) Pluripotent stem cells progressing to the clinic. Nat Rev Mol Cell Biol 17:194–200. doi:10.1038/nrm.2016.10
30. Varma AK et al (2013) Spinal cord injury: a review of current therapy, future treatments, and basic science frontiers. Neurochem Res 38:895–905. doi:10.1007/s11064-013-0991-6
31. Irvine KA, Blakemore WF (2008) Remyelination protects axons from demyelination-associated axon degeneration. Brain 131:1464–1477. doi:10.1093/brain/awn080
32. Faulkner J, Keirstead HS (2005) Human embryonic stem cell-derived oligodendrocyte progenitors for the treatment of spinal cord injury. Transpl Immunol 15:131–142. doi:10.1016/j.trim.2005.09.007
33. Nistor GI, Totoiu MO, Haque N, Carpenter MK, Keirstead HS (2005) Human embryonic stem cells differentiate into oligodendrocytes in high purity and myelinate after spinal cord transplantation. Glia 49:385–396. doi:10.1002/glia.20127
34. Yasuda A et al (2011) Significance of remyelination by neural stem/progenitor cells transplanted into the injured spinal cord. Stem Cells 29:1983–1994. doi:10.1002/stem.767
35. All AH et al (2015) Early intervention for spinal cord injury with human induced pluripotent stem cells oligodendrocyte progenitors. PLoS One 10:e0116933. doi:10.1371/journal.pone.0116933
36. Lebkowski J (2011) GRNOPC1: the world's first embryonic stem cell-derived therapy. Interview with Jane Lebkowski. Regen Med 6:11–13. doi:10.2217/rme.11.77
37. Baker M (2011) Stem-cell pioneer bows out. Nature 479:459. doi:10.1038/479459a
38. de Lau LM, Breteler MM (2006) Epidemiology of Parkinson's disease. Lancet Neurol 5:525–535. doi:10.1016/S1474-4422(06)70471-9
39. Hely MA et al (1999) The sydney multicentre study of Parkinson's disease: progression and mortality at 10 years. J Neurol Neurosurg Psychiatry 67:300–307
40. Barker RA, Drouin-Ouellet J, Parmar M (2015) Cell-based therapies for Parkinson disease-past insights and future potential. Nat Rev Neurol 11:492–503. doi:10.1038/nrneurol.2015.123
41. Kefalopoulou Z et al (2014) Long-term clinical outcome of fetal cell transplantation for Parkinson disease: two case reports. JAMA Neurol 71:83–87. doi:10.1001/jamaneurol.2013.4749
42. Kriks S et al (2011) Dopamine neurons derived from human ES cells efficiently engraft in animal models of Parkinson's disease. Nature 480:547–551. doi:10.1038/nature10648
43. Grealish S et al (2014) Human ESC-derived dopamine neurons show similar preclinical efficacy and potency to fetal neurons when grafted in a rat model of Parkinson's disease. Cell Stem Cell 15:653–665. doi:10.1016/j.stem.2014.09.017
44. Barker RA, Studer L, Cattaneo E, Takahashi J (2015) G-Force PD: a global initiative in coordinating stem cell-based dopamine treatments for Parkinson's disease. Npj Parkinson's Disease 1:15017. doi:10.1038/npjparkd.2015.17
45. Li W et al (2016) Extensive graft-derived dopaminergic innervation is maintained 24 years after transplantation in the degenerating parkinsonian brain. Proc Natl Acad Sci U S A 113:6544–6549. doi:10.1073/pnas.1605245113
46. Morizane A, Takahashi J (2016) Cell therapy for Parkinson's disease. Neurol Med Chir (Tokyo) 56:102–109. doi:10.2176/nmc.ra.2015-0303
47. Scudellari M (2016) How iPS cells changed the world. Nature 534:310–312. doi:10.1038/534310a
48. Barker RA et al (2016) Are stem cell-based therapies for Parkinson's disease ready for the clinic in 2016? J Parkinsons Dis 6:57–63. doi:10.3233/JPD-160798
49. McKeown SJ, Stamp L, Hao MM, Young HM (2013) Hirschsprung disease: a developmental disorder of the enteric nervous system. Wiley Interdiscip Rev Dev Biol 2:113–129. doi:10.1002/wdev.57
50. Sasselli V, Pachnis V, Burns AJ (2012) The enteric nervous system. Dev Biol 366:64–73. doi:10.1016/j.ydbio.2012.01.012
51. Lake JI, Heuckeroth RO (2013) Enteric nervous system development: migration, differentiation, and disease. Am J Physiol Gastrointest Liver Physiol 305:G1–24. doi:10.1152/ajpgi.00452.2012
52. Burns AJ et al (2016) White paper on guidelines concerning enteric nervous system stem cell therapy for enteric neuropathies. Dev Biol 417:229–251. doi:10.1016/j.ydbio.2016.04.001
53. Burns AJ, Thapar N (2014) Neural stem cell therapies for enteric nervous system disorders. Nat Rev Gastroenterol Hepatol 11:317–328. doi:10.1038/nrgastro.2013.226
54. Bondurand N, Natarajan D, Thapar N, Atkins C, Pachnis V (2003) Neuron and glia generating progenitors of the mammalian enteric nervous system isolated from foetal and postnatal gut cultures. Development 130:6387–6400. doi:10.1242/dev.00857
55. Cooper JE et al (2016) In vivo transplantation of enteric neural crest cells into mouse gut; engraftment, functional integration and long-term safety. PLoS One 11:e0147989. doi:10.1371/journal.pone.0147989
56. Fattahi F et al (2016) Deriving human ENS lineages for cell therapy and drug discovery in Hirschsprung disease. Nature 531:105–109. doi:10.1038/nature16951
57. Workman MJ et al (2017) Engineered human pluripotent-stem-cell-derived intestinal tissues with a functional enteric nervous system. Nat Med 23:49–59. doi:10.1038/nm.4233

58. Xu B et al (2013) Non-linear elasticity of core/shell spun PGS/PLLA fibres and their effect on cell proliferation. Biomaterials 34:6306–6317. doi:10.1016/j.biomaterials.2013.05.009
59. Burridge PW et al (2014) Chemically defined generation of human cardiomyocytes. Nat Methods 11:855–860. doi:10.1038/nmeth.2999
60. Lippmann ES, Estevez-Silva MC, Ashton RS (2014) Defined human pluripotent stem cell culture enables highly efficient neuroepithelium derivation without small molecule inhibitors. Stem Cells 32:1032–1042. doi:10.1002/stem.1622
61. Bao X, Lian X, Palecek SP (2016) Directed endothelial progenitor differentiation from human pluripotent stem cells via Wnt activation under defined conditions. Methods Mol Biol 1481:183–196. doi:10.1007/978-1-4939-6393-5_17
62. Cheung C, Bernardo AS, Trotter MW, Pedersen RA, Sinha S (2012) Generation of human vascular smooth muscle subtypes provides insight into embryological origin-dependent disease susceptibility. Nat Biotechnol 30:165–173. doi:10.1038/nbt.2107
63. Jonsson MK et al (2012) Application of human stem cell-derived cardiomyocytes in safety pharmacology requires caution beyond hERG. J Mol Cell Cardiol 52:998–1008. doi:10.1016/j.yjmcc.2012.02.002
64. van den Berg CW et al (2015) Transcriptome of human foetal heart compared with cardiomyocytes from pluripotent stem cells. Development 142:3231–3238. doi:10.1242/dev.123810
65. Berger DR, Ware BR, Davidson MD, Allsup SR, Khetani SR (2015) Enhancing the functional maturity of induced pluripotent stem cell-derived human hepatocytes by controlled presentation of cell-cell interactions in vitro. Hepatology 61:1370–1381. doi:10.1002/hep.27621
66. Hrvatin S et al (2014) Differentiated human stem cells resemble fetal, not adult, beta cells. Proc Natl Acad Sci U S A 111:3038–3043. doi:10.1073/pnas.1400709111
67. Cornacchia D, Studer L (2017) Back and forth in time: directing age in iPSC-derived lineages. Brain Res 1656:14–26. doi:10.1016/j.brainres.2015.11.013
68. Wu H et al (2007) Integrative genomic and functional analyses reveal neuronal subtype differentiation bias in human embryonic stem cell lines. Proc Natl Acad Sci U S A 104:13821–13826. doi:10.1073/pnas.0706199104
69. Nishizawa M et al (2016) Epigenetic variation between human induced pluripotent stem cell lines is an indicator of differentiation capacity. Cell Stem Cell 19:341–354. doi:10.1016/j.stem.2016.06.019
70. Gu E, Chen WY, Gu J, Burridge P, Wu JC (2012) Molecular imaging of stem cells: tracking survival, biodistribution, tumorigenicity, and immunogenicity. Theranostics 2:335–345. doi:10.7150/thno.3666
71. van Laake LW, Passier R, Doevendans PA, Mummery CL (2008) Human embryonic stem cell-derived cardiomyocytes and cardiac repair in rodents. Circ Res 102:1008–1010. doi:10.1161/CIRCRESAHA.108.175505
72. Zhang YW, Denham J, Thies RS (2006) Oligodendrocyte progenitor cells derived from human embryonic stem cells express neurotrophic factors. Stem Cells Dev 15:943–952. doi:10.1089/scd.2006.15.943
73. Lui KO et al (2014) Tolerance induction to human stem cell transplants with extension to their differentiated progeny. Nat Commun 5:5629. doi:10.1038/ncomms6629
74. Figueiredo C, Blasczyk R (2015) A future with less HLA: potential clinical applications of HLA-universal cells. Tissue Antigens 85:443–449. doi:10.1111/tan.12564
75. Goldring CE et al (2011) Assessing the safety of stem cell therapeutics. Cell Stem Cell 8:618–628. doi:10.1016/j.stem.2011.05.012
76. Draper JS et al (2004) Recurrent gain of chromosomes 17q and 12 in cultured human embryonic stem cells. Nat Biotechnol 22:53–54. doi:10.1038/nbt922
77. Baker D et al (2016) Detecting genetic mosaicism in cultures of human pluripotent stem cells. Stem Cell Rep 7:998–1012. doi:10.1016/j.stemcr.2016.10.003
78. Garber K (2015) RIKEN suspends first clinical trial involving induced pluripotent stem cells. Nat Biotechnol 33:890–891. doi:10.1038/nbt0915-890
79. Chakradhar S (2016) An eye to the future: researchers debate best path for stem cell-derived therapies. Nat Med 22:116–119. doi:10.1038/nm0216-116
80. Cyranoski D (2014) Japanese woman is first recipient of next-generation stem cells. Nature. doi:10.1038/nature.2014.15915

Gene Therapy in the Nervous System: Failures and Successes

13

Jayanth S. Chandran, Joseph M. Scarrott, Pamela J. Shaw, and Mimoun Azzouz

Abstract

Genetic disorders, caused by deleterious changes in the DNA sequence away from the normal genomic sequence, affect millions of people worldwide. Gene therapy as a treatment option for patients is an attractive proposition due to its conceptual simplicity. In principle, gene therapy involves correcting the genetic disorder by either restoring a normal functioning copy of a gene or reducing the toxicity arising from a mutated gene. In this way specific genetic function can be restored without altering the expression of other genes and the proteins they encode. The reality however is much more complex, and as a result the vector systems used to deliver gene therapies have by necessity continued to evolve and improve over time with respect to safety profile, efficiency, and long-term expression. In this chapter we examine the current approaches to gene therapy, assess the different gene delivery systems utilized, and highlight the failures and successes of relevant clinical trials. We do not intend for this chapter to be a comprehensive and exhaustive assessment of all clinical trials that have been conducted in the CNS, but instead will focus on specific diseases that have seen successes and failures with different gene therapy vehicles to gauge how preclinical models have informed the design of clinical trials.

Keywords

Adeno-associated virus • Gene therapy • CNS • Neurodegenerative disease • Antisense oligonucleotides

13.1 Introduction

More than 25 years have passed since two key clinical trials demonstrated the potential of gene therapy: (1) In 1989, five patients with melanoma safely tolerated an infusion of tumour-infiltrating

J.S. Chandran • J.M. Scarrott • P.J. Shaw
M. Azzouz (✉)
Sheffield Institute for Translational Neuroscience, University of Sheffield,
385a Glossop Road, Sheffield S10 2HQ, UK
e-mail: m.azzouz@sheffield.ac.uk

S. El-Khamisy (ed.), *Personalised Medicine*, Advances in Experimental Medicine and Biology 1007,
DOI 10.1007/978-3-319-60733-7_13

lymphocytes that had been conferred resistance to neomycin with a retrovirus [1]; (2) In 1990, two children with severe combined immune deficiency (SCID) were treated with a retrovirally-mediated transfer of adenosine deaminase which resulted in stabilized number of blood T cells [2]. The intervening years have seen a massive increase in gene therapy clinical trials, with more than 2200 clinical trials approved as of 2016 (http://www.wiley.co.uk/genmed/clinical), and at least three gene therapies (Glybera (uniQure), Imlygic (Amgen), Strimvelis (Glaxosmithkline)) were approved by government regulatory commissions. We will solely focus on gene therapy alternatives for treating diseases of the central nervous system (CNS), and would recommend several other excellent reviews describing gene therapy outcomes in other tissues [3, 4].

The brain provides an added layer of complexity with respect to targeting due to the presence of the blood-brain barrier (BBB), composed of dynamic tight junctions formed between adjacent endothelial cells, which restricts particles from diffusing into the brain from the blood [5]. This barrier is a major roadblock to any gene therapy treatment option since it blocks >98% of all therapeutics [6] and effectively forces gene therapy vehicles to either be administered directly to the CNS, or have the ability to cross the BBB when infused systemically. A range of delivery vectors, which fall into two major classes (viral and non-viral) continue to be developed to more efficiently target the CNS (Fig. 13.1).

13.2 Viral Vectors

Viral vectors have always been a natural focal point with regards to gene therapy since viruses have evolved over millions of years to efficiently deliver genetic material to a host cell. The majority (~65%, http://www.wiley.co.uk/genmed/clinical) of all clinical trials employ a viral vector for gene delivery, with adenovirus (21.4%) and retrovirus (18.2%) used in more than half of the viral gene therapies. For targeting the CNS, however, adeno-associated viruses (AAVs) have emerged as a strong option due to their minimal toxicity, very low rate of genomic integration [7], and ability to transduce both dividing and post-mitotic cells. Each of the major viral vectors have individual strengths and limitations which make them more or less appropriate for specific therapeutic strategies:

13.2.1 Retrovirus

Retroviruses are a family of enveloped RNA viruses that stably integrate into a host genome following reverse-transcription of the RNA into a double-stranded DNA intermediate. Retroviruses can be classified into seven distinct genera, although only γ-retrovirus (derived from Moloney murine leukaemia virus; MoMLV) and lentivirus (derived from Human immunodeficiency virus 1; HIV-1) are routinely used in gene therapy clinical trials targeting CNS disorders [8]. Retroviral vectors based on MoMLV were among the first used in gene therapy clinical trials, and have a clear advantage over currently used DNA viruses in that they offer sustained expression of a transgene due to host genome integration. Their packaging capacity (between 7 and 9 kb) is restricted in comparison to adenoviruses (which can tolerate more than 30 kb) [9], but larger than AAVs (packaging capacity of 4 kb) [10, 11], making them suitable for a range of genetic targets.

There are, however, several major disadvantages to retroviral vectors that preclude them from being used extensively for CNS therapy. Firstly, MoMLV derived retroviral vectors only transduce dividing cells, which makes them a poor option for modifying post-mitotic cells like neurons. Secondly, retroviral vectors are produced at low titers (10^8 infectious units (IU)/ml) [10] relative to adenoviruses (10^{12} IU/ml) [10, 11] and AAVs (10^9 IU/ml) [12], making them less efficient and increasing the risk of off-target effects arising from high dosages. The biggest drawback, however, is the risk of oncogenesis stemming from the virus randomly integrating into a proto-oncogene promoter or close to a tumour suppressor gene in the host genome, a condition termed *insertional mutagenesis*. A

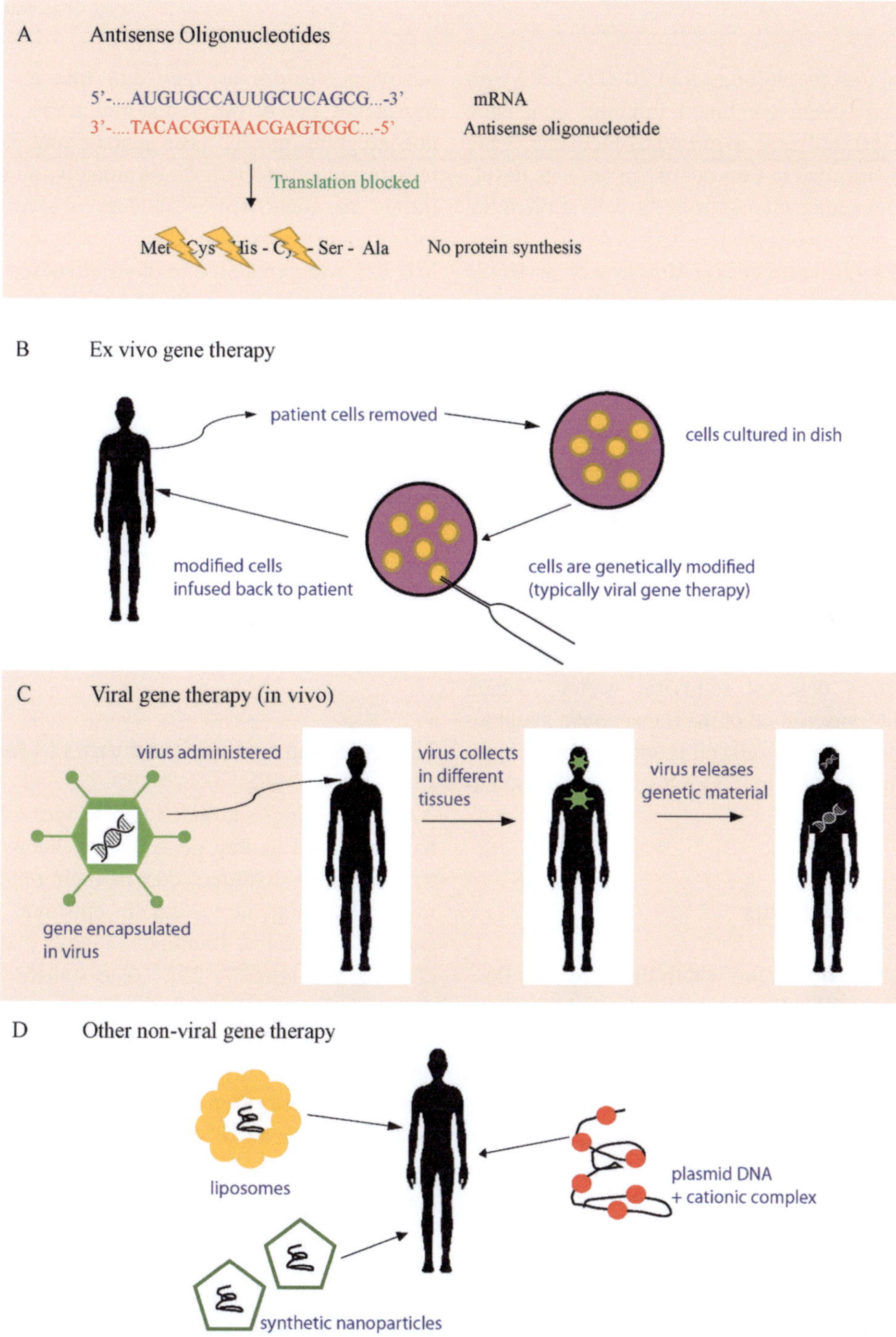

Fig. 13.1 Gene therapy options currently in preclinical and/or clinical trials. (**a**) Antisense oligonucleotides have become increasingly popular due to the ease of synthesis, and the specificity of the target. Antisense DNA is synthesized to bind to an mRNA target to either block protein synthesis, prevent mis-splicing events, or activate synthesis by binding to the promoter. (**b**) Ex-vivo gene therapies are frequently used in clinical trials and typically utilize a two-step process involving extraction of patient cells and modification of the cellular genome mediated by a virus, followed by administration of 'corrected' cells back to the patient. (**c**) In-vivo viral gene therapies can utilize a variety of viral vectors which contain a therapeutic gene of interest and are delivered to the patient allowing the virus to release the therapeutic genetic material inside the cell. (**d**) An increasing number of other non-viral gene therapy approaches continue to be developed to avoid toxicity associated with viral options. Such alternative vehicles include liposomes encasing the therapeutic genetic material, naked DNA directly injected into patients when in a complex with a cationic polymer such as PEI (polyethylenimine), and synthetic nanoparticles which are assembled around the gene.

clinical trial for children from 2000 to 2002 with X-linked severe combined immune deficiency (X-SCID) utilizing γ-retroviral-mediated gene therapy resulted in four out of ten patients developing leukemia, arising from the activation of the *LM02* proto-oncogene [13–15]. A similar activation of proto-oncogenes (*LM02* as well as *MDS1* and *MN1*) occurred more recently, however, in a clinical trial for Wiskott-Aldrich syndrome [16] again using γ-retrovirus, and seven out of 10 patients developed an acute leukemia. Several modifications of retroviral vectors have been introduced to enhance its safety profile. Engineering self-inactivating (SIN) retroviral vectors, which only transcribe the target gene with an internal promoter once the virus integrates into the genome and thereby minimize activation of endogenous oncogenes, may attenuate the onset of leukemogenesis [17]. The use of replication deficient retroviral vectors, which prevent transcription of the transgene in daughter cells of the transduced cell is another safety modification intended to reduce the oncogenic potential of the virus.

13.2.2 Lentivirus

While lentiviruses are within the retrovirus family, they can mediate gene transfer to both dividing and post-mitotic cells, and can be purified to higher titers (1×10^{10} TU/ml) than γ-retrovirus when pseudotyped with vesicular stomatitis virus G envelope protein (VSV-G) [18]. There are two key disadvantages to using lentiviral vectors in CNS therapies: (1) lentiviral particles do not diffuse across long distances limiting their applications in vivo [19]; (2) lentiviruses integrate within the host genome which poses a risk of oncogenesis, although the safety profile continues to improve through SIN vectors and mapping of lentiviral integration sites [20].

13.2.3 Adenovirus

Adenoviruses, which are double-stranded DNA viruses, offer several major advantages over retroviral vectors as they can tolerate large transgenes, can be purified at high titers, and do not integrate into the host genome and instead remain episomal [10]. Unfortunately, administration of adenoviruses induces a significant inflammatory response leading to cytotoxicity [21, 22], which resulted in the death of a patient in a clinical trial for ornithine transcarbamylase deficiency [23]. Developing modifications of the adenoviral particles either through peptide conjugation to the capsid or deletion of select transcription factors to reduce the immune response is an active area of research which will hopefully yield a safer next-generation set of vectors [24]. Adenoviruses, however, remain an important gene therapy vector for treating brain cancers such as gliomas (discussed later in this chapter) in which tumours can be targeted through an immune response.

13.2.4 Adeno-associated Virus (AAV)

AAVs are single-stranded DNA viruses that have emerged as key gene therapy vectors for treating CNS disorders due to their relatively minimal pathogenicity, largely episomal replication, and the low immune response that they elicit in the host [7, 25]. Gene transfer from AAV vectors occurs in both mitotic and post-mitotic cells, and while transgene expression remains stable in the brain for at least 10 years, it is diluted away from mitotic cells. The strongest point in favor of AAV usage in CNS gene therapy is that at least eight different serotypes can cross the blood-brain barrier when administered intravenously, which obviates the need for invasive delivery into the brain [26]. The key limitation of AAV vectors is the packaging capacity, as single stranded vectors can tolerate only 4.5 kb, with the more efficient self-complementary vectors restricted to 2.2 kb [27]. This excludes many simple gene replacement options, though with the advent of CRISPR/Cas9 genome editing [28, 29] it may be possible to correct loss-of-function mutations through homology-directed recombination of a corrected mutation mediated by AAVs.

13.3 Non-viral Vectors

13.3.1 Antisense Oligonucleotides

Antisense oligonucleotides (ASOs) are short sequences that are chemically modified to enhance stability and binding to an mRNA target, and as a result can activate gene expression by binding to a promoter [30, 31], prevent an unwanted splicing event, or degrade an mRNA target, thereby preventing protein synthesis [32]. Additionally, they are inexpensive to synthesize and purify, and can theoretically be tailored to an infinite range of genetic manipulations. The principal safety issues arising from the use of ASOs are toxicity associated with off-target effects [33] and thrombocytopenia [34], which has been noted in a few clinical trials. ASOs do not cross the blood-brain barrier, and therefore must be delivered directly into the CNS [32] for treating CNS disorders, which when coupled with the likely need for multiple ASO administrations over the course of the therapy increases the risk to the patient.

13.3.2 Naked DNA

An increasing number of gene therapy trials have opted to simply inject naked plasmid DNA with or without a cationic polymer directly into tissue. Naked uncomplexed DNA is the simplest system, but technically challenging to achieve widespread transduction as a gene therapy tool, since high pressure has to be applied to force the DNA into cells. Forming chemical complexes between the naked DNA and cationic polymers such as polyethylenimine (PEI), however, enhances cell entry as the polymer condenses the DNA, enabling it to endocytose into the cell as a DNA:polymer complex before the DNA is released from the complex in the cytoplasm [35, 36]. The low cost and simplicity of the method are obvious advantages to using naked DNA, and intranasal and intramuscular delivery routes to achieve CNS expression are feasible [37, 38]. The disadvantages include toxicity associated with high concentrations of PEI [39] and poor overall transgene expression.

13.3.3 Liposomes and Synthetic Nanoparticles

Liposomes are lipids that self-assemble with negatively charged DNA, and are a significant delivery vehicle in current gene therapy clinical trials. The majority of liposomes used in clinical trial gene therapies are based on cationic lipids, which promote fusion with cell plasma membranes and allow DNA to diffuse into the cell [40]. Nanoparticles consisting of synthetic polymers act in a similar way to liposomes as they can self-assemble around DNA and form a complex akin to a micelle which can fuse with cell membranes [41]. The advantage of these synthetic self-assembled complexes are that they are inexpensive to generate relative to viral vectors, and can be targeted to specific cell types by fusing peptide ligands onto the surface of the lipid/polymer. A similar approach can also be used to promote diffusion across the blood-brain barrier and avoid the intracranial administration of these particles. The disadvantage of the liposomes and nanoparticle polymers is that transfection efficiency is much lower than viral vector options and that liposomes induce a significant innate immune response [42].

13.4 Lessons from Clinical Trials

13.4.1 Gliomablastoma Multiforme

Glioblastoma multiforme (GBM) is the most common and most malignant tumour found in the CNS [43]. GBM has a poor prognosis, with only 3% of diagnosed patients surviving longer than 5 years [44, 45]. Therapy is normally restricted to tumour excision followed by intensive chemotherapy and radiation. Occasionally a subpopulation of cells in the tumour microenvironment, which behave as stem cells and are often referred to as cancer stem cells, can resist the effects of radiation and chemotherapy and proliferate at a later time to form secondary tumours [46–49]. As a consequence, there is an increasing emphasis on targeting these drug resistant cells through either pharmacological or genetic therapies. The genetic and epigenetic heterogeneity of GBM across all patients has precluded simple gene replacement therapy approaches, and several trials have instead focused on killing tumours by expressing the suicide gene Herpes Simplex Virus-1 Thymidine Kinase (HSV-TK), originally proposed by Moolten more than 30 years ago [50]. The premise of such a therapy is simple: destroy a tumour while sparing the CNS. The majority of the first wave of gene therapy clinical trials for glioma expressed the HSV-TK in an adenovirus or a retrovirus. The first large scale trial (248 patients) showed that the retroviral mediated HSV-TK expression was well tolerated and without adverse effects, but did not show any significant improvements in survival compared to controls, likely due to poor transgene expression within the tumour [51]. A similar overall conclusion was reached in several other clinical trials employing a retrovirus to express HSV-TK, although there were patients in each study that did appear free of recurring tumours several years later [52–54]. Of concern, however, were adverse effects observed in patients in two separate trials that ranged from seizures to serious neurological episodes, and which may have been related to the choice to carry out two intracranial injections of retroviral particles separated by a duration of 1 week [52, 55]. The major caveat of retroviral based glioma therapy appears to be the difficulty of achieving a high transduction efficiency in the tumours.

Adenoviral vector mediated suicide therapy has been used extensively since the first trial in 2000 with 21 patients, which directly compared HSV-TK gene transfer from a non-replicating adenovirus with a retrovirus and showed a significantly longer survival time with the adenoviral therapy [56]. A larger study with 36 patients showed that the HSV-TK gene transfer with a similar adenovirus extended the median life span of patients by an average of 6 months compared to standard surgery and radiation therapy suggesting that adenoviral vectors were capable of targeting intracranial tumours more efficiently than retroviral vectors [57]. Poor transgene expression with the non-replicative adenovirus restricts their potential in patients, however, and makes it more difficult to target all the cells within a tumour. Additionally, tumour cells express a low level of coxsackievirus and adenovirus receptor (CAR), which the adenovirus uses to bind to and enter the host cell, reducing transduction efficiency [58, 59].

Conditionally replicative adenoviruses (CRAds) are a gene therapy tool developed with the aim of selectively transducing and replicating within tumour cells, destroying them through cytolysis whilst leaving healthy cells unaffected. Two widely studied CRAds, ONYX-015 and Ad5-Delta24, were developed to target more cells within a tumour, though their mechanisms are distinct. Loss-of-function mutations in the tumour suppressors Retinoblastoma protein (Rb) and protein 53 (p53) lead to GBM due to uncontrolled proliferation. Adenovirus E1A and E1B proteins normally bind to and inactivate Rb and p53, and therefore prevent cellular apoptosis. ONYX-015 replicates in tumours deficient in p53 by lacking a functional adenovirus E1B gene, preventing translation of a 55 kda protein (E1B-55 K) that inactivates p53 and inhibits apoptosis [60, 61], though the specific relationship between E1B-55K and p53 remain unclear [62]. Delta24 replicates in tumours with impaired retinoblastoma (Rb) function due to a 24-bp deletion in the adenovirus E1 protein that disrupts binding to Rb protein [63, 64].

The first clinical trials utilizing ONYX-015 showed that intratumoural injection of the CRAd was tolerated by 24 patients without serious adverse effects [65], which has been supported by other studies using ONYX-015 to treat advanced sarcomas [66] and colorectal cancer [67]. A clinical trial has recently completed with the Ad5-Delta24 therapy to treat glioma, and although data from the phase 1 trial remains unpublished, the company running the trial (DNAtrix, Inc) was recently awarded a $2 million grant from the Food Drugs Administration (FDA) Orphan Products Development to support a phase 2 trial suggesting a favourable outcome from phase 1. In this trial, a short Arg-Gly-Asp (RGD) peptide was inserted onto the adenoviral capsid to diversify the binding sites on the host tumour cells and bias the CRAd towards αV integrin receptors that are abundant on the cell surface, which had been shown in preclinical models to enhance tumour cell death [68–70].

Several trials using other viruses that are modified to become conditionally replicative (termed oncolytic viruses; OVs) have been used to target glioma tumours. The best characterized of these OVs, known as G207, is an HSV-1 vector genetically altered to remove most of the virulent domains and induce replication in solely mitotic cells. G207 appears to be well tolerated in patients but has only modest effects as a therapy [71–74].

There have also been several clinical trials using non-viral gene therapy options to target GBM which are attractive options since they do not necessarily depend on a poorly expressed host receptor. A focal delivery through a small diameter catheter inserted intratumourally of an HSV-TK plasmid packaged within cationic liposomes was tolerated by patients in a small study, with half (4/8 patients) showing at least a 50% reduction in tumour volume [75]. A replication incompetent Semliki forest virus vector (SFV) carrying the human interleukin 12 (*IL*-12) gene packaged within cationic liposomes (LSFV-IL12) is in a phase I/II clinical trial for GMB, and based on previous use of LSFV-IL12 to treat melanoma and renal carcinoma is likely to be well tolerated [76]. Antisense oligonucleotides designed to inhibit transforming growth factor-beta 2 (TGF-β2), a cytokine that promotes tumour metastasis, have shown a promising median survival extension in patients with grade III glioma but has not been beneficial to patients with GBM [77, 78]. What is especially promising, however, is that patients in both the grade III glioma group and the GBM group reacted less adversely to their chemotherapy treatment when it was administered along with these convection-enhanced delivery ASOs, indicating that the ASOs may exert a positive secondary effect even if the median survival benefit is minimal [77].

13.4.2 Motor Neuron Disease

Motor neuron disease, otherwise known as amyotrophic lateral sclerosis (ALS), is a neurodegenerative disease that involves the selective degeneration of the upper and lower motor neurons, leading to progressive muscle atrophy [79]. ALS is unfailingly fatal, with no significant therapeutic options available, and death typically occurs 3–5 years from onset of disease. The current frontline treatment for ALS is riluzole, an anti-glutamatergic drug that extends survival by ~3–4 months [80]. The majority of ALS cases (90%) are sporadic in nature with the remaining 10% having a hereditary component [79].

A number of gene therapy approaches have been proposed regarding the treatment of ALS. One extensively explored avenue has been the use of neurotrophic factors – endogenous biomolecules which exert a protective or beneficial effect on neuron growth and survival – which when delivered to the CNS may rescue the neuronal degeneration seen in ALS. Neurotrophic factors have been a common theme in ALS research primarily due to the promising data generated by their use in animal and cell models. Factors such as glial cell line-derived neurotrophic factor (GDNF), brain derived neurotrophic factor (BDNF), vascular endothelial growth factor (VEGF) and ciliary neurotrophic factor (CNTF), have shown strong results when tested in disease models both in vitro and in vivo [81–86].

Unfortunately for patients, these encouraging results have so far failed to carry through to the clinic. Neurotrophic factors are commonly administered systemically in the form of a drug, but several trials have used gene therapy techniques in their methodology for the treatment of ALS. A 2010 phase II clinical trial (NCT00748501) used SB-509, an intramuscularly injected plasmid that encodes a zinc finger protein transcription factor (ZFP-TP), to upregulate endogenous VEGF. A 2010 press release by the developers of SB-509, Sangamo Biosciences (now Sangamo Therapeutics), found an acceptable safety tolerance in patients as well as some encouraging data demonstrating a delayed deterioration in muscle strength in treated patients, however no study data was published and no further trials involving SB-509 use in ALS were conducted. A recently published phase I/II open-label clinical trial (NCT02039401) assessing the safety of an intramuscular administration of VM202, a plasmid encoding hepatocyte growth factor (HGF), in ALS patients found it to be well tolerated but due to the small sample size and design of the experiment no conclusions could be drawn on treatment effect [87]. CNTF has been administered to patients ex vivo by the use of intrathecally implanted polymer capsules containing baby hamster kidney cells genetically engineered to release CNTF. A 1996 phase I study showed that detectable levels of CNTF could be delivered in this way without the dose-related adverse effects that had been observed in a contemporaneous study using systemic delivery [88, 89].

Meta-analyses of clinical trials involving the systemic administration of the neurotrophic factors recombinant human insulin-like growth factor I (rhIGF-I), CNTF and BDNF as drugs have all shown no effects in terms of patient survival [90–92].

Other gene therapy approaches targeting ALS involve post-transcriptional gene regulation by RNA interference, utilising either ASOs or virally delivered short RNA constructs. The first gene to be linked to ALS was superoxide dismutase 1 (SOD1), a ubiquitously expressed gene that encodes for an antioxidant protein important for the metabolism of free radical superoxide species [93]. Toxic gain-of-function mutations in SOD1 lead to ALS by an as yet undetermined mechanism [94]. The lack of motor neuron loss in SOD1 knockout mice suggest the feasibility of a treatment whereby SOD1 protein is reduced in patients [95]. Various RNAi approaches to reduce toxic mutant SOD1 protein levels by targeting mRNA have been widely tested in cell and animal models, particularly the G93A mutant mouse model [96, 97], with short hairpin RNA (shRNA), artificial micro RNA (amiRNA) and ASO technologies all showing substantial survival increases when delivered either virally in the case of sh- and amiRNAs or by direct delivery to the CNS in the case of ASOs [32, 98–100]. With respect to clinical trials, of the previous approaches only the use of ASOs has been administered to patients. A phase I/II clinical trial (NCT01041222) of Ionis-SOD1Rx, a SOD1 mRNA-targeting ASO, showed it to be tolerable when delivered intrathecally in patients but due to the low doses used in the study there was no indication of its efficacy in reducing SOD1 protein levels in the CNS [101]. ASOs have also been used in the treatment of spinal muscular atrophy (SMA), a monogenic disease in which mutations in the survival motor neuron 1 gene (SMN1) result in a loss-of-function that causes neuronal death and progressive muscle atrophy. A paralog of SMN1, SMN2, carries a single base pair change that affects correct splicing of exon 7, resulting in SMN2 contributing only 10–20% of the total amount of endogenous full length SMN protein. An ASO therapy (SPINRAZA™) has been developed that alters the splicing of SMN2, resulting in the inclusion of exon 7, the increased production of full-length SMN protein, and a subsequent amelioration of disease pathology [102, 103]. This therapy has been successfully approved by regulatory agencies in both the US and EU where it is used for the treatment of both paediatric and adult SMA. SMA is also a target for a gene transfer study involving the delivery of a full-length SMN transcript by a self-complementary AAV9 viral vector. Currently in phase I, the ongoing trial (NCT02122952) is assessing the safety and efficacy of intravenous delivery of the gene therapy, AVXS-101. This approach has the benefit of several successful preclinical studies using SMN gene replacement in SMN animal models [104–106].

13.4.2.1 Parkinson's Disease

Parkinson's disease (PD) is caused by the loss of dopaminergic neurons in the substantia nigra, and while disease etiology remains unclear, a minority of PD cases are familial and arise due to monogenic mutations in several dominantly and recessively inherited genes [107, 108]. Gene therapy strategies have not directly targeted the familial PD genes so far in clinical trials, but instead have looked at ways of attenuating the damage exerted by the onset of PD by providing trophic support, enhancing dopamine synthesis, and reducing hyperactive neurotransmitters. Neurturin is a functional analogue of GDNF that protects dopaminergic neurons in preclinical animal PD models [109–113]. A small 12 patient trial with neurturin packaged into AAV2 particles (known as CERE-120; Ceregene, San Diego, CA) and delivered directly to the putamen was well tolerated and offered a degree of clinical benefit warranting a larger clinical trial [114]. In the first set of double-blinded phase I clinical trials, CERE-120 was stereotaxically injected into the putamen of 38 PD patients (with 20 sham injections). Disappointingly, there were no clinical benefits noted in the CERE-120 treated patients after 1 year, and of greater concern, 13 out of the 38 CERE-120 treated individuals and 4 out of 20 sham treated reacted adversely to the injection, suggesting that more needs to be done to minimize toxicity associated with intrastriatal delivery [114, 115]. After assessing risks associated with injecting unilaterally or bilaterally into the putamen and/or substantia nigra with preclinical models [116], a new set of clinical trials began with bilateral injections of CERE-120 into six patients as a pilot study, which was tolerated without any serious adverse effects [117]. In a larger double-blind phase I study, bilateral infusion of CERE-120 into the putamen and substantia nigra of 24 PD patients was tolerated safely, but showed no significant improvement in PD diagnostic criteria compared to the 27 sham treated controls. A long-term (post 5 years) follow up of some of these studies with additional patients added also confirmed that intrastriatal administration of AAV2-neurturin was safe, although patients did not see a major clinical benefit as a result of the gene transfer [118].

An alternative set of strategies aimed at enhancing dopamine synthesis to prevent or delay dopaminergic cell degeneration have also utilized viral gene therapy vectors. To augment dopamine production in the CNS, PD patients are typically given L-DOPA, which is decarboxylated by aromatic L-amino acid decarboxylase (AADC), producing dopamine. The advantage with L-DOPA administration is that it can cross the blood-brain barrier, however not all patients are responsive to L-DOPA treatment. It is also associated with serious side effects and can lose efficacy over time, possibly as a consequence of endogenous AADC concentration decreasing as the disease progresses [119]. Elevating AADC, the rate-limiting step in dopamine production, is therefore a target for restoring dopamine levels. Preclinical PD animal models demonstrated that intrastriatal delivery of AAV2-AADC was tolerated and capable of enhancing long-term dopamine synthesis in the CNS [120–124]. Two different phase I clinical trials have assessed the tolerance and efficacy of a similar AAV2-AADC therapy with some modest benefits reported. In the first trial, which was followed-up several years after the initial experimental design and tolerability analysis, ten patients received stereotactic infusions of AAV2-AADC in the putamen at either a low or high vector dosages. All ten patients tolerated the treatment well, aside from some side effects that are not believed to be linked to the viral gene therapy, and showed a dose-dependent improvement in dopamine synthesis that most likely warrants the recruitment of patients for a larger trial [125–127]. In the second trial six patients received intrastriatal injections of AAV2-AADC, which was safely tolerated and showed modest improvements in motor coordination after 6 months, though the trial was unblinded and the efficacy may have been due to a placebo effect [128].

An experimental approach to expand the range of enzymes catalysing dopamine synthesis was carried out by packaging three genes into one lentiviral vector. This gene therapy based on lentivector, known as ProSavin (Oxford BioMedica, Oxford, UK) expresses tyrosine-hydroxylase, AADC and cyclohydrolase-1, and delivery of this vector in a rat PD model augmented dopamine synthesis in striatal neurons [129]. Bilateral injections of varying dosages of Prosavin in a Phase I/II clinical trial in a total of 15 patients were safely tolerated, and though the effects of the therapy were modest, patients with higher doses of Prosavin subsequently required a lower dose of dopamine medication suggesting enhanced dopamine production [130]. Current progress in viral vectors capable of further increasing dopamine synthesis [131] may enable the next clinical trial to show a more robust outcome.

The loss of dopaminergic neurons in the substantia nigra (Sn) has profound effects on other regions of the basal ganglia that give and receive inputs to and from the Sn, resulting in hyperexcitation of select neuronal populations, including glutamatergic neurons [132, 133]. One therapeutic option, therefore, is to suppress the overstimulated glutamatergic neurons and restore the balance between inhibitory and excitatory networks within the basal ganglia. Glutamic acid decarboxylase (GAD), the rate limiting enzyme catalysing the synthesis of the inhibitory neurotransmitter GABA, is a good candidate for suppressing excitatory neurons. GAD protected dopaminergic neurons and rescued behavioural deficits in a rat PD model when packaged into AAV2 particles and injected stereotaxically into the Sn [134]. In an unblinded phase I trial, twelve patients received varying dosages of AAV2-GAD infused into the subthalamic nucleus, which was safely tolerated and resulted in modest improvements in motor performance [135]. In a follow up double-blinded trial, 22 patients received the bilateral infusion of AAV2-GAD into the subthalamic nucleus with another 23 patients receiving the sham treatment [136]. Aside from a single adverse event that was not linked to the AAV2-GAD, patients tolerated the treatment well, and promisingly the AAV2-GAD cohort showed improvements at 6 months as measured on the unified Parkinson's disease rating scale (UPDRS). This suggests that this type of gene therapy may be a genuine therapeutic alternative for PD patients, though more trials and a longer follow-up will be necessary to better interpret its efficacy.

13.4.3 Huntington's Disease

Huntington's disease (HD) is a dominantly inherited monogenic neurodegenerative disease caused by repeat CAG expansions in huntington (*HTT*) that lead to the generation of abnormal toxic HTT protein [137]. Animal models of HD have shown a consistent improvement in behavioural and pathological abnormalities following suppression of both the healthy and mutant HTT protein [138–140]. Preclinical mouse models of HD show a reversal of disease symptoms and amelioration of disease pathology following ASOs inducing HTT mRNA degradation [138, 141], which has led to phase I clinical trials (NCT02519036) that are now recruiting for a similar gene therapy approach in HD patients. An alternative therapeutic approach is to express ciliary neurotrophic factor (CNTF), which exerts a neuroprotective effect on neurons typically compromised in HD [142]. The technical challenge in administering CNTF, which is inefficient at crossing the BBB [143] and is toxic at high doses [144], can be overcome by packaging baby hamster kidney (BHK) fibroblasts modified to secrete ciliary neurotrophic factor (CNTF) into semi-permeable polymers that slowly release between 5 and 25 ng/ml CNTF per hour [145–147]. In a primate HD model, these encapsulated BHK cells secreted sufficient CNTF to protect several populations of striatal neurons and prevent neurodegeneration [145]. In a small phase I trial of six patients using a similar approach which included several repeated implants of the CNTF expressing capsules, patients tolerated the encapsulated polymers for several years, although the therapy did not achieve significant clinical benefits despite improved function of intracerebral circuits [146, 147].

13.4.4 Alzheimer's Disease

Alzheimer's disease (AD) is a debilitating neurodegenerative disorder characterized behaviourally by impaired memory and cognition and by disease pathology consisting of neurofibrillary tangles, amyloid plaques, and extensive cell loss. Mutations in Amyloid beta (A4) precursor protein (*APP*), Presenilin 1 (*PSEN1*), and Presenilin 2 (*PSEN2*) cause early-onset AD by directly increasing production of Abeta peptides that promote amyloid plaque formation [148–150]. Initial cleavage of APP by beta-secretase 1 (BACE1) is a requirement for generating soluble Abeta that is subsequently cleaved by gamma-secretase to form the toxic Abeta peptide [151]. Reducing BACE1 activity is therefore a strategy for preventing Abeta production, and is an active focus of clinical AD therapy [152–154].

Postmortem AD brains have a reduction in PPARγ-coactivator-1α (PGC-1α), a regulator of mitochondrial function, oxidative phosphorylation and metabolism, and an inhibitor of BACE1 [155, 156]. A preclinical AD mouse model demonstrates that reducing BACE1 activity through lentiviral-mediated gene transfer of PGC-1α confers neuroprotection in the mice and reduces Abeta deposition [156]. Resveratrol, an active component of red wine that crosses the BBB [157], activates PGC-1α [158], and has been used to reduce Abeta expression in AD rodent models [159, 160]. As a large (119 patients) phase I clinical trial examining tolerance of AD patients to resveratrol was recently completed without any major adverse reactions [161], it is likely that there will be gene transfer strategies of PGC-1α in AD patients in the future.

A strategy to express nerve growth factor (NGF), a neurotrophin that supports cholinergic neurons [162]- a subpopulation of cells that are found to degenerate at early stages of AD [163] – has been utilized in two distinct clinical trials. Fibroblasts genetically modified to overexpress NGF were implanted into ten AD patients, and post-mortem analysis occurred between 1 and 10 years after treatment [164, 165]. All the patients safely tolerated the phase I therapy, and notably several brains showed evidence of trophic support such as axonal sprouting. Treatment of preclinical rodent models with AAV2 mediated expression of NGF (known as CERE-110) yielded promising evidence of trophic support [166], and a phase I clinical trial of CERE-110 was safe and well tolerated in patients [167]. A phase II trial (NCT00876863) which was also safely tolerated by patients, appears to have been ineffective, leading to the termination of the trial by Sangamo therapeutics. Further testing may be necessary to determine the best conditions for optimal delivery of NGF to AD patients.

13.5 Conclusions

The number of gene therapy clinical trials continues to increase every year illustrating the potential of both viral and non-viral strategies to treat a diverse array of diseases [168–170]. The reasons for the relative lack of efficacy of many of the gene therapies in patients is unclear but are a stark reminder of the difficulties in translating encouraging results in the lab into successful human clinical trials. A continuing focus on developing novel technologies that maintains and improve safety standards while enhancing the specificity and expression of gene transfer in patients will hopefully lead to a better outcome in future clinical trials.

Acknowledgements MA and JSC are supported by an ERC Advanced Investigator Award. JMS is supported by University of Sheffield studentship. PJS is supported as an NIHR Senior Investigator.

References

1. Rosenberg SA et al (1990) Gene transfer into humans – immunotherapy of patients with advanced melanoma, using tumor-infiltrating lymphocytes modified by retroviral gene transduction. N Engl J Med 323:570–578. doi:10.1056/NEJM199008303230904
2. Blaese RM et al (1995) T lymphocyte-directed gene therapy for ADA- SCID: initial trial results after 4 years. Science 270:475–480
3. Hedman M, Hartikainen J, Yla-Herttuala S (2011) Progress and prospects: hurdles to cardiovascular gene therapy clinical trials. Gene Ther 18:743–749. doi:10.1038/gt.2011.43
4. Kumar SR, Markusic DM, Biswas M, High KA, Herzog RW (2016) Clinical development of gene therapy: results and lessons from recent successes. Mol Ther Methods Clin Dev 3:16034. doi:10.1038/mtm.2016.34
5. Reese TS, Karnovsky MJ (1967) Fine structural localization of a blood-brain barrier to exogenous peroxidase. J Cell Biol 34:207–217
6. Pardridge WM (2002) Drug and gene targeting to the brain with molecular Trojan horses. Nat Rev Drug Discov 1:131–139. doi:10.1038/nrd725
7. McCarty DM, Young SM Jr, Samulski RJ (2004) Integration of adeno-associated virus (AAV) and recombinant AAV vectors. Annu Rev Genet 38:819–845. doi:10.1146/annurev.genet.37.110801.143717
8. Barquinero J, Eixarch H, Perez-Melgosa M (2004) Retroviral vectors: new applications for an old tool. Gene Ther 11(Suppl 1):S3–S9. doi:10.1038/sj.gt.3302363
9. Volpers C, Kochanek S (2004) Adenoviral vectors for gene transfer and therapy. J Gene Med 6(Suppl 1):S164–S171. doi:10.1002/jgm.496

10. Howarth JL, Lee YB, Uney JB (2010) Using viral vectors as gene transfer tools (Cell Biology and Toxicology Special Issue: ETCS-UK 1 day meeting on genetic manipulation of cells). Cell Biol Toxicol 26:1–20. doi:10.1007/s10565-009-9139-5
11. Choudhury SR et al (2016) Viral vectors for therapy of neurologic diseases. Neuropharmacology. doi:10.1016/j.neuropharm.2016.02.013
12. Negrete A, Kotin RM (2007) Production of recombinant adeno-associated vectors using two bioreactor configurations at different scales. J Virol Methods 145:155–161. doi:10.1016/j.jviromet.2007.05.020
13. Hacein-Bey-Abina S et al (2003) LMO2-associated clonal T cell proliferation in two patients after gene therapy for SCID-X1. Science 302:415–419. doi:10.1126/science.1088547
14. Hacein-Bey-Abina S et al (2008) Insertional oncogenesis in 4 patients after retrovirus-mediated gene therapy of SCID-X1. J Clin Invest 118:3132–3142. doi:10.1172/JCI35700
15. Hacein-Bey-Abina S et al (2010) Efficacy of gene therapy for X-linked severe combined immunodeficiency. N Engl J Med 363:355–364. doi:10.1056/NEJMoa1000164
16. Braun CJ et al (2014) Gene therapy for Wiskott-Aldrich syndrome – long-term efficacy and genotoxicity. Sci Transl Med 6:227ra233. doi:10.1126/scitranslmed.3007280
17. Maetzig T, Galla M, Baum C, Schambach A (2011) Gammaretroviral vectors: biology, technology and application. Virus 3:677–713. doi:10.3390/v3060677
18. Sena-Esteves M, Tebbets JC, Steffens S, Crombleholme T, Flake AW (2004) Optimized large-scale production of high titer lentivirus vector pseudotypes. J Virol Methods 122:131–139. doi:10.1016/j.jviromet.2004.08.017
19. Davidson BL, Breakefield XO (2003) Viral vectors for gene delivery to the nervous system. Nat Rev Neurosci 4:353–364. doi:10.1038/nrn1104
20. Sinn PL, Sauter SL, McCray PB Jr (2005) Gene therapy progress and prospects: development of improved lentiviral and retroviral vectors – design, biosafety, and production. Gene Ther 12:1089–1098. doi:10.1038/sj.gt.3302570
21. Kiang A et al (2006) Multiple innate inflammatory responses induced after systemic adenovirus vector delivery depend on a functional complement system. Mol Ther 14:588–598. doi:10.1016/j.ymthe.2006.03.024
22. Hartman ZC et al (2007) Adenovirus infection triggers a rapid, MyD88-regulated transcriptome response critical to acute-phase and adaptive immune responses in vivo. J Virol 81:1796–1812. doi:10.1128/JVI.01936-06
23. Wilson JM (2009) Lessons learned from the gene therapy trial for ornithine transcarbamylase deficiency. Mol Genet Metab 96:151–157. doi:10.1016/j.ymgme.2008.12.016
24. Capasso C, Garofalo M, Hirvinen M, Cerullo V (2014) The evolution of adenoviral vectors through genetic and chemical surface modifications. Virus 6:832–855. doi:10.3390/v6020832
25. Asokan A, Schaffer DV, Samulski RJ (2012) The AAV vector toolkit: poised at the clinical crossroads. Mol Ther 20:699–708. doi:10.1038/mt.2011.287
26. Zhang H et al (2011) Several rAAV vectors efficiently cross the blood-brain barrier and transduce neurons and astrocytes in the neonatal mouse central nervous system. Mol Ther 19:1440–1448. doi:10.1038/mt.2011.98
27. McCarty D, Self-complementary M (2008) AAV vectors; advances and applications. Mol Ther 16:1648–1656. doi:10.1038/mt.2008.171
28. Zhang F (2015) CRISPR-Cas9: prospects and challenges. Hum Gene Ther 26:409–410. doi:10.1089/hum.2015.29002.fzh
29. Haurwitz RE, Jinek M, Wiedenheft B, Zhou K, Doudna JA (2010) Sequence- and structure-specific RNA processing by a CRISPR endonuclease. Science 329:1355–1358. doi:10.1126/science.1192272
30. Younger ST, Corey DR (2009) The puzzle of RNAs that target gene promoters. Chembiochem 10:1135–1139. doi:10.1002/cbic.200900015
31. Janowski BA et al (2007) Activating gene expression in mammalian cells with promoter-targeted duplex RNAs. Nat Chem Biol 3:166–173. doi:10.1038/nchembio860
32. Smith RA et al (2006) Antisense oligonucleotide therapy for neurodegenerative disease. J Clin Invest 116:2290–2296. doi:10.1172/JCI25424
33. Bennett CF, Swayze EE (2010) RNA targeting therapeutics: molecular mechanisms of antisense oligonucleotides as a therapeutic platform. Annu Rev Pharmacol Toxicol 50:259–293. doi:10.1146/annurev.pharmtox.010909.105654
34. Chi X, Gatti P, Papoian T (2017) Safety of antisense oligonucleotide and siRNA-based therapeutics. Drug Discov Today. doi:10.1016/j.drudis.2017.01.013
35. Longo PA, Kavran JM, Kim MS, Leahy DJ (2013) Transient mammalian cell transfection with polyethylenimine (PEI). Methods Enzymol 529:227–240. doi:10.1016/B978-0-12-418687-3.00018-5
36. Luo D, Saltzman WM (2000) Enhancement of transfection by physical concentration of DNA at the cell surface. Nat Biotechnol 18:893–895. doi:10.1038/78523
37. Han IK et al (2007) Enhanced brain targeting efficiency of intranasally administered plasmid DNA: an alternative route for brain gene therapy. J Mol Med (Berl) 85:75–83. doi:10.1007/s00109-006-0114-9
38. Lu QL, Bou-Gharios G, Partridge TA (2003) Non-viral gene delivery in skeletal muscle: a protein factory. Gene Ther 10:131–142. doi:10.1038/sj.gt.3301874
39. Lv H, Zhang S, Wang B, Cui S, Yan J (2006) Toxicity of cationic lipids and cationic polymers in gene delivery. J Control Release 114:100–109. doi:10.1016/j.jconrel.2006.04.014

40. Allen TM, Cullis PR (2013) Liposomal drug delivery systems: from concept to clinical applications. Adv Drug Deliv Rev 65:36–48. doi:10.1016/j.addr.2012.09.037
41. Panyam J, Labhasetwar V (2003) Biodegradable nanoparticles for drug and gene delivery to cells and tissue. Adv Drug Deliv Rev 55:329–347
42. Audouy SA, de Leij LF, Hoekstra D, Molema G (2002) In vivo characteristics of cationic liposomes as delivery vectors for gene therapy. Pharm Res 19:1599–1605
43. Wen PY, Kesari S (2008) Malignant gliomas in adults. N Engl J Med 359:492–507. doi:10.1056/NEJMra0708126
44. Rouse C, Gittleman H, Ostrom QT, Kruchko C, Barnholtz-Sloan JS (2016) Years of potential life lost for brain and CNS tumors relative to other cancers in adults in the United States, 2010. Neuro-Oncology 18:70–77. doi:10.1093/neuonc/nov249
45. Grossman SA et al (2010) Survival of patients with newly diagnosed glioblastoma treated with radiation and temozolomide in research studies in the United States. Clin Cancer Res 16:2443–2449. doi:10.1158/1078-0432.CCR-09-3106
46. Westphal M, Lamszus K (2011) The neurobiology of gliomas: from cell biology to the development of therapeutic approaches. Nat Rev Neurosci 12:495–508. doi:10.1038/nrn3060
47. Cuddapah VA, Robel S, Watkins S, Sontheimer H (2014) A neurocentric perspective on glioma invasion. Nat Rev Neurosci 15:455–465. doi:10.1038/nrn3765
48. Osuka S, Van Meir EG (2017) Overcoming therapeutic resistance in glioblastoma: the way forward. J Clin Invest 127:415–426. doi:10.1172/JCI89587
49. Chen J et al (2012) A restricted cell population propagates glioblastoma growth after chemotherapy. Nature 488:522–526. doi:10.1038/nature11287
50. Moolten FL (1986) Tumor chemosensitivity conferred by inserted herpes thymidine kinase genes: paradigm for a prospective cancer control strategy. Cancer Res 46:5276–5281
51. Rainov NG (2000) A phase III clinical evaluation of herpes simplex virus type 1 thymidine kinase and ganciclovir gene therapy as an adjuvant to surgical resection and radiation in adults with previously untreated glioblastoma multiforme. Hum Gene Ther 11:2389–2401. doi:10.1089/104303400750038499
52. Ram Z et al (1997) Therapy of malignant brain tumors by intratumoral implantation of retroviral vector-producing cells. Nat Med 3:1354–1361
53. Klatzmann D et al (1998) A phase I/II study of herpes simplex virus type 1 thymidine kinase "suicide" gene therapy for recurrent glioblastoma. Study Group on Gene Therapy for Glioblastoma. Hum Gene Ther 9:2595–2604. doi:10.1089/hum.1998.9.17-2595
54. Shand N et al (1999) A phase 1-2 clinical trial of gene therapy for recurrent glioblastoma multiforme by tumor transduction with the herpes simplex thymidine kinase gene followed by ganciclovir. GLI328 European-Canadian Study Group. Hum Gene Ther 10:2325–2335. doi:10.1089/10430349950016979
55. Prados MD et al (2003) Treatment of progressive or recurrent glioblastoma multiforme in adults with herpes simplex virus thymidine kinase gene vector-producer cells followed by intravenous ganciclovir administration: a phase I/II multi-institutional trial. J Neuro-Oncol 65:269–278
56. Sandmair AM et al (2000) Thymidine kinase gene therapy for human malignant glioma, using replication-deficient retroviruses or adenoviruses. Hum Gene Ther 11:2197–2205. doi:10.1089/104303400750035726
57. Immonen A et al (2004) AdvHSV-tk gene therapy with intravenous ganciclovir improves survival in human malignant glioma: a randomised, controlled study. Mol Ther 10:967–972. doi:10.1016/j.ymthe.2004.08.002
58. Asaoka K, Tada M, Sawamura Y, Ikeda J, Abe H (2000) Dependence of efficient adenoviral gene delivery in malignant glioma cells on the expression levels of the Coxsackievirus and adenovirus receptor. J Neurosurg 92:1002–1008. doi:10.3171/jns.2000.92.6.1002
59. Bergelson JM et al (1997) Isolation of a common receptor for Coxsackie B viruses and adenoviruses 2 and 5. Science 275:1320–1323
60. Blackford AN, Grand RJ (2009) Adenovirus E1B 55-kilodalton protein: multiple roles in viral infection and cell transformation. J Virol 83:4000–4012. doi:10.1128/JVI.02417-08
61. Yew PR, Berk AJ (1992) Inhibition of p53 transactivation required for transformation by adenovirus early 1B protein. Nature 357:82–85. doi:10.1038/357082a0
62. O'Shea CC et al (2004) Late viral RNA export, rather than p53 inactivation, determines ONYX-015 tumor selectivity. Cancer Cell 6:611–623. doi:10.1016/j.ccr.2004.11.012
63. Gomez-Manzano C et al (2004) A novel E1A-E1B mutant adenovirus induces glioma regression in vivo. Oncogene 23:1821–1828. doi:10.1038/sj.onc.1207321
64. Fueyo J et al (2000) A mutant oncolytic adenovirus targeting the Rb pathway produces anti-glioma effect in vivo. Oncogene 19:2–12. doi:10.1038/sj.onc.1203251
65. Chiocca EA et al (2004) A phase I open-label, dose-escalation, multi-institutional trial of injection with an E1B-Attenuated adenovirus, ONYX-015, into the peritumoral region of recurrent malignant gliomas, in the adjuvant setting. Mol Ther 10:958–966. doi:10.1016/j.ymthe.2004.07.021
66. Galanis E et al (2005) Phase I-II trial of ONYX-015 in combination with MAP chemotherapy in patients with advanced sarcomas. Gene Ther 12:437–445. doi:10.1038/sj.gt.3302436
67. Reid TR, Freeman S, Post L, McCormick F, Sze DY (2005) Effects of Onyx-015 among metastatic

colorectal cancer patients that have failed prior treatment with 5-FU/leucovorin. Cancer Gene Ther 12:673–681. doi:10.1038/sj.cgt.7700819
68. van Beusechem VW et al (2003) Conditionally replicative adenovirus expressing a targeting adapter molecule exhibits enhanced oncolytic potency on CAR-deficient tumors. Gene Ther 10:1982–1991. doi:10.1038/sj.gt.3302103
69. Lamfers ML et al (2002) Potential of the conditionally replicative adenovirus Ad5-Delta24RGD in the treatment of malignant gliomas and its enhanced effect with radiotherapy. Cancer Res 62:5736–5742
70. Suzuki K et al (2001) A conditionally replicative adenovirus with enhanced infectivity shows improved oncolytic potency. Clin Cancer Res 7:120–126
71. Whisenhunt TR Jr, Rajneesh KF, Hackney JR, Markert JM (2015) Extended disease-free interval of 6 years in a recurrent glioblastoma multiforme patient treated with G207 oncolytic viral therapy. Oncolytic Virother 4:33–38. doi:10.2147/OV.S62461
72. Markert JM et al (2014) A phase 1 trial of oncolytic HSV-1, G207, given in combination with radiation for recurrent GBM demonstrates safety and radiographic responses. Mol Ther 22:1048–1055. doi:10.1038/mt.2014.22
73. Markert JM et al (2009) Phase Ib trial of mutant herpes simplex virus G207 inoculated pre-and post-tumor resection for recurrent GBM. Mol Ther 17:199–207. doi:10.1038/mt.2008.228
74. Markert JM et al (2000) Conditionally replicating herpes simplex virus mutant, G207 for the treatment of malignant glioma: results of a phase I trial. Gene Ther 7:867–874. doi:10.1038/sj.gt.3301205
75. Voges J et al (2003) Imaging-guided convection-enhanced delivery and gene therapy of glioblastoma. Ann Neurol 54:479–487. doi:10.1002/ana.10688
76. Ren H et al (2003) Immunogene therapy of recurrent glioblastoma multiforme with a liposomally encapsulated replication-incompetent Semliki forest virus vector carrying the human interleukin-12 gene – a phase I/II clinical protocol. J Neuro-Oncol 64:147–154
77. Bogdahn U et al (2011) Targeted therapy for high-grade glioma with the TGF-beta2 inhibitor trabedersen: results of a randomized and controlled phase IIb study. Neuro-Oncology 13:132–142. doi:10.1093/neuonc/noq142
78. Han J, Alvarez-Breckenridge CA, Wang QE, Yu J (2015) TGF-beta signaling and its targeting for glioma treatment. Am J Cancer Res 5:945–955
79. Renton AE, Chiò A, Traynor BJ (2014) State of play in amyotrophic lateral sclerosis genetics. Nat Neurosci 17:17–23. doi:10.1038/nn.3584
80. Bensimon G, Lacomblez L, Meininger V (1994) A controlled trial of riluzole in amyotrophic lateral sclerosis. N Engl J Med 330:585–591. doi:10.1056/NEJM199403033300901
81. Azzouz M et al (2004) VEGF delivery with retrogradely transported lentivector prolongs survival in a mouse ALS model. Nature 429:413–417
82. Ikeda K et al (1995) Effects of brain-derived neurotrophic factor on motor dysfunction in wobbler mouse motor neuron disease. Ann Neurol 37:505–511. doi:10.1002/ana.410370413
83. Krakora D et al (2013) Synergistic effects of GDNF and VEGF on lifespan and disease progression in a familial ALS rat model. Mol Ther: J Am Soc Gene Ther 21:1602–1610. doi:10.1038/mt.2013.108
84. Sagot Y et al (1995) Polymer encapsulated cell lines genetically engineered to release ciliary neurotrophic factor can slow down progressive motor neuronopathy in the mouse. Eur J Neurosci 7:1313–1322. doi:10.1111/j.1460-9568.1995.tb01122.x
85. Storkebaum E et al (2005) Treatment of motoneuron degeneration by intracerebroventricular delivery of VEGF in a rat model of ALS. Nat Neurosci 8:85–92. doi:10.1038/nn1360
86. Suzuki M et al (2008) Direct muscle delivery of GDNF with human mesenchymal stem cells improves motor neuron survival and function in a rat model of familial ALS. Mol Ther: J Am Soc Gene Ther 16:2002–2010. doi:10.1038/mt.2008.197
87. Sufit RL, Ajroud-Driss S, Casey P, Kessler JA (2017) Open label study to assess the safety of VM202 in subjects with amyotrophic lateral sclerosis. Amyotroph Lateral Scler Frontotemporal Degeneration 0:1–10. doi:10.1080/21678421.2016.1259334
88. Miller RG et al (1996) Toxicity and tolerability of recombinant human ciliary neurotrophic factor in patients with amyotrophic lateral sclerosis. Neurology 47:1329–1331
89. Aebischer P et al (1996) Intrathecal delivery of CNTF using encapsulated genetically modified xenogeneic cells in amyotrophic lateral sclerosis patients. Nat Med 2:696–699. doi:10.1038/nm0696-696
90. Bongioanni P, Reali C, Sogos V (2004) Ciliary neurotrophic factor (CNTF) for amyotrophic lateral sclerosis or motor neuron disease. Cochrane Database Syst Rev…
91. Group, T. B. S (1999) A controlled trial of recombinant methionyl human BDNF in ALS. Neurology 52:1427–1427. doi:10.1212/WNL.52.7.1427
92. Beauverd M, Mitchell JD, Wokke JH, Borasio GD (2012) Recombinant human insulin-like growth factor I (rhIGF-I) for the treatment of amyotrophic lateral sclerosis/motor neuron disease. Cochrane Database Syst Rev, N.PAG-N.PAG, doi:10.1002/14651858.CD002064.pub3.www.cochranelibrary.com
93. Rosen DR et al (1993) Mutations in Cu/Zn Superoxide dismutase gene are associated with familial amyotrophic lateral sclerosis. Nature 362:59–62. doi:10.1038/362059a0
94. Wong PC, Cai H, Borchelt DR, Price DL (2001) Genetically engineered models relevant to neurodegenerative disorders: their value for understanding disease mechanisms and designing/testing experimental therapeutics. J Mol Neurosci 17:233–257. doi:10.1385/JMN:17:2:233
95. Saccon RA, Bunton-Stasyshyn RKA, Fisher EMC, Fratta P (2013) Is SOD1 loss of function involved

in amyotrophic lateral sclerosis? Brain J Neurol 136:2342–2358. doi:10.1093/brain/awt097
96. Gurney ME et al (1994) Motor neuron degeneration in mice that express a human Cu,Zn superoxide dismutase mutation. Science (New York, N.Y.) 264:1772–1775. doi:10.1126/science.8209258
97. Tu P-hH et al (1996) Transgenic mice carrying a human mutant superoxide dismutase transgene develop neuronal cytoskeletal pathology resembling human amyotrophic lateral sclerosis lesions. Proc Natl Acad Sci 93:3155–3160
98. Foust KD et al (2013) Therapeutic AAV9-mediated suppression of mutant SOD1 slows disease progression and extends survival in models of inherited ALS. Mol Ther: J Am Soc Gene Ther 21:2148–2159. doi:10.1038/mt.2013.211
99. Ralph GS et al (2005) Silencing mutant SOD1 using RNAi protects against neurodegeneration and extends survival in an ALS model. Nat Med 11:429–433. doi:10.1038/nm1205
100. Raoul C et al (2005) Lentiviral-mediated silencing of SOD1 through RNA interference retards disease onset and progression in a mouse model of ALS. Nat Med 11:423–428. doi:10.1038/nm1207
101. Stoica L et al (2016) Adeno-associated virus-delivered artificial microRNA extends survival and delays paralysis in an amyotrophic lateral sclerosis mouse model. Ann Neurol 79:687–700. doi:10.1002/ana.24618
102. Miller TM et al (2013) An antisense oligonucleotide against SOD1 delivered intrathecally for patients with SOD1 familial amyotrophic lateral sclerosis: a phase 1, randomised, first-in-man study. Lancet Neurol 12:435–442. doi:10.1016/S1474-4422(13)70061-9
103. Finkel RS et al (2016) Treatment of infantile-onset spinal muscular atrophy with nusinersen: a phase 2, open-label, dose-escalation study. Lancet 6736:2–11. doi:10.1016/S0140-6736(16)31408-8
104. Passini MA et al (2011) Antisense Oligonucleotides delivered to the mouse CNS ameliorate symptoms of severe spinal muscular atrophy. Science Transl Med 3:72ra18–72ra18. doi:10.1126/scitranslmed.3001777
105. Foust KD et al (2010) Rescue of the spinal muscular atrophy phenotype in a mouse model by early postnatal delivery of SMN. Nat Biotechnol 28:271–274. doi:10.1038/nbt.1610
106. Passini MA et al (2010) CNS-targeted gene therapy improves survival and motor function in a mouse model of spinal muscular atrophy. J Clin Invest 120:1253–1253. doi:10.1172/JCI41615DS1
107. Valori CF et al (2010) Systemic delivery of scAAV9 expressing SMN prolongs survival in a model of spinal muscular atrophy. Sci Transl Med 2:35ra42–35ra42. doi:10.1126/scitranslmed.3000830
108. Cookson MR, Bandmann O (2010) Parkinson's disease: insights from pathways. Hum Mol Genet 19:R21–R27. doi:10.1093/hmg/ddq167
109. Dauer W, Przedborski S (2003) Parkinson's disease: mechanisms and models. Neuron 39:889–909
110. Herzog CD et al (2007) Striatal delivery of CERE-120, an AAV2 vector encoding human neurturin, enhances activity of the dopaminergic nigrostriatal system in aged monkeys. Mov Disord 22:1124–1132. doi:10.1002/mds.21503
111. Gasmi M et al (2007) Striatal delivery of neurturin by CERE-120, an AAV2 vector for the treatment of dopaminergic neuron degeneration in Parkinson's disease. Mol Ther 15:62–68. doi:10.1038/sj.mt.6300010
112. Gasmi M et al (2007) AAV2-mediated delivery of human neurturin to the rat nigrostriatal system: long-term efficacy and tolerability of CERE-120 for Parkinson's disease. Neurobiol Dis 27:67–76. doi:10.1016/j.nbd.2007.04.003
113. Horger BA et al (1998) Neurturin exerts potent actions on survival and function of midbrain dopaminergic neurons. J Neurosci 18:4929–4937
114. Kotzbauer PT et al (1996) Neurturin, a relative of glial-cell-line-derived neurotrophic factor. Nature 384:467–470. doi:10.1038/384467a0
115. Marks WJ Jr et al (2008) Safety and tolerability of intraputaminal delivery of CERE-120 (adeno-associated virus serotype 2-neurturin) to patients with idiopathic Parkinson's disease: an open-label, phase I trial. Lancet Neurol 7:400–408. doi:10.1016/S1474-4422(08)70065-6
116. Marks WJ Jr et al (2010) Gene delivery of AAV2-neurturin for Parkinson's disease: a double-blind, randomised, controlled trial. Lancet Neurol 9:1164–1172. doi:10.1016/S1474-4422(10)70254-4
117. Herzog CD et al (2013) Enhanced neurotrophic distribution, cell signaling and neuroprotection following substantia nigral versus striatal delivery of AAV2-NRTN (CERE-120). Neurobiol Dis 58:38–48. doi:10.1016/j.nbd.2013.04.011
118. Bartus RT et al (2013) Safety/feasibility of targeting the substantia nigra with AAV2-neurturin in Parkinson patients. Neurology 80:1698–1701. doi:10.1212/WNL.0b013e3182904faa
119. Marks WJ Jr, Baumann TL, Bartus RT (2016) Long-term safety of patients with Parkinson's disease receiving rAAV2-Neurturin (CERE-120) gene transfer. Hum Gene Ther 27:522–527. doi:10.1089/hum.2015.134
120. Mercuri NB, Bernardi G (2005) The 'magic' of L-dopa: why is it the gold standard Parkinson's disease therapy? Trends Pharmacol Sci 26:341–344. doi:10.1016/j.tips.2005.05.002
121. Sanftner LM et al (2005) AAV2-mediated gene delivery to monkey putamen: evaluation of an infusion device and delivery parameters. Exp Neurol 194:476–483. doi:10.1016/j.expneurol.2005.03.007
122. Sanchez-Pernaute R, Harvey-White J, Cunningham J, Bankiewicz KS (2001) Functional effect of adeno-associated virus mediated gene transfer of aromatic L-amino acid decarboxylase into the striatum of 6-OHDA-lesioned rats. Mol Ther 4:324–330. doi:10.1006/mthe.2001.0466

123. Bankiewicz KS et al (2000) Convection-enhanced delivery of AAV vector in parkinsonian monkeys; in vivo detection of gene expression and restoration of dopaminergic function using pro-drug approach. Exp Neurol 164:2–14. doi:10.1006/exnr.2000.7408
124. Forsayeth JR et al (2006) A dose-ranging study of AAV-hAADC therapy in Parkinsonian monkeys. Mol Ther 14:571–577. doi:10.1016/j.ymthe.2006.04.008
125. Bankiewicz KS et al (2006) Long-term clinical improvement in MPTP-lesioned primates after gene therapy with AAV-hAADC. Mol Ther 14:564–570. doi:10.1016/j.ymthe.2006.05.005
126. Mittermeyer G et al (2012) Long-term evaluation of a phase 1 study of AADC gene therapy for Parkinson's disease. Hum Gene Ther 23:377–381. doi:10.1089/hum.2011.220
127. Christine CW et al (2009) Safety and tolerability of putaminal AADC gene therapy for Parkinson disease. Neurology 73:1662–1669. doi:10.1212/WNL.0b013e3181c29356
128. Eberling JL et al (2008) Results from a phase I safety trial of hAADC gene therapy for Parkinson disease. Neurology 70:1980–1983. doi:10.1212/01.wnl.0000312381.29287.ff
129. Muramatsu S et al (2010) A phase I study of aromatic L-amino acid decarboxylase gene therapy for Parkinson's disease. Mol Ther 18:1731–1735. doi:10.1038/mt.2010.135
130. Azzouz M et al (2002) Multicistronic lentiviral vector-mediated striatal gene transfer of aromatic L-amino acid decarboxylase, tyrosine hydroxylase, and GTP cyclohydrolase I induces sustained transgene expression, dopamine production, and functional improvement in a rat model of Parkinson's disease. J Neurosci 22:10302–10312
131. Palfi S et al (2014) Long-term safety and tolerability of ProSavin, a lentiviral vector-based gene therapy for Parkinson's disease: a dose escalation, open-label, phase 1/2 trial. Lancet 383:1138–1146. doi:10.1016/S0140-6736(13)61939-X
132. Stewart HJ et al (2016) Optimizing transgene configuration and protein fusions to maximize dopamine production for the gene therapy of Parkinson's disease. Hum Gene Ther Clin Dev 27:100–110. doi:10.1089/humc.2016.056
133. Conn PJ, Battaglia G, Marino MJ, Nicoletti F (2005) Metabotropic glutamate receptors in the basal ganglia motor circuit. Nat Rev Neurosci 6:787–798. doi:10.1038/nrn1763
134. Shepherd GM (2013) Corticostriatal connectivity and its role in disease. Nat Rev Neurosci 14:278–291. doi:10.1038/nrn3469
135. Luo J et al (2002) Subthalamic GAD gene therapy in a Parkinson's disease rat model. Science 298:425–429. doi:10.1126/science.1074549
136. Kaplitt MG et al (2007) Safety and tolerability of gene therapy with an adeno-associated virus (AAV) borne GAD gene for Parkinson's disease: an open label, phase I trial. Lancet 369:2097–2105. doi:10.1016/S0140-6736(07)60982-9
137. LeWitt PA et al (2011) AAV2-GAD gene therapy for advanced Parkinson's disease: a double-blind, sham-surgery controlled, randomised trial. Lancet Neurol 10:309–319. doi:10.1016/S1474-4422(11)70039-4
138. Ross CA, Tabrizi SJ (2011) Huntington's disease: from molecular pathogenesis to clinical treatment. Lancet Neurol 10:83–98. doi:10.1016/S1474-4422(10)70245-3
139. Kordasiewicz HB et al (2012) Sustained therapeutic reversal of Huntington's disease by transient repression of huntingtin synthesis. Neuron 74:1031–1044. doi:10.1016/j.neuron.2012.05.009
140. Franich NR et al (2008) AAV vector-mediated RNAi of mutant huntingtin expression is neuroprotective in a novel genetic rat model of Huntington's disease. Mol Ther 16:947–956. doi:10.1038/mt.2008.50
141. Rodriguez-Lebron E, Denovan-Wright EM, Nash K, Lewin AS, Mandel RJ (2005) Intrastriatal rAAV-mediated delivery of anti-huntingtin shRNAs induces partial reversal of disease progression in R6/1 Huntington's disease transgenic mice. Mol Ther 12:618–633. doi:10.1016/j.ymthe.2005.05.006
142. Ostergaard ME et al (2013) Rational design of antisense oligonucleotides targeting single nucleotide polymorphisms for potent and allele selective suppression of mutant Huntingtin in the CNS. Nucleic Acids Res 41:9634–9650. doi:10.1093/nar/gkt725
143. Anderson KD, Panayotatos N, Corcoran TL, Lindsay RM, Wiegand SJ (1996) Ciliary neurotrophic factor protects striatal output neurons in an animal model of Huntington disease. Proc Natl Acad Sci U S A 93:7346–7351
144. Poduslo JF, Curran GL (1996) Permeability at the blood-brain and blood-nerve barriers of the neurotrophic factors: NGF, CNTF, NT-3, BDNF. Brain Res Mol Brain Res 36:280–286
145. Emerich DF et al (1997) Protective effect of encapsulated cells producing neurotrophic factor CNTF in a monkey model of Huntington's disease. Nature 386:395–399. doi:10.1038/386395a0
146. Bachoud-Levi AC et al (2000) Neuroprotective gene therapy for Huntington's disease using a polymer encapsulated BHK cell line engineered to secrete human CNTF. Hum Gene Ther 11:1723–1729. doi:10.1089/10430340050111377
147. Bloch J et al (2004) Neuroprotective gene therapy for Huntington's disease, using polymer-encapsulated cells engineered to secrete human ciliary neurotrophic factor: results of a phase I study. Hum Gene Ther 15:968–975. doi:10.1089/hum.2004.15.968
148. Haass C, Selkoe DJ (2007) Soluble protein oligomers in neurodegeneration: lessons from the Alzheimer's amyloid beta-peptide. Nat Rev Mol Cell Biol 8:101–112. doi:10.1038/nrm2101
149. Selkoe DJ, Podlisny MB (2002) Deciphering the genetic basis of Alzheimer's disease. Annu Rev

Genomics Hum Genet 3:67–99. doi:10.1146/annurev.genom.3.022502.103022
150. Hardy J, Selkoe DJ (2002) The amyloid hypothesis of Alzheimer's disease: progress and problems on the road to therapeutics. Science 297:353–356. doi:10.1126/science.1072994
151. Cai H et al (2001) BACE1 is the major beta-secretase for generation of Abeta peptides by neurons. Nat Neurosci 4:233–234. doi:10.1038/85064
152. Laird FM et al (2005) BACE1, a major determinant of selective vulnerability of the brain to amyloid-beta amyloidogenesis, is essential for cognitive, emotional, and synaptic functions. J Neurosci 25:11693–11709. doi:10.1523/JNEUROSCI.2766-05.2005
153. Yan R, Vassar R (2014) Targeting the beta secretase BACE1 for Alzheimer's disease therapy. Lancet Neurol 13:319–329. doi:10.1016/S1474-4422(13)70276-X
154. Vassar R (2014) BACE1 inhibitor drugs in clinical trials for Alzheimer's disease. Alzheimers Res Ther 6:89. doi:10.1186/s13195-014-0089-7
155. Sweeney G, Song J (2016) The association between PGC-1alpha and Alzheimer's disease. Anat Cell Biol 49:1–6. doi:10.5115/acb.2016.49.1.1
156. Katsouri L et al (2016) PPARgamma-coactivator-1alpha gene transfer reduces neuronal loss and amyloid-beta generation by reducing beta-secretase in an Alzheimer's disease model. Proc Natl Acad Sci U S A 113:12292–12297. doi:10.1073/pnas.1606171113
157. Braidy N et al (2016) Resveratrol as a potential therapeutic candidate for the treatment and management of Alzheimer's disease. Curr Top Med Chem 16:1951–1960
158. Lagouge M et al (2006) Resveratrol improves mitochondrial function and protects against metabolic disease by activating SIRT1 and PGC-1alpha. Cell 127:1109–1122. doi:10.1016/j.cell.2006.11.013
159. Wang R, Zhang Y, Li J, Zhang C (2017) Resveratrol ameliorates spatial learning memory impairment induced by Abeta1-42 in rats. Neuroscience 344:39–47. doi:10.1016/j.neuroscience.2016.08.051
160. Kim D et al (2007) SIRT1 deacetylase protects against neurodegeneration in models for Alzheimer's disease and amyotrophic lateral sclerosis. EMBO J 26:3169–3179. doi:10.1038/sj.emboj.7601758
161. Turner RS et al (2015) A randomized, double-blind, placebo-controlled trial of resveratrol for Alzheimer disease. Neurology 85:1383–1391. doi:10.1212/WNL.0000000000002035
162. Triaca V, Calissano P (2016) Impairment of the nerve growth factor pathway driving amyloid accumulation in cholinergic neurons: the incipit of the Alzheimer's disease story? Neural Regen Res 11:1553–1556. doi:10.4103/1673-5374.193224
163. Coyle JT, Price DL, DeLong MR (1983) Alzheimer's disease: a disorder of cortical cholinergic innervation. Science 219:1184–1190
164. Tuszynski MH et al (2015) Nerve growth factor gene therapy: activation of neuronal responses in Alzheimer disease. JAMA Neurol 72:1139–1147. doi:10.1001/jamaneurol.2015.1807
165. Tuszynski MH et al (2005) A phase 1 clinical trial of nerve growth factor gene therapy for Alzheimer disease. Nat Med 11:551–555. doi:10.1038/nm1239
166. Bishop KM et al (2008) Therapeutic potential of CERE-110 (AAV2-NGF): targeted, stable, and sustained NGF delivery and trophic activity on rodent basal forebrain cholinergic neurons. Exp Neurol 211:574–584. doi:10.1016/j.expneurol.2008.03.004
167. Rafii MS et al (2014) A phase1 study of stereotactic gene delivery of AAV2-NGF for Alzheimer's disease. Alzheimers Dement 10:571–581. doi:10.1016/j.jalz.2013.09.004
168. Ginn SL, Alexander IE, Edelstein ML, Abedi MR, Wixon J (2013) Gene therapy clinical trials worldwide to 2012 – an update. J Gene Med 15:65–77. doi:10.1002/jgm.2698
169. Edelstein ML, Abedi MR, Wixon J (2007) Gene therapy clinical trials worldwide to 2007 – an update. J Gene Med 9:833–842. doi:10.1002/jgm.1100
170. Edelstein ML, Abedi MR, Wixon J, Edelstein RM (2004) Gene therapy clinical trials worldwide 1989–2004-an overview. J Gene Med 6:597–602. doi:10.1002/jgm.619

Index

S. El-Khamisy (ed.), *Personalised Medicine*, Advances in Experimental Medicine and Biology 1007,
DOI 10.1007/978-3-319-60733-7

MIX
Papier aus verantwortungsvollen Quellen
Paper from responsible sources
FSC® C105338

FSC
www.fsc.org

If you have any concerns about our products,
you can contact us on
ProductSafety@springernature.com

In case Publisher is established outside the EU,
the EU authorized representative is:
Springer Nature Customer Service Center GmbH
Europaplatz 3, 69115 Heidelberg, Germany

Printed by Libri Plureos GmbH
in Hamburg, Germany